D0734342

WORKING WITH ADOLESCENTS

SOCIAL WORK PRACTICE
WITH CHILDREN AND FAMILIES

Nancy Boyd Webb, Series Editor

WORKING *with* ADOLESCENTS

A GUIDE FOR PRACTITIONERS

Julie Anne Laser
Nicole Nicotera

Series Editor's Note by Nancy Boyd Webb

Foreword by Jeffrey M. Jenson

THE GUILFORD PRESS
New York   London

© 2011 The Guilford Press
A Division of Guilford Publications, Inc.
72 Spring Street, New York, NY 10012
www.guilford.com

Printed in the United States of America

This book is printed on acid-free paper.

Last digit is print number: 9   8   7   6   5   4   3   2   1

Library of Congress Cataloging-in-Publication Data

Laser, Julie Anne.
   Working with adolescents : a guide for practitioners / by Julie Anne Laser
and Nicole Nicotera.
      p. cm. — (Social work practice with children and families)
   Includes bibliographical references and index.
   ISBN 978-1-60918-035-5 (hardcover : alk. paper)
   1. Social work with teenagers.   2. Adolescent psychology.   3. Teenagers—
Counseling of.   4. Teenagers—Family relationships.   I. Nicotera, Nicole.
II. Title.
   HV1421.L373 2011
   362.7—dc22

                                                              2010040073

To Tom Luster, who died during the writing of this book

I have learned to be a scholar, a professor, and a better human being through knowing Tom.

He taught me how to think critically, to scrutinize the details, but to always try to find the meaning of the results in the "big picture." He taught me how to use research results to improve human functioning for children, youth, and society.

He taught me that one needed to always push oneself to know more, to think more deeply, to question one's own ideas, and to humbly share those ideas with others.

He taught me that learning happens in- and outside of the "ivory towers" of the academic world and that one can learn equally from theoretical geniuses like Uri Bronfenbrenner or from Sismayo and the other "Lost Boys of the Sudan" who were "found" by Tom and his wife, Carol.

He taught me how to run a graduate classroom, to expect the highest level of performance, but to always respect the student for who he or she was and where he or she was coming from, and to want each student to succeed to his or her highest potential. Tom taught me, by example, that even though he had a million things to do, he had time for each student's questions and to sit with him or her until he or she understood. Throughout the dissertation process with my students, I try to channel what Tom taught me to my students, and thereby his knowledge that was shared with me lives on in many others whom he never met.

He taught me that academia was a place where you could both be a scholar and a great parent. Though I had met them only briefly, he kept me abreast of his children's academic, athletic, and life pursuits. He was so proud of Anna's and Ben's accomplishments and the adults they had become.

He taught me that even though we were studying serious issues, there was always time to laugh, especially at ourselves.

He taught me what to expect from the academic world as a professor and gave me great counsel when it did not act as expected.

He is and will be sorely missed.

—Julie Anne Laser

About the Authors

Julie Anne Laser, PhD, MSW, LCSW, is Associate Professor in the Graduate School of Social Work at the University of Denver, where she coordinates the high-risk youth track of the MSW curriculum as well as teaches in the clinical and research series. Dr. Laser's research focus is on adolescent resiliency, particularly the relevance of specific ecological and internal protective and risk factors by culture and gender. She recently completed large studies of resilience in Japanese, Korean, Chinese, and Senegalese youth and homeless teens in the United States. Projects are under way to evaluate resilience in Latin American youth. Dr. Laser has more than 20 years of clinical social work experience and has worked in Mexico, Switzerland, Japan, and China, as well as a variety of urban and rural settings in the United States. She is particularly interested in school social work.

Nicole Nicotera, PhD, MSW, LICSW, is Associate Professor in the Graduate School of Social Work at the University of Denver, where she teaches clinical practice theories and skills and a doctoral research course in qualitative analysis. Dr. Nicotera's research and scholarship focus on measuring civic development in children, interventions to enhance civic leadership and positive youth development, the influences of neighborhood collective socialization and social cohesion on young people, and issues of unearned privilege and oppression in social work practice, education, and research. Her recent research with young people in public housing neighborhoods examines civic engagement and the capacity of youth to act as agents of neighborhood change. As a clinical social worker, Dr. Nicotera worked with children, youth, and families in a community mental health center, where she used art, play, and sand-tray therapies, as well as other intervention modalities. She also has extensive school social work experience with seriously emotionally and behaviorally challenged children.

Contributing Authors

Douglas Davies, PhD, MSW, is Lecturer at the School of Social Work, University of Michigan, Ann Arbor. Dr. Davies is an infant mental health specialist who was trained at the Child Development Project at the University of Michigan (Selma Fraiberg, Director). From 1979 to 1995 he was a Clinical Social Worker/Social Work Specialist in the Child and Adolescent Psychiatry Outpatient and Infant Psychiatry Programs in the Department of Psychiatry at the University of Michigan. From 1991 to 2000 he was Lecturer in Psychiatry at the University of Michigan Medical School. In 2005 he was elected to the National Academies of Practice, Washington DC, as a "Distinguished Social Work Practitioner," and in 2007 received a lifetime award, the Selma Fraiberg Award, from the Michigan Association for Infant Mental Health. His clinical research interests are in intervention with toddlers and parents, treatment of trauma in young children, therapy of young cancer survivors, and child care consultation. He has published several clinical articles on these topics. His 2010 book, *Child Development: A Practitioner's Guide,* Third Edition (Guilford Press), describes how to apply child development theory to clinical practice. In his practice, Dr. Davies works with children, adolescents, and parents; supervises clinicians individually and in groups; and consults to mental health agencies and child care centers.

Jeffrey M. Jenson, PhD, is the Philip D. and Eleanor G. Winn Professor for Children and Youth at Risk and Associate Dean for Research in the Graduate School of Social Work at the University of Denver. Dr. Jenson's teaching and research interests focus on the etiology, prevention, and treatment of childhood and adolescent aggression, juvenile delinquency, and substance abuse. He has published three books and numerous articles on the topic of adolescent problem behavior. His recent book, *Social Policy for Children and Youth: A Risk and Resilience Perspective* (with Mark Fraser), was the 2008 recipient of the Society for Research on Adolescence Social Policy Award for Best Edited Book. Dr. Jenson is currently principal investigator of the Youth Empowerment Project, an investigation aimed at improving academic and behavioral outcomes among youth residing in four Denver public housing communities. He was recently principal investigator of the Youth Matters Denver Public Schools Prevention Project, a randomized trial assessing the effects of a structured curriculum on aggression and substance use among elementary school students in 28 Denver public schools. Dr. Jenson received the University of Denver Distinguished Scholar Award in 2003 and the University Lecturer Award in 2007. He was Editor-in-Chief of the journal *Social Work Research* from 2004 to 2008 and received the Society for Social Work and Research Aaron Rosen Award for his scholarly contributions in 2009.

George Stuart Leibowitz, PhD, MSW, LCSW, is Assistant Professor at the University of Vermont, where he teaches family systems therapy, clinical theory and practice, and substance abuse. Dr. Leibowitz is a licensed clinical and forensic social worker, with more than 15 years of experience as a clinical supervisor and psychotherapist treating trauma and sexual behavior problems among male adolescents in a variety of inpatient and outpatient settings in New York City, New Mexico, and Colorado. His current research focus involves an understudied area of trauma, understanding dissociation and attachment among diverse groups of offending adolescents.

Tom Luster, PhD, was Professor in the Department of Family and Child Ecology at Michigan State University. His research focused primarily on three areas: (1) risk and resilience, (2) adolescent mothers and their children, and (3) influences on parenting behavior. His latest research included a 9-year longitudinal study of adolescent mothers and their children in Flint, Michigan, and an ongoing study of the Sudanese refugees known as the "Lost Boys," who lived for most of their lives in refugee camps in Ethiopia and Kenya without contact with their parents. Dr. Luster's recent edited books include *Parenting: An Ecological Perspective*, Second Edition (2005), and *Disorders in Adolescence*, Volume 2 in *Crisis in Youth Mental Health: Critical Issues and Effective Programs* (2006). He was working on a book chronicling the experiences of Sisimayo Faki Henry, one of the "Lost Boys," when he died in March 2009. This book also examines factors that contributed to resilient outcomes among these youth who grew up in extraordinarily difficult circumstances as a result of the 20-year civil war in Sudan. Dr. Luster was an extraordinary scholar and an exceptional human being.

Shannon Sainer, MSW, is Director of Evaluation and Community Programs at the Colorado Organization on Adolescent Pregnancy, Parenting, and Prevention. Ms. Sainer began her career in adolescent sexual health as a Peace Corps volunteer working with the Nicaraguan Ministry of Health in HIV/AIDS prevention. Returning to the United States, she received an MSW from the University of Denver. For the last several years she has worked on a national project funded by the Centers for Disease Control and Prevention to advise local and state health organizations and schools in the use of evidence-based adolescent sexual health approaches and programs.

Series Editor's Note

Adolescence is a see-saw time of excitement and danger. This eventful period of development, roughly between the ages of 13 and 19, offers simultaneously the possibility of finding oneself and of losing oneself. The adolescent body is mature and attractive, but the frontal lobe of the adolescent brain is, as yet, not fully developed, resulting in impaired judgment about risk taking that the youth may consider exciting, but not dangerous. The idea that a 16-year-old can obtain a driver's license terrifies many grandparents who see the full-page ads in the *New York Times* that expose the frequency with which teenagers have fatal car accidents. Practitioners and counselors who work with young people are dealing with individuals who may have very high ideals and aspirations for society and themselves, but whose motivation to reach their goals may waver because of the necessary effort involved in doing so. The youth between childhood and adulthood can experience a roller coaster of emotions, including depression, rage, and high anxiety, as well as great happiness and satisfaction. To say that it is a challenge to work with these young people is an extreme understatement.

Working with Adolescents employs a multifaceted, ecological perspective through which practitioners can understand both normal adolescent development and those young people who are having serious difficulties coping with their lives. Laser and Nicotera convey the complexity of this topic and systematically walk the reader through the numerous contexts in which an adolescent functions and which can help or hinder his or her struggle for identity. Assessment of risk and protective factors that influence development can offer clues as to appropriate types of intervention when the youth is off course. The book is admirable in its approach, which juggles several balls at once and helps the reader comprehend the complexity and the relative influence of a variety of factors on the teen's behavior.

Separate chapters discuss the family, the school, the neighborhood, and the media, with attention to the specific risk and protective factors that apply in each sphere. The issues of sexual and gender identity, teen sexual activity, substance abuse, mental health, and adolescent delinquency all receive careful attention, with cases illustrating clinical applications for each topic. Despite this roster of problematic possibilities, the authors consistently convey an attitude of respect for their adolescent clients, and draw readers into the fascinating challenge of how to help them most effectively.

The book is carefully organized and the format helpfully provides a useful framework for clinical assessment and intervention. All of the chapters end with questions for discussion, thereby ensuring fascinating and stimulating classroom and workshop dialogues.

As editor of Guilford's Social Work Practice with Children and Families series, I knew that a book on adolescent development was needed to provide a valuable complement to Douglas Davies's book *Child Development: A Practitioner's Guide.* Laser and Nicotera have succeeded in shaping their own appealing views of this developmental stage that many practitioners find daunting. Their work offers many guideposts toward the final chapter, titled "The Joys of Working with Adolescents." I hope this book will succeed in converting many students, practitioners, and educators who may have approached this work with trepidation into clinicians who are fascinated by the many intriguing facets of this exciting time of life.

NANCY BOYD WEBB, DSW

Foreword

Adolescents face enormous developmental challenges in American society. At no time in the country's history have young people been confronted simultaneously by such a wide array of positive and negative influences and opportunities. Fortunately, most young people become healthy adults who participate in positive life activities. For some adolescents, however, the path to adulthood is characterized by involvement in problem behaviors like dropping out of school, delinquency, violence, or substance abuse. Other youth experience significant individual or mental health impairments that hinder their opportunity to live a healthy adult life. The prospect of a successful future for adolescents who become involved in antisocial conduct or suffer from adverse mental health conditions is limited.

Unraveling the causes of adolescent problems and designing effective social interventions for young people is a complicated endeavor. Experts from criminology, psychology, public health, education, and social work agree that there is no single pathway leading to problem behavior. In fact, there are numerous theoretical explanations from each of these disciplines that seek to explain the onset and persistence of childhood and adolescent problems. Frameworks such as life course theory (Farrington & Welsh, 2006; Moffitt, 1993), positive youth development (Catalano, Hawkins, Berglund, Pollard, & Arthur, 2002; Lerner, Fisher, & Weinberg, 2000), and social learning-based models (Catalano & Hawkins, 1996) have been applied widely to adolescent behavior in the past several decades. These and other theories have contributed greatly to our understanding of the many factors affecting adolescent development. Yet despite these theoretical advances, many explanatory frameworks in the adolescent literature focus solely on individual or social factors and fail to consider the multiple levels of risk and protection that influence a young person's behavior.

This book will help practitioners and educators recognize the importance of understanding principles of risk and protection across multiple levels of influence. The authors' commitment to a systemic view of adolescent development is rooted in the early work of Bronfenbrenner (1979, 1986) and other developmental psychologists who recognized that a complex set of individual, family, social, and environmental factors impact young people's behavior. This evidence provides an important foundation to material presented in the book and to the larger topic of understanding the risk, protective, and promotive factors that are associated with typical adolescent problems.

Awareness of the risk and protective influences in young people's lives reveal, a critical piece of the puzzle pertaining to adolescent development. However, frameworks of problem behavior based solely on risk and protection fall short of explaining why some adolescents thrive in the face of individual, social, and environmental adversity. Therefore, it is critical that practitioners, policymakers, and researchers understand the characteristics of young people who are resilient in the face of considerable risk exposure. Explaining why some adolescents persevere and become successful adults, when logic tells us they have little chance to prosper and thrive, lies at the heart of this volume.

Part I of the volume helps us understand the complexities associated with elements of risk, protection, and resilience in the lives of adolescents. In these chapters, Laser and Nicotera examine the ever-changing nature of adolescent development. Importantly, they suggest that a multisystemic–ecological approach is necessary to understand key developmental phases among young people. Further, they identify appropriate intervention approaches to target the multiple levels of influence identified in their ecological framework. Case examples illustrate how a multisystemic–ecological model is applicable to a variety of practice settings. Collectively, the chapters in the first section equip readers with the knowledge to understand the multiple levels of influence that affect adolescent development. The authors also identify key intervention points and principles that correspond to different levels of risk, protective, and promotive factors.

Part II examines adolescent development and behavior from a variety of contexts. The multisystemic–ecological theme is carried across separate chapters that probe the individual, family, peer, school, neighborhood, and media influences on adolescent development. Each chapter is a significant contribution and, together, this section demonstrates the importance of viewing risk, protective, and promotive factors in the context of an adolescent's daily life. In Chapter 9, the authors use a very detailed case study to illustrate the multisystemic–ecological model. This is a unique and compelling way to articulate complex material presented in earlier chapters.

Prior studies of adolescent development and behavior reveal that many of the same protective, risk, and promotive factors are associated with a number of common adolescent problems (e.g., Rutter, 2001). For example, longitudinal studies reveal that adolescents who participate in delinquent conduct, use illegal drugs, or engage in early sexual activity often experience very similar risk and protective traits in their family, school, and neighborhood environments. Designing, implementing, and testing interventions that consider the influence of such traits across multiple problems is a challenging task for any theoretical model. Fortunately, the authors meet this challenge in Part III. In the book's final chapters, efficacious interventions aimed at substance abuse and delinquency highlight the importance of clinical strategies that address both risk and protection among adolescents. Additional entries identify effective strategies for helping adolescents who are experiencing gender identity questions or mental health problems. The authors note correctly that the infusion of risk- and protection-based strategies in programs aimed at adolescents has improved the efficacy of prevention and treatment efforts with young people (Hawkins, 2006; Jenson, in press; Woolf, 2008). In fact, intervention strategies guided by knowledge of risk and protective factors associated with adolescent problems are now widely recognized by state and federal government agencies and other public and private entities as the dominant approach to preventing and treating childhood and adolescent problems (Center for the Study and Prevention of Violence, 2010; Centers for Disease Control and Prevention, 2008; National Institute on Drug Abuse, 1997; Substance Abuse and Mental Health Services Administration, 2010).

This book highlights the importance of recognizing ways in which individual, family, social, and environmental factors influence adolescent development and behavior. Today's young people experience a more diverse set of positive and negative influences than perhaps any group of adolescents in history. Rapid developments in technology and information management, to name a few, have significantly changed the way in which young people think, feel, and behave. The authors' approach to posing and answering key questions of adolescent development and behavior from a multisystemic–ecological approach is timely and important. Evidence gained in the past two decades suggests that empirically based and theoretically sound interventions can prevent the onset and reduce the persistence of many adolescent problems (Foxcroft, Ireland, Lister-Sharp, Lowe, & Breen, 2003; Gottfredson & Wilson, 2003; Wilson & Lipsey, 2007). The authors' emphasis on understanding key interactions among individual, social, and environmental influences on adolescent development and behavior provides a solid foundation to help all young people become successful adults.

I would be remiss if I did not acknowledge the outstanding contributions made to this volume by Professor Tom Luster. Sadly, Tom passed away during the preparation of the manuscript. The importance of human and social ecology in adolescent development was a constant theme of Tom's illustrative career. His important work in adolescent development will be long revered by the many practitioners, students, and researchers whose lives and careers he so deeply affected.

JEFFREY M. JENSON, PhD

References

Bronfenbrenner, U. (1979). *The ecology of human development: Experiments by nature and design.* Cambridge, MA: Harvard University Press.

Bronfenbrenner, U. (1986). Ecology of the family as a context to human development: Research perspectives. *Developmental Psychology, 22,* 723–742.

Catalano, R. F., & Hawkins, J. D. (1996). The social development model: A theory of antisocial behavior. In J. D. Hawkins (Ed.), *Delinquency and crime: Current theories* (pp. 149–197). New York: Cambridge University Press.

Catalano, R. F., Hawkins, J. D., Berglund, L., Pollard, J. A., & Arthur, M. W. (2002). Prevention science and positive youth development: Competitive or cooperative frameworks? *Journal of Adolescent Health, 31,* 230–239.

Center for the Study and Prevention of Violence. (2010). *Blueprints for violence prevention.* Retrieved from *www.colorado.edu/cspv.*

Centers for Disease Control and Prevention. (2008). *Understanding youth violence.* Fact sheet. Atlanta: Centers for Disease Control and Prevention, National Center for Injury Prevention and Control.

Farrington, D. P., & Welsh, B. C. (2006). *Saving children from a life of crime: Early risk factors and effective interventions.* New York: Oxford University Press.

Foxcroft, D. R., Ireland, D., Lister-Sharp, D. J., Lowe, G., & Breen, R. (2003). Longer-term primary prevention for alcohol misuse in young people: A systematic review. *Addiction, 98,* 397–411.

Gottfredson, D. C., & Wilson, D. B. (2003). Characteristics of effective school-based substance abuse prevention. *Prevention Science, 4,* 27–38.

Hawkins, J. D. (2006). Science, social work, prevention: Finding the intersection. *Social Work Research, 30,* 137–152.

Jenson, J. M. (in press). Advances in preventing childhood and adolescent problem behavior. *Research on Social Work Practice.*

Lerner, R. M., Fisher, C. B., & Weinberg, R. A. (2000). Toward a science for and of the people: Promoting civil society through the application of developmental science. *Child Development, 71,* 11–20.

Moffitt, T. E. (1993). Adolescence-limited and life-course-persistent antisocial behavior: A developmental taxonomy. *Psychological Review, 100,* 674–701.

National Institute on Drug Abuse. (1997). *Preventing drug use among children and adolescents: A research guide to what works* (National Institutes of Health Pub. No. 97-4212). Bethesda, MD: National Institutes of Health.

Rutter, M. (2001). Psychosocial adversity: Risk, resilience, and recovery. In J. M. Richman & M. W. Fraser (Eds.), *The context of youth violence: Resilience, risk, and protection* (pp. 13–41). Westport, CT: Praeger.

Substance Abuse and Mental Health Services Administration. (2010). National Registry of Effective Programs. Retrieved from *www.nrepp.samhsa.gov.*

Wilson, S. J., & Lipsey, M. W. (2007). School-based interventions for aggressive and disruptive behavior: Update of a meta-analysis. *American Journal of Preventive Medicine, 33,* S130–S143.

Woolf, S. H. (2008). The power of prevention and what it requires. *Journal of the American Medical Association, 299,* 2437–2439.

Acknowledgments

We want to express our gratitude for the support and assistance we have received writing the book. We thank our guest authors, Douglas Davies, George Stuart Leibowitz, Tom Luster, and Shannon Sainer, and Jeffrey Jenson for the Foreword. We are also indebted to Series Editor Nancy Boyd Webb for her careful review of every chapter and the suggestions she offered throughout the process. We have great appreciation for Guilford Senior Editor Jim Nagcotte, who also read and provided important suggestions for chapter revisions and insight into the "ins and outs" of getting the book completed. We thank Elizabet Covarrubias and Megan Yoder, our research assistants, for their meticulous attention to detail, as well as the many adolescents in our lives who shared their experiences with us, especially Ariana, Orion, and Haily. Last, but not least, we appreciate our respective partners, Paul Stephens and Ellen Winiarczyk, who endured the highs and lows of the entire writing process from conceptualization to completion.

Contents

PART III. CLINICAL INTERVENTIONS
FOR PROBLEMATIC ADOLESCENT BEHAVIOR

WORKING WITH ADOLESCENTS

PART I

THEORETICAL FRAMEWORK

CHAPTER 1

Challenges in Clinical Work with Adolescents

AN OVERVIEW

What Is Adolescence?

Youth are on a voyage of self-discovery. They are beginning to understand who they are and who they are not. This is a process that takes many years to complete and may be arduous at times. During this period of self-discovery, they consider who they want to become—first ideally, and then later more realistically.

The term *adolescence* is not universally defined. In some cultures, adolescence is the period when the child obtains the necessary education or ceremonial rituals to be prepared for the adult world. Therefore, in some cultures this period of adolescence is relatively short. However, in mainstream American culture adolescence lasts longer, spanning 10 or more years. Youth-oriented practitioners usually consider it to span 12–21 years of age. Some youth workers, due to their involvement in the legal system, consider adolescence as ending at 18. However, others suggest that adolescence ends only when the youth is fully independent and has completed his or her education or started on a career, which could occur as early as 18 years or not until the early to mid-20s. We define adolescence as including young people whose ages range from about 13 years old to about 20 years old.

Most credit G. Stanley Hall (1904) with coining the term *adolescence*. He called this a period of "stress and storm." Later theorists proposed that adolescence is not necessarily a tumultuous stage of development. The "rebel without a cause" perception of youth is a myth that has been perpetuated in movies and literature, but not in fact (Bandura, 1964). Certainly, new issues confront youth as they leave childhood, but contemporary theorists believe adolescence should not be a uniquely stressful time. Jessor, Turbin, and Costa (1998) found that youth who had high aspirations and positive self-esteem when they entered high school were likely to be well adjusted upon leaving high school. Frequently, our adolescent clients have had inadequate support and resources, and few caring adults in their lives. For these clients the passage through to adulthood can be risky and difficult.

Adolescence is a time of amazing growth and vitality. Adolescents can think in new and exciting ways, they are usually in the peak of health, and they are often involved with a wide network of people—from the family, neighborhood, and school to after-school activities, work, and religious affiliations. It can be an exciting, satisfying, and happy time. However, for some youth, adolescence can be a period of profound loneliness, depression, and ostracism. These youth may feel they do not fit in with their peers; others may feel the experiences they have had keep them from meaningful relationships. They may feel no one could really understand them or the events they have endured. They fear rejection if they reveal their "true selves." For the casual observer, these youth may scoff at and deride others who hold more conventional views. But frequently this voiced disdain covers feelings of inadequacy, vulnerability, and pain.

Adolescence in Context

Young people grow up in particular contexts including the family, school, and neighborhood. In turn, the media influences each of these contexts. This book offers clinical strategies to assess teens and create interventions that are appropriate in these different contexts. Additionally, the book focuses on both positive influences (*protective factors*) and negative influences (*risk factors*) in each of the environments or contexts in which the youth develops. We promote a holistic assessment of the youth, one that enables you to become familiar with him or her in multiple contexts, and the strengths and challenges he or she experiences in each context. From that perspective, we discuss how to support growth in each context, as well as appropriate interventions to employ.

A Multisystemic–Ecological Approach

The multisystemic–ecological approach to practice with teens accounts for the numerous contexts described above in combination with the psychological and social factors that affect youth. Throughout the book we use the term *M-E approach* as shorthand for the multisystemic–ecological approach. Ecological theory is the foundation for the M-E approach, which requires practitioners to consider not only clients' psychological experiences, but also the sociopolitical influences that create context and meaning.

Consider an adolescent who is acting out—say, vandalizing his or her school. The M-E approach leads practitioners to assess not only psychological reasons for the acting out (such as a behavioral disorder), but also broader systems as influences on the youth's behavior (such as experiences of racism, bullying, or homophobia). Acknowledging and understanding the impact of these broader systems does not mean condoning the acting-out behavior. But it does lead to a more thorough evaluation of the presenting problem, which then has a greater chance of guiding interventions that will be effective.

Consider the following case example, which was developed and embellished from a news story (St. John, 2007). Shahir is a 14-year-old refugee from Afghanistan who has been living in Clarkson, Georgia, for the past 4 years. He lives with his 16-year-old sister, his grandparents, and his father. His mother died during the war in Afghanistan. Shortly after her death, the family feared further persecution and escaped their home for a refugee camp in northern India, where they lived for 1 year. Later, the family immigrated to the United States. Shahir is now a member of a local soccer team in Clarkson that consists of players from all over the world who also came to the town as refugees. Clarkson has become a major U.S. refugee resettlement center. Given this common history of refugee status, and having a tongue-in-cheek sense of humor, the team chose to name itself the "Fugees." The team practices and plays their games in the park that is centrally located in downtown Clarkson. The team looks forward to possibly becoming regional champions in the next season.

Shahir's family life is loving and supportive. He loves and admires his grandfather who was a champion soccer player when he was a young man in Afghanistan. His family interacts with some of the other families of the boys on the soccer team. Shahir is in the ninth grade at the local high school, where his teammates are also students. While his grades continue to be above average and his social skills on par with other ninth-grade boys, the school social worker meets with him because of recent behaviors: refusing to answer questions in class, the disappearance of his usually sunny disposition and smiles, and a fight with a boy he barely knows. Recently, the mayor of Clarkson declared, "There will be nothing but football and baseball down there [the park] so long as I am mayor," adding, "Those fields weren't made for soccer." Many of the long-time town residents of Clarkson support this declaration. As a result, the Fugees team has not been able to practice for 3 weeks, and one of the most important games of the season takes place next week.

A traditional approach to the assessment of Shahir tends toward exploration of the psychological factors that might be influencing Shahir's current behavioral challenges. These could include behavioral reactions to depressive or anxious thoughts:

- If the anniversary of his mother's death is not far off.
- If Shahir and is worried about disappointing his father or grandfather as he becomes more Americanized.
- If Shahir is anxious because of disagreements that arise with teammates now that they are no longer allowed to hold practice sessions.

In contrast, the M-E approach expands assessment to include Shahir's behavior in different contexts and the sociopolitical factors that may be influencing his behavioral changes. As such, the ecological practitioner would explore ramifications of the local mayor's decree that no soccer team can use the field in the local park. The practitioner will consider how Shahir, his peers, and his family view the mayor's decree, and assist in considering whether there are any connections to the frustration over not being able to practice and Shahir's current behavior. The practitioner will also consider the mayor's decree in the context of post-9/11 attitudes, which have left some Americans fearing and having bias against (even discriminating against) persons from the Middle East and South Asia. Additionally, the practitioner needs to consider how the community welcomed Shahir's family and other refugee families to Clarkson. In this light, some of the questions the M-E practitioner will pose include:

- "Are school and community members targeting the Fugees with racial and religious bias in the aftermath of the mayor's decree?"
- "Are there any youth from Afghanistan or other refugee youth who play on the local baseball and football teams?"
- "Are longtime Clarkson residents interacting positively with immigrants from Afghanistan and other countries?"

This expanded assessment has the potential to open up multiple options for intervention aimed at changing the psychological *and* sociopolitical influences on Shahir's current behaviors. For example, the practitioner may collaborate with the Fugee teammates and their families to contact their neighborhood councilperson and to speak at a City Council meeting. The practitioner might also intervene at the school level if peers are taunting the Fugee teammates with racial and religious slurs. Shahir's experience illustrates the complexity and multiple contexts that may influence clients' behaviors and feelings. It is our hope that the M-E approach to understanding teen clients will increase your ability to build cross-system relationships that lead to positive outcomes for youth.

How Ecological Theory Illuminates Adolescent Development

Human ecology is the science of interrelationships between living organisms and between organisms and their natural, built, and social environments (Bubolz & Sontag, 1993; Hayword, 1994). Ecological theory proposes that the characteristics of the individual interacting with characteristics of the environment over time influences development (Barrows, 1995; Bubolz & Sontag, 1993; Griffore & Phenice, 2001). Bronfenbrenner (1979), the originator of the term *human ecology*, speaks of the developing person "as a growing dynamic entity that progressively moves into and restructures the milieu in which it resides" (p. 21). The environment transforms and accommodates the individual and the individual transforms and accommodates the environment. Neither the environment nor the individual is the same due to the interaction. (Bronfenbrenner, 1979, 1986, 1989). A human ecological perspective allows the practitioner to assess and intervene at the multilevel interactions between a teen and his or her environments.

Time is an important ingredient in ecological theory. Bronfenbrenner (1979) uses the term *chronosystem* to denote generational influences affecting the individual, critical events, and everyday stresses that contribute to human development. *Generational influences* become more apparent during adolescence and young adulthood. The environmental factors of an era have an impact on that generation for the rest of their lifespan. In the United States such generational influences include the Great Depression, World War II, the Cold War, the Vietnam War, the Civil Rights Movement, the Women's Movement, the fall of the Berlin Wall, September 11, and the War on Terrorism. These events change the nature of society and have an impact on the developing teen. For example, ideas about who is safe and how to secure safety in post-9/11 America may be the reason why Shahir's team cannot practice soccer in the park.

Critical events are particular life events that influence an individual, though not necessarily his or her contemporaries. They include events such as death or incarceration of a parent, serious illness, moving to a better neighborhood, the birth of a sibling, or graduating from high school. Such events have an enormous impact on the development of the individual, but not on the wider society in which that person is developing. Practitioners who ask teen clients to make timelines of their lives can assess for the effects of critical events. As a youth plots his or life events, ask what each event meant to him or her and what he or she learned from the event. As the intervention continues, ask how the critical events he or she experienced shaped him or her to be the person he or she is today.

Everyday stresses refer to the daily issues individuals face such as financial insecurity, traffic, time pressure, sleeping patterns, family coping methods, relationship struggles, friendship quarrels, and dietary issues. The ability to cope with these frequent and sometimes chronic issues helps to mold the individual. Asking the youth "What hassles do you have to deal with every day?" can begin to give some insight into his or her everyday stresses.

The chronosystem has a profound effect on the development of the adolescent. It also helps to form his or her identity through the connection to his or her generation, personal experiences, and life stresses. The chronosystem helps define his or her worldview and the understanding of his or her place in that world.

The Microsystem

The individual develops in a number of different contexts. The initial structure where development occurs is the microsystem. It involves the reciprocal interplay among people, objects, and symbols. The microsystem has been defined "as a pattern of activities, roles, and interpersonal relations experienced by the developing person in a given face-to-face setting with particular physical and material features and containing other persons with distinctive characteristics of temperament, personality, and systems of belief" (Bronfenbrenner, 1989, p. 227). The initial microsystem that the infant inhabits is the home, where the majority of interaction is between the infant and the parent, or primary caregiver. As the child grows and enters other microsystems he or she has interactions with different people and objects. Examples of these other microsystems include day care, church, synagogue, mosque, school, the neighborhood, and the peer network. In adolescence, youth participate in a multitude of microsystems. We address youth development and resilience in the family, school and neighborhood microsystems.

Development is bidirectional; that is, the family and school influence development and the teen, in turn, influences the family and school. As the teen moves from one setting to another, relationships may change. One microsystem, such as neighborhood, may be a venue where he or she flourishes and another, such as the school, may be a location where he or she feels stifled, lost, or stigmatized. Understanding youth in the clinical context requires information about activities, roles, and relationships in each microsystem. This knowledge provides insight into social and emotional functioning.

The Mesosystem

The mesosystem is the interface between two microsystems. The mesosystem refers to the interrelations among two or more settings in which the developing adolescent actively participates. An example of a mesosystemic interface is the relationship between home and school. The connections between these settings provide continuity for the developing person and insight for all members of the microsystems to understand the adolescent and how he or she develops in the other context. For example, positive functioning increases when there is interaction between the multiple settings where the youth resides (Bunting, 1996; Deslandes, Royer, & Turcotte, 1997; Fuller & Olsen, 1998; Pipher, 1994). The positive interface of these spheres is a source of support for the adolescent. Fuller and Olsen discuss the importance of the home–school interface at the middle school and high school levels. They state that students whose parents are involved in their schools have higher aspirations and commitments to lifelong education. These students are more likely to avoid high-risk behaviors, are more involved in school or community activities, and are more likely to avoid school problems (Rolande, Royer, & Turcotte, 1997). The adolescent needs the interaction between these two important spheres of his or her life to achieve a greater degree of adjustment.

If the important people in the adolescent's life know each other, he or she feels more secure and more supported. For instance, if the parent and the teacher come together to discuss the student's academic progress with the student present, the student is aware not only that these important players in his or her life care about and are interested in him or her, but also that these individuals hold him or her accountable. This is especially important if the student has tried in the past to triangulate parent and teacher, so that they were at odds with each other, instead of working together as a team. The adolescent now understands that there will be the possibility for ongoing discussion, information sharing, and dialogue between these members of the two microsystems.

Another mesosystemic interface that is important for the adolescent is the family and peer microsystem interaction. Pipher (1994), stresses the importance of the adolescent to invite friends into the home so that members of each microsystem know each other and the roles that each has in the developing person's life. Adolescents are happier when friends are comfortable with the family and the family is at ease with his or her friends. Understanding and support promote communication between a teen's microsystems and avoid possible distrust, animosity, or disregard for members from separate microsystems. Greater knowledge and trust across each microsystem enhances adolescent functioning. For example, the adolescent's adjustment improves by strengthening both the family–school interaction and the family–peer interaction.

Practitioners conduct enhanced assessments and interventions when they assess the varied activities, roles, and relationships a teen has in one microsystem and how these activities, roles, and relationships support or undermine his or her development in another microsystem. For example, how the adolescent makes and retains friends in the neighborhood microsystem may be quite different from how he or she makes and retains friends in the school microsystem. Helping the youth understand the similarities and differences in how he or she "operates" in each microsystem will improve his or her social functioning. Additionally, modifying the environment can help the individual be successful in a different or new microsystem.

The Exosystem

The exosystem does not involve the developing person as a participant. The adolescent does not influence events in the exosystem, but nonetheless the events affect his or her development. Some examples of the exosystem are mom's or dad's work, mom's or dad's school or extrafamilial activities, the local board of education, the state and federal legislature, Immigration and Naturalization Services (INS), and Medicaid. For example, decisions to lay off employees at a parent's workplace can have profound effects on family finances and in turn a teen's options for present and future choices. Additionally, parent stress due to job loss can filter down to the teen resulting in strained parent–child relations.

The Macrosystem

The macrosystem is the cultural environment that permeates the microsystem, mesosystem, and exosystem. It is the cultural setting that includes social expectations for individual and group behavior. Macrosystems include tenets of behavior; rules (both spoken and unspoken); morals of a particular time, place, generation, and environment; and attitudes toward diversity and civil rights. Macrosystem expectations can be universal or pertain to a particular subset of any population. A society's biases and prejudices undergird these expectations. As a result, some values and behaviors are the "norm" while others are aberrant. For example, traditional gender role norms suggest that men ought to be the major breadwinners in a family. Hence, men who elect to be a stay-at-home parent are an oddity and even shunned in certain circles as "playing mom."

The adolescent perspective on expectations of the macrosystem is often in flux. He or she may subscribe to rules, morals, and tenets of behavior that differ somewhat or drastically from parent and society expectations. Youth ostracize peers who exhibit behaviors and attitudes that differ from macrosystem norms. Youth may feel a great deal of tension between the expectations and norms of behavior in the family as compared to the neighborhood or school. For example, when recent immigrant youth attend school in a new country they often feel tension because teachers are not able to fully appreciate their home cultures and languages. Practitioners who understand the effects of macrosystems and the pressure youth experience from these effects will have a greater appreciation about the adolescent's sense of identity, purpose, and values.

Case Study: Applying Ecological Theory and the M-E Approach

Ecological theory and the M-E approach highlight the multiple systems that influence an individual's relationships and the myriad opportunities for assessment and intervention beyond a teen's psychological status. The following case example challenges you to apply the ideas and concepts presented in this chapter.

Ramona is a 16-year-old African American. She resides in Chicago with her two brothers, Carlos, 18, and Juan, 14, and her mother Alfreda, 46. The children's father and Alfreda's husband, George, 49, resides in Detroit, Michigan. Alfreda and George grew up in Detroit where they each have extensive family networks. When the children were young, George's mother provided child care so that George could work and Alfreda could attend university. George worked at a major automotive plant and the family finances suffered because of the boom and bust nature of that industry. On the completion of her degree, Alfreda believed that a move to Chicago would create a more stable future for the family since the auto industry had cycled through bad times in the past. However, George believed that they would stay in Detroit forever and that the depressed economy would turn around so that Alfreda could find a local teaching job. However, schools were closing, teachers lost jobs, and teaching opportunities in Detroit seemed remote.

When George was out of work for 12 months, Alfreda suggested that the family move to Chicago where there were more teaching jobs and possibilities for his employment. However, George did not want to give up hope on the work he had done for most of his adult life. Also, his parents were aging now and he wanted to be available to them. This difference of opinion caused conflict between the couple. However, when Alfreda obtained a teaching job in Chicago and the auto industry took further hits, George finally agreed that he would move. The couple agreed that George would stay in Detroit until they sold their home. Alfreda and the children moved to Chicago, but 12 months later they still had not sold their home and George's parents' health declined rapidly. It has now been 4 years since the original move and the couple is despondent about ever having the family live in the same city. George's parents need his help and their home still has not sold. In contrast, Alfreda adores her work with the students and has many friends at school where she teaches.

Ramona was 12 when she left Detroit. She has a circle of friends in Chicago at her high school. She sings in the choir at her church, and has a small part in the musical at her school. Ramona passes by her mom's elementary school on her way home. Frequently she walks home with her mom. Ramona misses her grandmother in Detroit and all of her cousins. Her dad used to come to visit at least twice a month, but recently his visits decreased to once a month because of caring for his parents.

Carlos's transition to life in Chicago has not been good. He had trouble in school when he first arrived, and was evaluated and placed in special education. Some of the other students in his classes do not value their education and would prefer to "run the streets." He has begun to question why he should stay in school since he is doing so poorly. He has frequent verbal fights with Ramona and has stolen money from both Ramona and his mom. Some of Carlos's friends have asked out Ramona, but she has not been interested. Carlos's friends are a little rough. On two occasions, one guy who is in school with Carlos followed Ramona home. This made her nervous, and now she always stops by her mom's school on her way home.

Juan is doing well in school, but his mother worries because he parrots some of Carlos's ideas. Juan is athletic and plays pick-up basketball on the playground of his mother's school. This is his last year in middle school. Next year he will be in high school.

QUESTIONS FOR THE REFLECTIVE PRACTITIONER

1. What microsystems does each adolescent in the family inhabit?
2. Describe each of the teen's roles, activities, and relationships in each microsystem.
3. How do Ramona's, Carlos's, and Juan's activities, roles, and relationships support or undermine development in their other microsystems?
4. What mesosystemic interfaces affect Ramona, Carlos, and Juan?
5. What exosystems influence their lives?
6. What macrosystemic influences are in Ramona's, Carlos's, and Juan's lives?
7. What generational issues are influencing Ramona's, Carlos's, and Juan's lives?

8. How are the generational influences of the parents different than the adolescents?

9. What critical events have been important in Ramona's, Carlos's, and Juan's lives?

10. What everyday stresses does each adolescent experience?

11. What do you miss about each adolescent if an ecological perspective is not used?

CHAPTER 2

The Push–Pull
of Adolescent Development

Chapter Overview

To better understand the world of adolescents, we first need to see how adolescents develop into adults. We can do so by investigating the different domains of adolescent development, which include physical development, cognitive development, moral development, emotional development, identity development, and social development. As adolescents mature, they grow in each of these domains, sometimes more effectively and healthfully in particular domains rather than across all domains. On occasion, when an adolescent is making great strides in one domain of development another domain of development is temporarily left by the wayside. Practitioners can assess where clinical intervention is needed for a client by having a firm understanding of normative adolescent development and where the client diverges from this. Some domains may seem stunted or need opportunities for growth and benefit from clinical intervention, whereas other domains may simply need more time to develop. In this chapter, we investigate adolescent risk taking and the major domains of adolescent development: physical, cognitive, brain, moral, emotional, identity, and social development.

Adolescent Physical Development

Puberty

The concept of adolescence may be defined biologically as the onset of puberty and the onset of sexual reproductive functioning. The age of puberty has been steadily declining among U.S. youth (Santrock, 2005).

Currently, the onset of puberty in the United States is approximately 12 years old for females, and 14 years old for males. There have been a number of theories about why there has been such a decline; some researchers point to an increase in health and nutrition (Kaplowitz, Slora, Wasserman, Pedlow, & Herman-Giddens, 2001). Others are concerned that an increase in hormones in food or childhood obesity may be the cause for earlier puberty. Nonetheless, the age of menarche (first period for females) has declined from the age of 17 in the 1840s to the age of 12 in the United States currently. There certainly does seem to be a relationship between the percentage of body fat in comparison to body weight and the onset of menstruation. Overweight girls are experiencing their first period earlier than other generations and, in female youth who have lost considerable weight due to anorexia or extreme participation in sports, cease to menstruate or delay the onset of menstruation.

Growth and Maturation

Part of the awkwardness of the early adolescent years is due to the adolescent *growth spurt*. This rapid growth happens 2 years earlier in females than it does in males, thereby creating a marked difference in height in females and males in the middle school years, with the females often towering over their male peers. Frequently, in the middle school years, females look much older than their biological age whereas males appear much younger.

Both males and females may face some difficult issues related to early or late maturation. Studies of maturation and popularity find that early-maturing males, because of their greater physical capability, have a competitive advantage over their peers and are therefore often very popular, more relaxed in social situations, and cooperative with adults (Meschke & Silbereisen, 1997). However, the same cannot be said for early-maturing females. For early-maturing females, their physical appearance of being a "Barbie" in a crowd of "Skippers" is initially a minus. The early-maturing females were at greater risk for eating disorder issues and depression until their later-maturing female peers caught up to them (Hayward et al., 1997). Late-maturing males had greater feelings of inadequacy, negative self-concept, and feelings of rejection than their on-time or early-maturing male peers (Sinkkonen, Anttila, & Siimes, 1998). However, late-maturing females were not characterized by negative psychological reactions. It is hypothesized that for late-maturing females, being childlike or waiflike is not negative, as long as they are not too extremely late maturing (Brooks-Gunn, 1988). An important topic of discussion between a practitioner and an adolescent involves understanding where the youth fits on this continuum from early to late maturing and how that impacts his or her self-esteem and self-concept.

The growth spurt is often *asynchronous*, resulting in dissimilar rates of growth in different parts of the body, thereby creating the appearance of some young adolescents as having enormous hands and feet and an overall gangly appearance. This rapid growth may cause younger adolescents to be somewhat uncoordinated as they learn to adjust to their larger body. The comical expression of "tripping over one's own feet" in early adolescence can actually be a source of embarrassment and humiliation. A clinician can help the youth to understand that this is a temporary event and this information may help to lessen the pain and embarrassment. I once had a client whose father told her "to look on the bright side of her size 10 shoes in that she could always get a summer job stomping out forest fires." The father was unable to see that poking fun at the girl's large feet only added more pain and shame about her self-image.

Adolescent Health Related to Risk Taking

Along with sexual development through puberty, the adolescent is experiencing increased muscle development, which creates greater strength and physical ability coupled with larger stature and the appearance of more adult physical characteristics. The combination of these physical changes often leads to greater independence and less adult monitoring. This may be a risky parental decision, especially with regard to males. Interestingly, Werner and Smith (1992) found that adolescent females faired best when they lived in homes where there was an emphasis on independence, emotional support, and less overprotection. However, adolescent males who lived in households that emphasized concrete structured rules, parental supervision, and adult role models functioned best. Therefore, in adolescence, females need increased independence over time while males need adult interaction and continued parameters for behavior regulation. Garbarino (1999, 2001) suggests that we, as a society, socialize our adolescent females and males very differently by protecting our teenage females to a greater extent than our teenage males, and supporting adolescent female emotional development better than we do adolescent male emotional development. By not allowing males to fully understand their emotions and not monitoring them as closely as our females, we do not give males the best tools for healthy development. Therefore, the lack of monitoring of boys may in fact lead to greater risk taking. Programs that help males bond to other men, preferably their own father, are extremely beneficial for healthy male development.

With greater independence, the experience of increased physical strength and vigor may lead to feelings of omnipotence that can create reckless behavior and risk taking. Additionally, the concept of death is extremely distant for youth, so they may perceive themselves as invulnerable. *Egocentrism*, feelings of being "special," the need to look good or augment oneself, and the conflict of values between self, parents, and peers can also lead to risk taking (Phenice & Griffore, 2000).

Others have suggested that risk-taking behavior is related to adolescent stress. Elkind (1984) discusses that the outward appearance of many sophisticated youth is merely a facade. Though the adolescent gives the appearance of being competent, the chinks in his or her armor are visible through closer scrutiny of his or her behavior. Many of the risk-taking behaviors of the adolescent, in fact, may constitute maladaptive methods of dealing with the stress in his or her life. Binge drinking, sexual acting out, disordered eating, cutting behavior, and truancy are a few of the ineffective ways adolescents may try to combat stress. If practitioners understand these behaviors as not simply problematic but symptoms of a greater issue, they can begin to treat the possible root cause as stress related.

It has also been suggested that adolescent risk taking is related to popularity (Mayeux, Sandstrom, & Cillessen, 2008), in that the quest for popularity leads to increases in alcohol use and sexual activity. There can be a cyclical phenomenon to this in that with greater notoriety there is increased popularity and a greater desire to continue to push the boundary to more risky behaviors.

Additionally, innovations in neuroscience have proposed that adolescent risk taking is a function of two systems of the brain developing at different times. These are the limbic system and the prefrontal cortex. The social-emotional brain, the limbic system, undergoes a change at about the time of puberty, 12–14 years old, which causes changes in the youth's attentiveness to rewards, sensation seeking, emotional arousal, short-term gratification, and attention to social norms. However, the cognitive control portion of the brain, the prefrontal cortex—responsible for impulse control, planning, self-regulation, anticipating future consequences, resistance to peer influences, and forethought—does not begin to mature until the mid-teens and does not fully mature until the mid-20s (Steinberg, 2009). Therefore, the social-emotional maturing brain is left unchecked until the cognitive control portion of the brain can "catch up." Thus adolescent risk behavior can be viewed as a function of timing of the growth of these different portions of the brain. Therefore, from a neuroscience perspective, cognitive interventions that change the youth's risk-taking behavior will not work because the behavior is a function of an incompletely developed brain. What will work from a neuroscience perspective to reduce risk taking is to change the environment where the youth lives. Hence, programs that support youth's healthy development until the cognitive control portion of the brain matures include those that involve parental monitoring, improved after-school programs (since research has shown that most risk-taking behavior is happening between 3 and 7 P.M.), and more organized school activities. Additionally, legislative initiatives such as graduated driver's licenses, disallowing cell phone texting while driving, reducing-off campus privileges to underclassmen, and enforcing curfews have been helpful in decreasing risk-taking behavior (Steinberg).

Adolescence and Disordered Eating

Disordered eating problems and body image affect many teenage females and some teenage males. A study of the eating behaviors of junior high school females found that many of the females had had concerns about their weight and body image beginning in the elementary school years. Over one-quarter of the subjects reported that they had first dieted at age 12 or younger and that 27% of the subjects were currently on diets (Moreno & Thelen, 1995). This is both a health issue, as well as a mental health issue. The perception that their body is somehow inadequate and needs changing speaks very strongly to these girls' lack of confidence in themselves. Practitioners must understand and help adolescent females feel more comfortable with their bodies. The following three nutritional issues are particularly deleterious to youth: anorexia nervosa, bulimia, and obesity.

Anorexia Nervosa

Anorexia nervosa is a disorder in which the individual perceives herself to be overweight and franticly controls calorie intake and increases exercise levels to reduce weight. Even though she may be extremely thin, perhaps even cadaverous, the anorexic adolescent considers herself not an ideal weight. Frequently, these young women are prone to perfectionism and feel that they have no control over their lives, other than their ability to control their calorie intake. They are often very high achievers, and come from families that are driven by success.

Practitioners who work with adolescent clients with eating disorders should collaborate with a registered dietician in order to work on both the emotional issues, as well as the nutritional issues. Clients with anorexia can suffer from brittle bones, skin discoloration, increased facial hair, discontinuation of menstruation, and depression. A physician should also be involved since this disorder can result in death in extreme circum-stances.

Most recently, Internet anorexia blogs have developed that support this disordered thinking by giving young women techniques to further restrict calories. These sites have been extremely destructive to young women with eating disorders. Practitioners should inquire where the ado-lescent is obtaining information about nutrition. Clients with anorexia who are struggling to control their weight may hide the extent of their weight loss by wearing baggy clothes and lie about the amount of food they are consuming, or the amount of time they are spending exercising. This may make it difficult for parents and concerned adults to really assess their behavior. Additionally, if the youth presents with a more advanced form of anorexia, a therapist who specializes in eating disorders should see the client because in severe cases anorexia can be life threatening and the client may be in such a danger to self that hospitalization may be necessary.

Bulimia

The adolescent with bulimia, like one with anorexia, sees her weight as problematic, but she is unable to restrict calories to lose weight and therefore goes through cycles of eating and then purging food through vomiting or the use of laxatives, enemas, or diuretics. As this behavior continues the clients with bulimia will become preoccupied with food, sometimes consuming a great deal of high-calorie food and then purging it from her system. The result of this seesaw behavior may include health issues such as ulcers, dental problems, hair loss, stomach complaints, and digestive problems. The client's physical appearance may vary from thin to normal weight.

The adolescent with bulimia feels an intense pressure to be thin and obsesses about food constantly by creating a cycle of preoccupation with food, overconsumption of food, disgust with self for the overconsumption, purging food from self, and renewed preoccupation with food. Frequently, the client's issues with food stems from depression and low self-esteem. Practitioners should work on enhancing the client's self-esteem and self-concept. Sometimes antidepressants are effective for treating bulimia.

Obesity

Many believe that obesity has become an epidemic in the United States. Some research has found that over a quarter of American adolescents are obese (Popkin & Urdery, 1998). This has long-term negative ramifications for their health in adulthood because eating patterns learned in childhood and adolescence continue in adulthood. A multitude of health disorders in adulthood have been linked to obesity such as diabetes, heart disease, and back and skeletal problems.

Additionally, these youth may be harassed by their peers for being overweight, feel uncomfortable socializing with their peers due to their weight, or unable to lead an active lifestyle due to their weight. They may feel a great deal of stigma and have trouble making and maintaining friendships.

Youth with issues of obesity need to explore their relationship to food and how they use food. Has food become a soother of difficult emotions, a suppressor of difficult memories, a comfort to loneliness, or a friend who does not judge them? If any of these issues are true for the young person, this suggests that food is no longer considered simply a means of sustenance. Collaboration between the practitioner, a registered dietician, and the young person must consider both the emotional issues, as well as the dietary, issues.

Though the youth may gain some notoriety for being "big" it often undermines his or her self-esteem by constantly being the brunt of derisive jokes. A recent client shared that he "did not want to be known as the 'fat kid' any longer; he wanted people to see past his physical self." Though he understood he was more than the "fat kid," he felt that many of his peers chose not to know who he really was. He said that he laughed with them when they joked about his weight but inside he cried. Through counseling, he was able to better know himself and convey that image to his schoolmates, while simultaneously with the help of a registered dietician reduce his weight and maintain a healthy diet. He became a more confident and happier 15-year-old.

Adolescent Cognitive Development and Brain Development

Adolescents according to Piaget (1952, 1970) are in the stage of *formal operations*, meaning that they can think abstractly, creatively, and in novel ways. Their brains can think scientifically and multidimensionally about a topic or a problem. When they choose to use this new cognitive ability, the result can be amazingly intellectually stimulating, scintillating, and enlightening. Of course not all youth spend a great deal of time thinking in formal operations. Some youth find themselves so very interesting and their thoughts and feelings so unique that they become self-absorbed. *Adolescent egocentrism* refers to this fascination with their new thinking process and often wanting to share their "pearls of wisdom" with their friends, siblings, parents, and teachers. They can often become self-engrossed in their own thinking, believing that they are the only ones who ever conceived of an issue in this manner and that they are the sole harbinger of the truth. Those around a youth with this "enlightenment" may consider it as an interesting time of self-discovery or a somewhat tedious time of self-absorption.

To highlight this point a youth I know very well told me, "Sometimes I have these great new ideas in my head and I need to tell someone before I forget them." This unfortunately was his rationale for his inability to keep his mouth shut in class! He truly believed his thoughts had never been conceived of before. His own fascination with the novelty of his thoughts and his fear of forgetting his thoughts before he could share them with others created a dilemma for him in class. After his third time of being written up for talking in class by the teacher, we discussed that he carry a little notebook titled "Smart Ideas" where he could write down his ideas down so they would not be lost and then when the time was appropriate he could share those smart ideas with others. This was a workable solution for him, his teacher, and his classmates. It also underscores the potency of the concept of formal operations on an adolescent mind.

Neurodevelopment begins *in utero* but continues through adolescence. The majority of brain development is completed before early childhood, though development in the neocortex of the brain continues through adolescence (Perry, 2001b). The neocortex is the part of the brain that encompasses the frontal lobes, parietal lobes, occipital lobes, and the corpus callosum (Perry, 2008). The neocortex is responsible for such cognitive functions as abstraction, self-image, socialization, and affiliation (Perry, 2005). Perry believes that brain development is affected by both genetics and environment (2001b, 2005). The initial expression of the genes begins shortly after conception in a patterned manner. However, as the individual grows and develops, the environment where the individual resides has a profound effect on how genes are expressed. Perry has found that children who have been exposed to neglect or childhood trauma (domestic violence, physical abuse, sexual abuse, physical injury, death of a loved one, or destruction of home, school, or community) can change the actual physical development of the brain (2001b, 2008). This underscores the need to support programs that target the prevention of child abuse and neglect. It also highlights the importance of early clinical intervention to minimize the effects of childhood trauma on developing brains. Perry's assertion that brain development continues through adolescence is an important and positive fact for practitioners, in that adolescent brains are not yet fully formed and with the proper nurturance and stimulation some growth is still possible.

Adolescent Moral Development

In childhood, moral judgment and behavior derives from wanting to avoid trouble and to be perceived by the adults in their life as doing what is right. This represents *externally* controlled behavior. By contrast, in adolescence, the youth learns to internalize "What would I want to see happen in this situation?" Adolescents begin to understand that they should do the "right thing" because it is the right thing to do and not to gain positive regard or avoid criticism from others. Therefore, the youth moves from the external control of childhood moral behavior to autonomy and internal control in adolescence. This progression, however, varies greatly among youth.

Moral reasoning is the outcome of the adolescent's new and novel ways of thinking. Based on formal operations (Piaget, 1952, 1970), the youth can think through a problem with *multifinality*, to imagine a variety of different outcomes for an event. Piaget believed that the strength of moral reasoning depends on the perception of reality. With enhanced perception of reality, the developing individual will improve his or her moral reasoning as he or she improves cognitive understanding. Similarly, with greater cognitive development and more life experience, the youth is more competent at organizing and evaluating his or her experiences. Along with this comes the ability to take another's point of view and to think abstractly.

Other theorists like Bandura (1982, 1989, 1995, 1997) believe that the developing person learns primarily about moral behavior from his or her direct experiences. Through his or her own life experiences the person learns to be moral. But he or she does not necessarily have to experience a situation him- or herself to develop morally; he or she can also learn moral behavior by observing others. *Vicarious experiences* are experiences that the developing person witnessed or heard about that had an influence on the developing person. A vicarious experience can help the developing person increase or decrease moral behavior. When the experience that is witnessed or heard about happens to someone with whom the developing person is close its impact is greater. An example of this would be a youth who witnesses another youth getting in trouble for cheating on an exam. The vicarious experience of seeing a friend being punished for his or her immoral behavior teaches the youth how important it is to be an honest test taker. The youth did not have to have the experience happen personally to learn from it. Thereby, witnessing an experience with a very positive or a negative outcome will affect the developing person's future moral behavior and development.

Kohlberg's (1963) theory of moral development is closely connected to Piaget's understanding of moral reasoning. Kohlberg believes, like Piaget, that moral reasoning develops in a particular sequence. Kohlberg has created three major stages of moral development that also have several substages. In adolescence, youth may have achieved the third major stage of moral development that he calls *postconventional*. Kohlberg believes that some adolescents and adults never get to the postconventional stage of moral development and others only make brief "forays" into it. Within the postconventional stage, the first substage is called the *social contract*, meaning that one chooses to act morally by considering the greatest good for the greatest number. The second substage of postconventional moral development and the highest level for Kohlberg is called *universal ethical principles.* These principles are strongly held beliefs in the right course of action even though it may put the individual in peril. These principles are held more closely than one's allegiance to a government, affiliation, or membership. The actions of Mahatma Gandhi, Martin Luther King Jr., and Nelson Mandela, whose adherence to their ethical principles were more important than their own personal safety, are examples of universal ethical principles. The achievement of this last stage of Kohlberg's moral development can be seen in some youth by their becoming very passionate about a cause or an issue and their willingness to make life changes to better live in accordance with those issues. Youth involvement in such activities as political demonstrations, environmental activism, Peace Corps, mission trips, or enlisting in the military are all possible activities where their moral ethical principles bring them to be involved in the activity.

Many have criticized Kohlberg's overreliance on concepts of justice. Other concepts such as responsibility, friendliness, and courage are of equal importance for moral development. In fact, there may be many moral actions that are more highly valued by females such as community building, consensus making, friendliness, courage, responsibility, and accommodation (Gilligan, Lyons, & Hamer, 1990). Others consider the role of gender in the individual's ability to regulate his or her emotions. In that, girls and boys are socialized differently to value different aspects of interpersonal interactions. Boys are frequently socialized to value competition, achievement orientation, and not to avoid conflicts. Girls are often socialized to nurture, have empathy, and comply with adult requests. Therefore, through different experiences different moral behaviors will be seen.

Moral development has also been understood as the development of specific emotions and the regulation of those emotions. Emotions that are important to moral development are embarrassment, guilt, shame, empathy, and sympathy (Eisenberg, 2000). The depth of these moral emotions will also determine how the individual will regard his or her own behavior. An individual can internalize an outcome, which means that the situation comes from his or her own making, or can externalize an outcome, which means that the situation was created by outside events beyond the individual's control (Eisenberg, 2000). Therefore, adolescents who are able to take responsibility for their actions by internalizing the outcomes are better adjusted and have greater emotional regulation. Additionally, youth have greater moral development if they are able to regulate their emotions and internalize their behavior. This is an important concept for practitioners because it means part of the work that must be done with youth in a clinical setting is helping them "own" their own behavior and emotional regulation of feelings.

Another theorist, Lickona (1991), views good character as the composite of moral knowing, moral feeling, and moral action. *Moral knowing* includes moral awareness, knowing moral values, perspective taking, moral reasoning, and decision making. Moral knowing is the component that is closest to the theories of Piaget, Kohlberg, and Gilligan, namely, the cognitive process that is involved in moral development. *Moral feeling* is the emotional component of good character. Moral feeling includes conscience, self-esteem, empathy, loving the good, self-control, and humility. Lickona includes the prosocial moral emotions of Eisenberg (2000): empathy and sympathy. He also uses the term *self-control*, which is similar to Eisenberg's term *emotional regulation*. Lickona believes that empathy can be gained as a vicarious experience similar to Bandura's understanding of moral development. Lickona sees the outcome of moral knowing and moral feeling to be moral action. *Moral action* includes competence, which is the ability to solve a conflict fairly; will, which is the desire and the energy to solve a conflict fairly; and habit, which consists of fair conflict resolution.

The case of David highlights the point of Lickona's (1991) triadic view of moral development. David was a 14-year-old who was caught shoplifting. In counseling, David was able to verbalize that his shoplifting was in fact stealing from another person and therefore wrong (moral thinking). Prior to that he had not been able to conceive of shoplifting as an offense against another and only thought of it as a manner of getting something he wanted, but did not have money to pay for. Through therapy, he was also able to explore his own feelings about theft, both as the perpetrator and the victim, thereby coming to better name and understand his own moral emotions. Finally, David was able to connect his moral thinking with his moral feeling by performing an act of reparation at the convenience store from which he had frequently pilfered. Through his moral action he was able to get to know the family from which he had been stealing and to realize how his behaviors and the shoplifting of others had a large affect on the family's livelihood. David was able to articulate these ideas to his friends, as well, so that they could begin to understand the ramifications of their actions. David's story exemplifies Lickona's understanding of moral development through growth in moral thinking, moral feeling, and moral actions.

Adolescent Emotional Development

Adolescents feel their emotions very strongly and intensely. Feelings of joy and sorrow can be felt in quick succession with equal vigor. This means that sometimes adolescents seem to be on an emotional "roller coaster" from profound happiness to despair and back.

Adolescents sometimes can communicate their feelings adequately or a particular event can trigger an extreme emotional response, thereby making them appear to be moody. It is often helpful for practitioners to give adolescents a vocabulary with which to talk about their emotions. Such simple techniques as naming the emotion and connecting the emotion to the action that caused the emotion are often very good first steps. Sometimes a youth will say that he or she is "mad" when in fact he or she is feeling frustrated, incompetent, lonely, embarrassed, or demeaned. By giving the adolescent a more ample vocabulary to talk about his or her emotions, the youth can better understand the power of the emotion and why it triggered the response that it did. Once adolescents can name and understand their emotions, they can begin to control those emotions that cause them to act in ways that they may later regret.

Emotional Intelligence

It has been suggested that the ability to understand one's emotions and use them effectively is more important than cognitive ability (Goleman, 1995, 1998, 2001). In fact, Goleman believes that emotional intelligence (EI) is a better predictor of success than IQ. He has separated EI into four components. The first is *self-awareness*; this includes emotional self-awareness, accurate self-assessment, and self-confidence. The second component is called *self-management*, which includes self-control, trustworthiness, conscientiousness, adaptability, achievement drive, and initiative. The third component is termed *social awareness* and focuses on the concepts of empathy, service orientation, and organizational awareness. The fourth component is called *relational management*, which includes the desire and practice to develop others' talents, exerting influence when needed, communication, conflict management, leadership, being a bridge between individuals, teamwork, collaboration, and being a catalyst of change. Goleman believes that excellence in any one of these four components is a key to success in almost any vocation (1998). He suggests that the ability to improve upon these components may be set by midadolescence. Others have suggested that EI may be different for females and males. Murray (1998) found females higher in empathy and social responsibility and males higher in tolerance and self-confidence.

Gender and Emotional Development

Females

Carol Gilligan has made the study of adolescent females' waning confidence in themselves her life work. She has found that many females in adolescence "lose their voice" (Gilligan et al., 1990, p. 25). By this she means that some females, as they go through adolescence, repress some of their knowledge and assertive behavior. They prefer to act as the "nice girl" who has no prickly or strong feelings. This illegitimate behavior causes the adolescent female to be in danger of losing her "voice" because it creates an inauthentic perception of herself in her mind and the minds of her friends. She is acting in a manner that jeopardizes her own development as an individual. She also enters into friendships by being someone she is not, which decreases her ability to have a meaningful authentic friendship. Pipher (1994) suggests that many bright and sensitive adolescent females become shy and doubting young women. She suggests that adolescent females need opportunities to "shine" and be acknowledged to increase their emotional development. Harter (2004) disagrees with the perceptions of Gillian and Pipher and believes that there is no such thing as "losing voice" in today's females; she has found females to be very verbal about their thoughts and feelings. Similarly, Kindlon (2006) writes about "Alpha Girls" who receive better grades, are leaders both in and out of school, and are entering the workforce with gusto.

Males

Males have different issues when it comes to emotional development. Pollack (1999) believes that males in adolescence choose to hide their emotional side, frequently believing they need to be "tough guys." Gurian (2006) believes that males need family, community support, and mentors to best develop in adolescence. He suggests that we allow males to leave the family system too early and therefore they do not receive important life information and emotional support from caring and connected adults, but instead receive incorrect information or a lack of information and inadequate emotional support from peers who are confronting their own development. These males are then stifled from fully developing their emotional self due to the lack of role models to help explain the complexity of emotions. Kindlon and Thompson (1999) suggest that the issues of violence are often related to the inability to understand the emotional life of males. They also believe that males would be more emotionally competent if they were not defined in such narrow terms by what is considered masculine behavior. Males need to be better educated in the art of communication, and the teaching of empathy needs to be implemented for all males (Kindlon & Thompson, 1999).

Practitioners such as school social workers can help boys become more emotionally literate by practicing a vocabulary that increases their emotional language and their connection of that vocabulary to the events of their own life. Through open communication that is honest and direct, the youth does not have to hide behind bravado or self-aggrandizement. He can connect in an authentic manner that reveals his true emotions or the confusion about understanding his conflicting emotions.

Adolescent Identity Development

The great issue for adolescents is coming to know "Who am I?" Am I the same person or a different person when I am around my parents, siblings, friends, schoolmates, or neighbors? Is it OK to be a different person in different situations? How much of me is the same in each of these situations? Erik Erikson (1959) termed adolescent psychosocial development as a struggle between "identity versus identity confusion." He sees the positive outcome of this stage to be *fidelity*, that is, one is true to oneself in any and all situations. The development of an integrated identity is the major task for adolescence, and in fact, Erikson believes that it is not fully congealed until early adulthood because of the conflict between being oneself and self-doubt of who one may be (identity vs. confusion).

Pieces of the Identity Puzzle

Pieces of the identity puzzle include plans for a vocation for the future and how one's work shapes who he or she is as an individual and how he or she is seen by society by the work that he or she does. Vocational aspirations often involve education, although vocational aspirations are also tied to family and socioeconomic influences as well. For example, in the Pacific Northwest region of the United States where families have been employed in the fishing and logging industries for generations, it was highly likely that their children would follow in their vocational footsteps. In recent years, as these industries have fallen away due to diminishing salmon populations and forest protection, young people have had to find new vocational paths to follow. As youth search for a vocation they may question: Do I want to do the same thing I have seen my parents do or do I want to try something new? Do I have the requisite skills to pursue education or training in the topic of interest? Will there be employment in my field when I have completed my studies and training? Can I withstand the years of education or training and apprenticeship to obtain the vocational goal I desire? Do I have the ambition to persevere when it is tedious or while my friends are involved in more enjoyable pursuits?

Other ingredients in the creation of an integrated identity are the core values of how to live life and what is most important and meaningful in life. Family, friends, religion, and environment often shape these values. Additionally, an ideology of the *idealized self*, which specifies who he or she wants to be and who the individual is if he or she makes a particular decision all contribute to an integrated identity. For example, "Am I the type of person who does this behavior or am I not the type of person who involves him- or herself in this behavior?" The concept of an idealized self is also tied to moral development.

Margaret Mead (1965) and others (G. Mead, 1934) have suggested that in more traditional societies, identity was easier to form since there was little generational change and socialization was mostly the responsibility of parents and other family members. However, in mainstream American society there are a myriad of influences and people who complicate the formation of coming to an integrated identity. Change in a youth's life and the unpredictability of identity development may delay the process. As mentioned already, multiple environments can complicate the process of identity formation.

Formation of sexual and gender identity is part of knowing oneself and having an integrated identity. Adolescents often question their sexual identity and orientation comparing themselves and others: Am I straight, gay, lesbian, or bisexual? A teen's biological gender and family and cultural values related to gender roles also affect identity development by giving the youth messages, though sometimes conflicting, about what it means to be a man or a woman in the society where he or she lives. Some teens experience the biological gender with which they were born as contrary to their inner feelings on whether they want to live as a young man or a young woman. They may ask, "Am I the biological gender to which I was assigned at birth?" "Do the male or female reproductive organs I was born with really fit who I am today?" Chapter 11 contains further discussion of sexual identity and gender identity development.

A cultural identity is also important for an integrated identity. "How does my race or ethnic group contribute to who I am as an individual and how I fit into society?" W. E. B. Du Bois (1903, 1996, p. 299), speaking of African American youth states that there is often a "Twoness, two hearts and minds" from the minority to the majority culture. "Do I have the same identity in the minority community as I do in the majority society?" Additionally, macro factors and micro interactions related to racism influence the racial identity development of teens of color (Cross, 1991; Tatum, 2003). This can lead to the struggles to which Du Bois refers in his statement about "two minds and two hearts." In contrast, many white adolescents live in ignorance of their white racial identity due to macro and micro interactions that presume whiteness as an assumed normality (Hardiman, 1994; Helms, 1990, 1995; Tatum, 2003). White teens who grow up in more racially homogeneous neighborhoods and schools tend to be most unaware of their whiteness and struggle when they are called to interact in the larger world that is decidedly multicultural. The identity statuses related to white identity development progress toward the acquisition of an antiracist, white identity.

Identity Statuses

James Marcia (1966, 1991, 1993) suggests that there are four identity statuses. These statuses are determined by the absence or presence of a *crisis*, a serious questioning and consideration of different and varied occupations and ideologies and an eventual *commitment* to a particular occupation and ideology. There is no order to these statuses; the youth simply exists in one of the four statuses.

The first status is called *identity moratorium*, in which the youth has considered many occupations and ideologies but has not made a commitment to any one. This youth is often a drifter, pursuing many different options, but not committing to any work or ideology. It is as if he or she continues to put on new hats but never finds one he or she likes. Because there is no commitment, the youth is often dissatisfied quickly and tries to find a new opportunity rather than having the perseverance to continue when the job gets difficult or boring or his or her ideas are tested by others.

Identity foreclosure is the second status. The youth has not contemplated other vocations or ideologies; he or she has instead committed to a job and an ideology. This is sometimes seen in youth who follow in the family business without evaluating their own desires for meaningful work or pursue a vocation to please their parents or unflinchingly support the family ideology. Without the meaningful conflict of self-discovery, the youth is not fully happy in his or her vocation or has not fully understood what it means to hold a particular ideology.

Marcia calls the third identity status *identity diffusion*. There has not been a crisis nor has there been a commitment to a vocation or an ideology. This youth is the proverbial "Peter Pan" who is not pursuing any activity that will lead to either meaningful work or a set of principles to live by. He or she is rudderless and in need of an opportunity to refocus.

Finally, the fourth identity status, called *identity achievement*, is when the youth has both gone through the difficult work of considering the options for his or her future work and values and has made a meaningful commitment to a particular occupation and a set of guiding principles. Marcia (1966, 1991, 1993) considers that this status is the best outcome for the youth.

So how can we best guide our adolescent clients to an identity achievement status? Some suggestions include the use of vocational aptitude tests, summer employment, internships, shadowing, and interviewing individuals in areas of employment interest. Youth should be encouraged to explore what they do not like about an occupation and what they do like about an occupation, and what they like with the realization that for all occupations there will be activities that one likes less than other activities. Additionally, is their desired occupation or ideology based in fantasy or reality? Ask the youth to describe what he or she sees him- or herself doing in 3 years, 5 years, and 10 years. Once he or she is done, ask whether he or she has a plan to make that a reality and what steps must be taken today to make it an opportunity for him or her in the future.

Racial identity statuses have been defined by theories of person of color identity development (Cross, 1991; Parham, 1989) and theories of white identity development (Hardiman, 1994; Helms, 1990, 1995). It is important to remember that these identity statuses are viewed as phases of identity development such that each may overlap with one another and a young person can be in one phase in one context and another phase in a different context. Additionally, identity development, on all fronts, is a lifelong endeavor that tends to be emphasized during adolescence, even though it may not be completed until early adulthood.

Person of color identity development is represented by five statuses: conformity, dissonance, immersion–emersion, internalization, and integrative awareness (Cross, 1991).*Conformity identity status* has two modes. The active mode results from the preponderance of images, often perpetuated by the media, that suggests a white model of lifestyle and beauty in the absence of images of people of color. This mode is also perpetuated when young people of color attend schools, for example, where the majority of teachers are white. These images may lead the young person of color to question, "If all of these images of beauty and success are of white people, what does that say about me?" Other young people of color in the conformity status may be in the passive mode: "No one will treat me different because I am African American or Latino." Whichever mode the young person is in, he or she enters the *dissonance status* when personal experiences of racism are acknowledged. This often happens for young people of color during their teen years if, for example, they are rejected by their white peers or the parents of their white peers by not being invited to parties or the differential treatment they may experience shopping at the mall with their white friends when store clerks treat them with suspicion, but not their white counterparts.

Experiences of the dissonance status can be followed by the *immersion–emersion status* THAT develops as the young person becomes justifiably angry about his or her experiences of racism. Some young people in this status may develop an "in-your-face" identity that shuns whatever they view as the "white normative standard." Many young people move beyond this to the *internalization status* in which they develop a more integrated identity. In this status, the teen remains very aware of how racism and other forms of oppression serve to exploit his or her self-image and works to deflect that exploitation. However, he or she may reject the formerly held view of certain behaviors, such as getting good grades in school, as part of a presumed "white normative standard." The *integrative awareness status* may follow during which the teen expresses positive feelings about his or her racial self, recognizes the illness of oppression, and works to combat it within him- or herself and the society around him or her. The process of movement within these identity statuses will depend on the cultural and ethnic heterogeneity of the contexts in which the young person is raised. This is not to suggest that there are some contexts in which racism is nonexistent, but that the experiences of racism may be buffered by other experiences a youth may have if he or she lives in a more racially mixed neighborhood or attends a school where many teachers share his or her racial identity.

The model of white identity development has six identity statuses: contact, disintegration, reintegration, pseudo-independence, immersion–emersion, and autonomy (Hardiman, 1994; Helms, 1990, 1995). Movement among the white identity statuses is also dependent on the level of heterogeneity of the contexts in which a young white person is being raised. As noted earlier, white people who are raised in predominantly white contexts have a greater tendency to be unaware of their white racial identity. In fact, the initial identity status in the model of white identity development is called *contact*. When the young white teen is in the contact status he or she lacks an awareness of his or her own whiteness and is naïve concerning people of color. As a result, the teen in this identity status often claims to be color blind and is likely to commit racist actions or have racist thoughts without recognizing them as racist.

At the point that the teen becomes aware that whites receive unearned, preferential treatment over people of color he or she enters the *disintegration status*. The teen in this status typically feels shame, guilt, and/or confusion about this differential and unearned preferential treatment. He or she often may have a sense of seeing racism everywhere, but may deny the reality of this experience for people of color. For example, the white teen's peer of color may question whether a white teacher's actions toward him or her are racist and the white teen may respond by telling his or her peer that the "teacher is just a jerk, because she treats everyone poorly."

The white teen begins to take on the *reintegration status* as he or she attempts to reduce the discomfort of the previous status. As a result, the teen in this status tends to view people of color as responsible for their experiences of racism and may excuse his or her own acts or thoughts of racism by pointing out to others, "I have friends who are people of color." If the white teen begins to take the awareness of racism from the previous status and more openly recognize it by questioning the stereotypes and assumptions he or she has about people of color, then he or she enters the *pseudo-independence status*. This status is labeled pseudo or artificial because the young white person in this status works to deny his or her white racial identity and is likely to point out, "Whites are racist, but not me. I might be more like Black people than you all even think!"

If the white teen moves beyond these attitudes toward a deeper awareness of racism, both cognitively and emotionally, then he or she is likely to enter the *immersion–emersion status*. In this status, the teen is able to acknowledge that he or she messes up sometimes and is unintentionally racist and works to make changes in him- or herself. The teen will seek out other white teens who share his or her cause to end racism as well as directly confront racism when he or she sees it. As the young white person enters the *autonomy status* he or she maintains the goals and changes from the immersion–emersion status and as a result becomes more capable of genuine relationships with people of color. As with all aspects of adolescent development, the white teen's movement through these identity statuses is influenced by the many contexts in which he or she is raised. In addition to the range of diversity in his or her school and neighborhood, his or her family's attitudes about race will also influence this aspect of the teen's identity development.

Adolescent Social Development

During adolescence, individuals outside of the family contribute to social development. Such social skills as making and maintaining friendships are first acquired in school-age children, but they are honed in adolescence. For the adolescent, friendships serve many functions such as companionship, stimulation, physical support, ego support, social comparison, intimacy, and affection (Santrock, 1998).

Peer Group Relations

Dunphy (1963) was the first to articulate the concept of the development of peer group relations in adolescence. He believes that males and females in the school-age years are in the *precrowd stage* where they primarily are in unisex groups isolated from other groups. The second stage is the *beginning of the crowd* where a unisex group of females interacts with a group of males, typical of the middle school years. The following stage is called *structural transition of the crowd*; unisex groups are forming heterosexual groups especially among upper-status members of the group, which happens in the later middle school years. The fourth stage is called the *fully developed crowd* where heterosexual groups are integrated, typical of the high school years. Later in high school, Dunphy calls it *the beginning of crowd disintegration* where couples from the various groups splinter into dyads.

Peer Influence

Peer influence and the susceptibility to peer influence is actually the strongest in preadolescence and early adolescence. This may be attributed to the lack of an integrated identity. As youth enter middle or later adolescence the influence declines. Additionally, boys generally are more susceptible to peer pressure than girls, although middle school girls can be legendary in their ability to organize cliques and be mean-spirited to those in and outside the cliques (Wiseman, 2003).

Parenting and the Adolescent

Friendships outside of the family also contribute to the beginning separation from family. However, it has been found that adolescents particularly value their parents' advice regarding future-oriented goals such as finances, education, and career plans, though peers have more influence over social-oriented activities such as fashion, music, and dating (Lau, Quadrel, & Hartman, 1990). Similarly, the need for youth autonomy has been overstated in pop culture. Youth are most resilient when their parents are aware of their goings-on and have continued involvement in their everyday activities.

However, there is a shift in the power equation, which can sometimes lead to role conflict for parents. Parents of adolescents must learn to "walk the thin line" between support and control. This is very difficult because the adolescent is both very dependent on his or her parents but is also striving for independence. This relationship is made more difficult if the relationship through the childhood years was strained.

Parents of adolescents should be encouraged to get in the habit of asking their youth his or her opinion. It is a great way of initiating conversation and gives the parent good insight into their daughter's or son's thinking and reasoning processes.

The parent must remember that actions speak louder than words. The adolescent is gaining an ever-increasing sense of a moral compass and is watching how the parent navigates his or her life. The parent's reasoning, morals, and choices are all being watched and considered vis-à-vis the youth's developing moral standards. The parent's choices can either support his or her own moral choices or contradict them.

Because adolescents are spending a lot of time trying to figure out what they want to do with their lives, they are looking for models of adulthood. Practitioners can help adolescents find these models within their family or within their community, either in informal or formal mentoring programs.

Parents should not be afraid to be the parent. Knowledge about how the parent feels about an issue or choice has been found to be an important deterrent for adolescent substance use and sexual activity. Parenting an adolescent can be confusing and filled with contradictory messages. The youth sometimes sends his or her parents the message that he or she desires to be left alone. The media has contributed to this perception of an adolescent needing a great deal of autonomy and freedom to wrangle with his or her metamorphosis into the adult world. However, the emancipation of youth before he or she is fully self-sufficient risks being counterproductive and sometimes even disastrous for the adolescent's emerging sense of self-identity and competence.

QUESTIONS FOR THE REFLECTIVE PRACTITIONER

1. How do you assess your adolescent client's physical development?
2. How do you assess your adolescent client's cognitive and brain development?
3. How do you assess your adolescent client's moral development?
4. How do you assess your adolescent client's identity development?
5. How do you assess your adolescent client's social development?
6. What information about adolescent development is important for your adolescent client to understand?
7. What information about adolescent development is important for your adolescent client's parents to understand?

Chapter Summary

In this chapter we have discussed the different domains of adolescent development, which include physical development, cognitive development, moral development, emotional development, identity development, and social development. Additionally, a variety of competing theories of adolescent risk have been presented. It is our hope that with a good understanding of adolescent development the practitioner can be most effective in understanding and evaluating adolescent behavior.

In the following chapter, we further deepen our understanding of adolescent development by using a resilience framework to gain a holistic assessment of adolescent development and adolescent risk behaviors across environments. The ecological approach allows a unique vantage point from which to examine youth from the inside out; it presents the intersection between internal characteristics and external factors in the adolescent's environment that influence youth resiliency or vulnerability.

CHAPTER 3

Resilience in Adolescence

Chapter Overview

How do some youth persevere amidst great adversity while others seem to fall apart when there is the slightest disturbance in their world? What are the factors that support this resolve or undermine healthy development? Such questions form the essence of the study of resilience in youth. This chapter investigates the development of resilience research and theory, defines resilience, presents the use of ecological theory as a means of conceptualizing resilience, and defines protective and risk factors that are important in adolescence across multiple microsystems.

The Development of Resilience Research and Theory

Historically, resilience research focused primarily on issues of risk and vulnerability. Risk factors in adolescent development were researched in much the same way as is done in the field of epidemiology, cataloging conditions or variables that compromised health or social functioning for the developing individual (Jessor, Van Den Bos, Vanderryn, Costa, & Turbin, 1995). Many investigators created lists of risks factors and then quantified the number of risks for any given individual or subset of the population. The individual's composite number of risk factors indicated the likelihood of the individual's attainment of a negative outcome. An abbreviated list of these risk factors for youth includes a history of physical or sexual abuse, parental marital discord, parental depression, lack of parent–child relationship, isolation from or intimidation by peers, and living in an unsafe neighborhood (Butler, 1997; Garmezy, 1993; McMillan & Reed, 1994; Rutter, 1987; Seilhamer & Jacob, 1990; Werner, 1985, 1989b). However, regardless of the myriad of risks that were found to reduce positive developmental outcomes in youth, the risk research was unable to explain the small but significant group of adolescents who still flourished under the yoke of these risk factors. Continuing to look at risks did not shed light into why these individuals were successful; it only made their ability to cope with risks more perplexing.

The focus on individual and environmental *protective factors* that promoted positive youth development and sometimes ameliorated negative events brought about a shift in the field, and the concept of resilience was created. Rutter (1987) explains "not only has there been a shift in focus from vulnerability to resilience, but also from risk variables to the process of negotiating risk situations" (p. 316). This shift allowed the researcher to view resilience as one of the outcomes that could result from stressful life events. Therefore an unfortunate life event in the youth's life could actually improve, not affect, or decrease functioning for that youth. This brought about a dramatic change in the conceptualization of adolescent development as well. No longer was youth development a liturgy of how to avoid risks that increased the chance of vulnerable outcomes, but rather the exploration of positive influences that supported healthy development. For the practitioner who read this research, it offered a more hopeful prognosis for clients who had experienced difficult events. These clients were no longer "doomed" to have the event undermine their growth and development; the event could trigger growth, have no influence on growth, or as previously thought make growth more difficult. Each of these options was possible.

Henderson and Milstein (1996) developed a model by adapting the earlier work of Richardson, Neiger, Jensen, and Kumpfer (1990), which discusses four possible outcomes in response to stressful life experiences. The first possible outcome was called *reintegration with resiliency*; the youth had survived and gained strength from the stressful life event. Through the experience, the youth developed healthy coping mechanisms to deal with the disruption. These healthy coping mechanisms were then available to the youth to use in the future. The youth had in fact become stronger because of the experience. The second possible outcome Henderson and Milstein called *homeostasis*; the youth retreated to a safe place. The life disruption was neither a strengthening life experience nor a detrimental experience. The third possible outcome was reintegration with loss that was termed *maladaption*. The youth was negatively affected by the disruption. The youth had decreased self-esteem and reduced healthy coping skills. This might not be a final prognosis, but the current life situation for the youth was compromised. The final and the most deleterious outcome was called *dysfunctional reintegration*; the youth was severely affected by the disruption. The major negative event had universally undermined the youth's growth and development and had deeply scarred the individual.

An example of the different possible outcomes to stressful life experiences can be seen in the alternative scenarios of a youth, Sarah who was involved with the judicial system after an act of graffiti tagging. The involvement with the judicial system and the subsequent responsibility to be involved in community service helped Sarah to understand that her behavior was incorrect and needed changing. Although the experience was anxiety producing for her, it made her revaluate and change her behavior so that she would never again be involved in tagging (*reintegration with resiliency*). Or Sarah may have had the same anxiety-producing experience with community service and decided she hated community service and would avoid tagging in the future; not necessarily that she had the epiphany that tagging was an inappropriate activity and hurt the community, but that she did not like what happened if she was caught for tagging (*homeostasis*). The third option was that through community service Sarah resented the work and considered how she might be able to tag without getting caught in the future and met others at community service who supported her desire to tag in the future (*maladaption*). The fourth option was that her community service only made Sarah angry and fueled her desire to increase her tagging behavior regardless of whether she was caught again (*dysfunctional reintegration*).

The concept of stress is also important to resilience. "Resilience refers to a dynamic process encompassing positive adaptation within the context of significant adversity. Implicit to this notion are two critical conditions: (1) exposure to significant threat or severe adversity, and (2) the achievement of positive adaption despite major assaults on the developmental process" (Luthar, Cicchetti, & Becker, 2000, p. 543). Therefore, resilience occurs when there is stress. Conversely, resilience cannot occur if there is no stress in one's environment. This is an important caveat because it means that protecting youth from all negative external influences, a virtually impossible endeavor anyway, undermines the youth's best development. Youth who are most resilient have had to negotiate some adversity in their lives. Figure 3.1 presents a model to help you understand resilience.

Current resilience research has concentrated on assessing protective and risk factors that can either promote or deter healthy growth and development. There have been a large number of scholars who have added a great deal to the field of resilience. Among the noteworthy resilience researchers are Werner (1985, 1986, 1989a, 1989b, 1994) and Smith (Werner & Smith, 1992, 1998, 2001), who continue to conduct longitudinal research that began in Hawaii in 1955. Werner's and Smith's ability to track this cohort, which began with careful scrutiny of prenatal and birth records

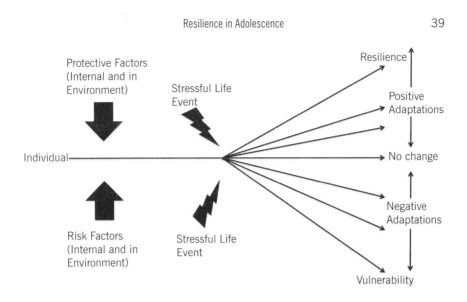

FIGURE 3.1. Laser's resilience model.

and then periodic interviews and testing that continues into midlife, has offered considerable insight into the subject of resilience.

Defining Resilience

Through the work of Werner and Smith, and the contributions of many other scholars, a large body of information has been gained regarding protective factors that the individual may possess or factors that are present in the developing person's environment that promote healthy development. Werner and Smith (1992) define the concept of resilience as "Resilience and protective factors are the positive counterparts to both vulnerability, which denotes an individual's susceptibility to a disorder, and risk factors, which are biological or psychosocial hazards that increase the likelihood of a negative developmental outcome in a group of people" (p. 3). Other resilience researchers have similar but distinct definitions; each adds a slightly different focus to better illuminate and conceptualize the subject.

Rutter (1987, 1989) describes resilience as a dynamic process that allows an individual to adapt to a particular given situation. Rutter (1987) states, "It requires some form of intensification (vulnerability) or amelioration (protection) of the reaction to a factor that in ordinary circumstances leads to a maladaptive outcome" (p. 317). Rutter (1987) acknowledges that certain behaviors may be adaptive for a particular situation, but may put the individual at greater risk in other circumstances. Therefore, a certain behavior in a particular context may afford survival at the present, but may be deleterious for future development. An example of this would be disassociation during a traumatic experience. The disassociative event may have helped the individual survive the traumatic experience, but using disassociation as a normal coping mechanism can undermine healthy functioning (Leibowitz, Laser, & Burton, in press).

Sameroff, another resilience expert, believes resilience is simply a matter of weighing the protective and the risk factors. Sameroff (2000) states, "The more risk factors the worse the outcomes; the more protective factors, the better the outcomes" (p. 20). Sameroff also discusses the contextual influences of the family, neighborhood, school, and the culture to either promote or inhibit child development. Therefore, resilience can be evaluated through an ecological framework where risk and protective factors are viewed in the context of the family microsystem, school microsystem, neighborhood microsystem where all are being influenced by the macrosystem.

Garmezy believes that the ability to "bounce back" by the individual is central to a conceptualization of resilience. Garmezy (1993) states that the central element of resilience "lies in the power of recovery and in the ability to return once again to those patterns of adaptation and competence that characterized the individual prior to the pre-stress period" (p. 129). Similarly, Cicchetti, Toth, and Rogosch (2000) discuss resilience as the process of "initiating their self-righting tendencies" (p. 409). Furthermore, Wang, Haertel, and Walberg (1994) discuss the importance of resiliency as an active event. It is the creation of strategies and the initiating of self-righting mechanisms that is important for understanding resiliency for these researchers. Therefore, resilience is not a passive event. The youth makes choices to persevere. Hence, if the youth is apathetic or defeated, the outcome is more likely to be vulnerability than resilience. The youth has to feel that he or she has some ability to control his or her own destiny in order to believe that he or she can "weather the storm."

The environment where the youth is developing is always a contributing factor in the success or the failure of that individual. Scarr and McCartney (1983) remark that resilient youth are active participants in their own environment. The resilient adolescents' ability to make the most of the environment that they currently inhabit increases their ability to withstand the negative effects of the environment. Kumpfer (1999) also considers environmental factors as important for resilience and has created a framework that is based on Bronfenbrenner's ecological theory. It begins with the flow of stressors and challenges that impact the environmental context of the microsystem of the developing individual where there are both protective and risk factors present. The microsystem then impacts the transaction of the person with his or her environment. This in turn impacts internal resiliency factors that the individual possesses that include cognitive, emotional, physical, spiritual, and behavioral factors. Finally, either adaptations that create resilient reintegration or maladaptive reintegration are created.

Luthar and colleagues (2000) stress the importance of specifying resilience in a particular domain and not across all areas of the individual's life. This allows for the investigation of success in a particular sphere, which they delineated as educational resilience, social resilience, and behavioral resilience. Therefore, the youth may maintain good grades in school, may be able to maintain good relationships with others, or act appropriately, but perhaps not all of those at the same time or all of the time. This is an important distinction in that resilience does not make a "super youth" in all spheres of his or her life. For example, if the youth has experienced street violence in his or her neighborhood microsystem, he or she may actively look to his or her school microsystem as an area of success and a venue where he or she feels safe. Or the youth may be successful in maintaining good friendships, even though he or she is experiencing a great deal of chaos and unhappiness in his or her family microsystem. In fact, his or her difficulty in one microsystem often acts as a catalyst for looking for and obtaining support in another microsystem of his or her life.

The criteria for labeling the adaptation as resilient are often determined by the magnitude of the traumatic experience. Depending on the incident, resilience can be interpreted as mere survival, maintenance of average functioning, or superior functioning (Luthar et al., 2000). For instance, the Lost Boys who traversed Sudan (Luster, Bates, & Johnson, 2004) into Kenya were resilient in their surviving the event (see Chapter 4 for further discussion). However, a youth who after the loss of a sibling learns a new appreciation for life and his or her family, or a youth who is able to successfully make a circle of new friends at a new school he or she is attending is also resilient. All outcomes denote resilience, but they are not similar in scope of the event or personal outcome. Luthar and colleagues strongly urge that future researchers operationalize specific criteria for establishing "successful adaptation" within each population, not across all populations. For the practitioner, he or she must dispel his or her own preconceptions of what it means to be resilient. He or she must consider how the client would define "coming out OK" from a particular experience. What does it mean to him or her to persevere?

Similarly, the adolescent's perception of risk may be quite different from the practitioner's or researcher's (Luthar et al., 2000). In other words, what the researcher or practitioner defines as a risk factor may not be interpreted as a risk factor by the teen. The perception of risk can be subject to *generational influences, critical events* the youth has experienced in his or her life, or *everyday stresses* (see Chapter 1). If the youth has experienced a particular risk previously, the reappearance of the risk may not be as alarming for the youth, especially if the youth has successfully negotiated the risk in the past.

Additionally, any individual is more competent negotiating risk on some days and less competent on other days. Individuals at high risk "rarely maintain consistent positive adjustments over a long period of time" (Luthar et al., 2000, p. 551). Resilience is not static and even the most resilient are prone to upward and downward adaptations. On any given day, an individual's ability to be resilient is related to the stresses and strains that he or she is experiencing.

The influence of the social and cultural context on protective and risk factors needs to be taken into account (Gore & Eckenrode, 1996; Laser, 2003; Laser, Luster, & Oshio, 2007a, 2007b). The individual is always imbedded in a community with a particular cultural context where they consider some behaviors normative and important for development, while trivializing other behaviors. Therefore, what may seem to be an insurmountable risk factor for one individual or community may be a minimal stress of daily living for another. Similarly, what is regarded as important for development may not be seen as pertinent to another culture or community. For instance, in the Hmong culture it is extremely important for a female to know how to cook, clean, and sew to attract a suitable mate. This domestic savvy is not a particularly critical characteristic for youth living on the north shore of Chicago to date.

Defining Protective Factors in Adolescence

In Frankl's (1963) seminal work *Man's Search for Meaning*, the author concludes that "we can predict an individual's future only within the large frame of a statistical survey referring to a whole group; the individual personality, however, remains essentially unpredictable. The basis for any predictions would be represented by biological, psychological or sociological conditions. Yet one of the main features of human existence is the capacity to rise above such conditions and transcend them" (p. 207). Protective factors or promotive factors are the characteristics of the individual and his or her environment that enable him or her to transcend negative experiences. It is not clear whether these factors *protect* the individual from negative consequences or merely *promote* the likelihood of more positive outcomes.

Garmezy (1985) sees three primary types of protective factors: personality factors, the nature of the early caregiving environment, and supportive others. Garmezy, Masten, and Tellegen (1984) says that "positive outcomes in the face of multiple adversities typically are not randomly distributed; they tend to be related systematically to positive characteristics of families, communities and children themselves" (p. 101). Garmezy (1985) has a strong belief in the influence of the context of the developing person in either improving or impeding healthy development.

Henderson and Milstein (1996) suggest that the child's reaction to the event and the path of reintegration for the child is determined by the child's individual and environmental protective factors. An increased number of protective factors will create better outcomes for the child. Henderson and Milstein also believe that the passage of time can be ameliorative. The strength of these protective factors can determine the child's reaction to the disruption, as well as how that disruption is reintegrated into the child's view. The stressors, adversities, or risks are buffered by individual and environmental protective factors.

Additionally, there are protective factors that support resilient processes at different stages of development. These may be more related to relationships or physical characteristics. For instance, in infancy the most resilient infants, who are often considered the *good babies*, are distinguished by such protective factors as a strong sense of attachment to a primary caregiver, trust in his or her environment, and easy temperament, coupled with the physical attributes of being alert, healthy, and active (Laser, 2003). In the preschool years, the young child being able to *help oneself and get help as needed* marks resilience. The most resilient young children are often attached to a special adult and have learned empathy and emotional cues, but are also physically attractive, have the ability to concentrate on a task, and are verbal (Laser). In middle childhood, these protective factors begin to become more characterized by the child's ability to successfully negotiate his or her social environment. He or she begins to *learn the art of interaction with the world around his him or her.* In middle childhood, particularly salient protective factors are once again attachment to a special adult, but also the ability to have social competence in the many microsystems he or she inhabits: if his or her home life is stressful, the child sees school as a haven. He or she exhibits good problem-solving skills, has expectations for the future, and initiates social support across age and gender (Laser). It is not only the possession of these particular protective factors that are important, but that the individual possesses these protective factors at the stage of development when they are needed.

Gore and Eckenrode (1996) found that individual protective factors helped to account for individual differences to both environmental and biological risks. However, protective factors were often related to each other. Furthermore, the presence of certain protective factors determined the emergence of future protective factors (Gore & Eckenrode). As an example, the child who has greater social competence is better at making and keeping friends and is therefore more likely to be able to obtain social support when needed.

The issues of time and timing also are important to protective factors (Gore & Eckenrode, 1996). Yule (1992) also found that the age and the level of development across the domains of development were important in the ability for the protective factor to be salient for the individual. As discussed in Chapter 2, a boy whose physical development is ahead of his peers has an advantage over his peers.

However, some protective factors seem to exert a special influence in edifying the individual in times of stress and difficulty. An example of this would be the protective factor of spirituality, which supports the youth during the good times, but can sustain the youth during the difficult times. Some of these factors are internal to the individual, while other protective factors are characteristics or relationships in the microsystems where the individual resides.

Internal Protective Factors

Many of the protective factors are beliefs, perceptions, and traits that help the individual to right oneself during times of turmoil or difficulty. Table 3.1 lists internal protective factors that are discussed in the resilience literature extensively and are more fully discussed in Chapter 4. Each of these internal characteristics of the individual helps to supports resilient outcomes.

TABLE 3.1. Internal Protective Factors

• Mental flexibility	• Sense of humor
• Cognitive ability	• Spirituality/faith/sense of purpose
• Gender	• Optimism
• Physical beauty	• Emotional intelligence
• Easy temperament	• Creation of a personal myth
• Perceive social support	• Moral development
• Self-efficacy	• Autonomy
• Internal locus of control	• Stick-to-it-ness/perseverance

The Development of Resilience Theory in an Ecological Framework

As the client can be viewed and better understood in each microsystem he or she inhabits, protective factors, as well as risk factors, can be organized by microsystem. Among the many protective factors within the family microsystem that support greater adolescent functioning are *family microsystem protective factors* (Table 3.2), more fully discussed in Chapter 5; *school microsystem protective factors* (Table 3.3), more fully discussed in Chapter 6; and *neighborhood microsystem protective factors* (Table 3.4), more fully discussed in Chapter 7.

TABLE 3.2. Family Microsystem Protective Factors

• Mother's level of education	• Parental transfer of positive values
• Family economic stability	• Required helpfulness/chores
• Parental marriage or commitment	• Extended family to offer support
• Maternal relationship with youth	• Sense of family belonging
• Paternal relationship with youth	• Family social economic status

TABLE 3.3. School Microsystem Protective Factors

• School mentor for youth	• Sense of being needed at school
• Sense of belonging at school	• School friendships
• Classroom size and school size	• Social networking
• Enjoyment of school	• Extracurricular sports or clubs

TABLE 3.4. Neighborhood Microsystem Protective Factors

• Sense of community	• Sense of belonging
• Community pride	• Safety
• Collective efficacy	• Social capital

Defining Risk Factors in Adolescence

The connotation of risk is used to discover which variables increase the probability of negative outcomes for the population. However, the mere absence of a risk does not necessarily equate to the presence of a protective factor.

Risks do not affect all people in the same manner. Sameroff (2000) sees that some risks affect all children in the family; however, other risks affect only certain children in the family. Furthermore, even when the age and the stage of development are controlled, children are not equally affected by the same risk (Gore & Eckenrode, 1996; Sameroff, 2000).

Rutter (1987) believes that the particular risk is not as pertinent as the accumulation of risk factors. Risks add up and more risks create a greater likelihood of a negative outcome. Rutter (1999) remarks that children, even in the same family, vary in their vulnerability to risks. Rutter (1987) has found that there is generally a positively correlated relationship between childhood behaviors and adult behaviors; however, the correlation generally is extremely low. It is only when an individual with multiple risks in childhood is later evaluated in adulthood where there is a greater correlation. Hence, it is the accumulation of risks over time that is more deleterious for development.

Rutter (1989) also believes that these risks act as a causal chain in which one negative event impacts the individual so that he or she becomes more susceptible to further risks. He describes both the school and the family microsystem as venues where the emergence of particularly deleterious risks can then create other future risks. In the school system, Rutter emphasizes the role of poor schooling and in the family microsystem the role of poor parenting. Both these occurrences create a variety of negative repercussions for the child or youth.

Risks seem to have a cumulative effect (Bogenschneider, 1998; Werner, 1994). Werner reports that two-thirds of the children in her study with four or more risk factors developed serious learning or behavioral problems by age 10. Similarly, Garmezy (1993) found a relation between the number of stressors and psychiatric disorder in children. He found that a single risk factor increased the probability of childhood psychiatric disorder by 1%; two stressors increased the probability of mental disorder by another 5% for a total of 6%; three stressors increased the rate by another 6% for a total of 12%, and finally, four or more stressors increased the probability of psychiatric disorder by an increment of 21% for a total of 33%.

Risks, however, may have some beneficial affects. Some level of risk may be necessary for growth (Gore & Eckenrode, 1996). In Elder's (1974) seminal research, he found that some risk actually improved social independence and greater functioning. Bandura (1997) believes that it is only through life's challenges that there is achievement. Likewise, Garmezy (1993) believes that some emotional distress does not nullify the presence of resilient behavior. It is the awareness that the world is an imperfect place that may in fact improve functioning. Therefore, children and youth who are overly protected by their caregivers from all negative outcomes may be less resilient.

Many risk factors have been evaluated by researchers as having a particularly deleterious impact on development. Included are some of the risk factors that are the most frequently cited in the resilience research: *developmental risk factors* (Table 3.5), which either are intrinsic to the individual or have happened in the course of his or her development and are more fully discussed in Chapter 4; *family microsystem risk factors* (Table 3.6), which are experienced in the family environment and are more fully discussed in Chapter 5; *school microsystem risk factors* (Table 3.7), which the youth experiences in the school setting and are more fully discussed in Chapter 6; and *neighborhood microsystem risk factors* (Table 3.8), which the youth experiences in his or her neighborhood and are discussed more fully in Chapter 7.

TABLE 3.5. Developmental Risk Factors

• Gender and age	• Difficult temperament
• History of physical abuse	• History of sexual abuse
• Low socioeconomic status	• Severe or chronic illness in childhood

TABLE 3.6. Family Microsystem Risk Factors

• Parental depression or mental illness	• Personality differences with parents
• Maternal level of education	• Parents not physically present
• Parents not emotionally present	• Lack of attached parental role
• Parents not aware of youth's activities	• Severe marital/partner discord
• Witness to domestic violence	• Family size
• Sibling spacing	• Living in a home that is overcrowded
• Parental drug and/or alcohol abuse	• Frequency of moving

TABLE 3.7. School Microsystem Risk Factors

• Poor academic success	• Attention difficulties
• Difficulty making or keeping friends	• Scapegoating by teacher
• Being bullied by peers	• Social isolation

TABLE 3.8. Neighborhood Microsystem Risk Factors

• Violence in the neighborhood	• Lack of role models in the neighborhood
• Gang activity in the neighborhood	• Lack of safety in the neighborhood
• Lack of repair and upkeep of homes/ buildings	• High rates of abandoned homes/ buildings

1. Is it possible to increase internal protective factors and decrease developmental risk factors?
2. As a practitioner, how do you increase family protective factors and decrease family risk factors?
3. As a practitioner, how do you increase school protective factors and decrease school risk factors?
4. As a practitioner, how do you increase neighborhood protective factors and decrease neighborhood risk factors?
5. How does using a resilience framework change a practitioner's way of understanding a problem?

Chapter Summary

Each of the protective and risk factors that have been discussed may be more or less pertinent to a particular individual in a particular situation at a particular time. It should be underscored that not all youth are susceptible to the same risk factors nor do they feel the support of all of the protective factors discussed. In fact, in recent research it has been found that there is no constellation of protective or risk factors that are universal for both females and males and not one is the same for all situations (Laser, 2003, 2008; Laser et al., 2007a, 2007b). Therefore, what may support a female's healthiest development may not support a male's development. In addition, the risk factors that seem to be most deleterious for delinquent behavior are different from the risk factors that are most deleterious for sexual acting-out behavior. We discuss specific protective and risk factors for many different adolescent behaviors in Chapters 10–14.

In the following chapter, we discuss particular internal characteristics of the adolescent that support or undermine healthy development. In the next chapters, we focus on each particular microsystem that the youth inhabits and the particular protective and risk factors in that environment: the family environment (Chapter 5), the school environment (Chapter 6), and the neighborhood environment (Chapter 7).

PART II

THE ADOLESCENT
IN CONTEXT

CHAPTER 4

Internal Assets and Individual Attributes Associated with Healthy Adolescent Outcomes

Tom Luster

Chapter Overview

Most of us have met someone or read about someone who is a competent, well-adjusted, upbeat, and caring individual despite exposure to significant adversity. Researchers have tried to understand this phenomenon and identify factors that contribute to positive outcomes in vulnerable youth. Many of the protective factors associated with resilient outcomes fall into one of three categories: (1) individual attributes or internal assets, (2) relationships, and (3) community resources and opportunities (Masten & Powell, 2003). This chapter focuses on the first of these three categories—individual attributes or internal assets. However, it is important to keep in mind that the protective factors in various categories are intertwined; adolescents' individual attributes develop in the context of relationships and the supports and opportunities available in their communities.

This chapter is divided into four sections. The first section describes the key internal assets and individual attributes that have been linked to positive outcomes in youth. The second section focuses on individual characteristics that have been identified as risk factors because they are associated with problem outcomes in youth. In addition, vulnerability, or one's susceptibility to succumb to the risk he or she faces, is considered in the second section. Two people who experience similar risk profiles may have different outcomes because of differences in vulnerability, much like two people may differ in terms of a health outcome even though they are the same age and have similar diets, exercise habits, and stress levels. Section three is concerned with intervention approaches designed to enhance the internal assets of youth. How can we help youth acquire the assets they need to thrive? Finally, the experiences of the Sudanese refugees, known in the media as *The Lost Boys of Sudan*, are used as an example of how important individual attributes can be in dealing with extremely adverse circumstances. The "Lost Boys" were separated from their parents in childhood by the civil war in Sudan, and subsequently lived in peer groups in refugee camps in Ethiopia and Kenya. The Sudanese youth spent much of middle childhood and adolescence without the support and guidance of their parents, in refugee camps that offered relatively little in terms of community supports and opportunities. Thus, they are an ideal group for thinking about the individual attributes that help youth cope with extreme adversity.

Internal Assets and Individual Attributes
That Are Protective Factors

An appropriate starting point is to define internal assets and individual attributes that are protective factors. The term *assets* refers to characteristics of the person (internal assets) or of the environment (external assets) that have been linked to positive development in children and youth regardless of the individual's risk status; in other words, these are characteristics and contextual supports that are viewed as important for optimal development of all youth. The Search Institute identified 40 developmental assets that were important for adolescent development and provided support for the importance of these assets using samples of adolescents from entire schools or communities (Scales & Leffert, 1999); a list of these 40 assets can be found at the Search Institute's website (*www.search-institute. org*). *Protective factors* have been defined as aspects of the person or environment that buffer or ameliorate the effects of adversity, thus allowing the person to be more successful than he or she would be without the protective factors (Werner & Smith, 2001). Unlike studies of assets, the samples used to identify protective factors typically involve children and youth who appear to be at high risk for problem outcomes because of their exposure to significant risks.

Are these two different names for the same thing? As evident in Table 4.1, there is considerable overlap in the list of internal assets and individual attributes that consistently have been identified as protective factors in various studies (Masten & Powell, 2003). Most things that are beneficial for youth in general are beneficial for youth exposed to significant risks.

TABLE 4.1. Internal Assets and Protective Factors: Comparison to the Lost Boys

Internal assets for adolescents—Search Institute	Protective factors: Individual Attributes—Masten and Powell (2003)	Protective factors: Individual attributes—The Lost Boys of Sudan
Commitment to learning • Achievement motivation • School engagement • Homework • Bonding to school • Reading for pleasure	Cognitive ability • IQ scores • Attentional skills • Executive functioning skills	• A commitment to education • Resourcefulness and problem-solving skills/decision-making skills
Positive identity • Personal power • Self-esteem • Sense of purpose • Positive view of personal future	Self-esteem and self-efficacy • Competence • Worth • Confidence	• Self-efficacy that develops from dealing successfully with adversity over and over again • Tempered sense of mastery
Social competences • Planning and decision making • Interpersonal competence • Cultural competence • Resistance skills • Peaceful conflict resolution	Temperament and personality • Adaptability • Sociability Self-regulation • Impulse control • Affect and arousal regulations	• Ability to elicit positive reactions and support from adults • Sociability and ability to maintain supportive peer relationships
Positive values • Caring • Equality and social justice • Integrity • Honesty • Responsibility • Restraint	Positive outlook on life • Hopefulness • Belief that life has meaning • Faith	• Ability to focus on the present and future rather than what they had lost; attending school in the refugee camps without parents to prod them • Religiosity—finding meaning in their experiences • A future orientation—a desire to help rebuild southern Sudan when the war is over • Hopefulness of being reunited with family members and having new opportunities in the United States • Personal coping strategies to deal with trauma, such as separation from families, and ambiguous loss—that is, not knowing if other members of their family were dead or alive • Emotion-focused strategies • Problem-focused strategies

Although the two concepts are closely related, in some cases a factor that is protective in a context of high risk may not be very useful for people at low risk. Rutter (2006a) provides a nice example of this. Being a carrier of the sickle cell gene is protective for people who live in an area where the risk for malaria is high, but it is not beneficial to people who live in areas free of malaria. Whereas conceptually assets are viewed as the building blocks that all youth need for positive development (Scales & Leffert, 1999), the individual attributes that are protective may depend on the risks youth are exposed to, their context, and the outcome of interest (Rutter).

Internal Assets

Since 1989, the Search Institute has conducted research on developmental assets (Scales & Leffert, 1999). The researchers initially identified 30 developmental assets that were thought to be important for positive youth development based on a review of child and adolescent development research, as well as studies of resilience and prevention. Additional research and focus groups with urban youth, youth in poverty, and youth of color resulted in an extended list of 40 assets for adolescents divided into eight categories, including four categories of internal assets and four categories of external assets. The four major categories of internal assets for adolescents are (1) commitment to learning, (2) positive identity, (3) social competence, and (4) positive values. These four categories include the 20 internal assets listed in Table 4.1.

Commitment to Learning

The commitment to learning assets includes beliefs, values, and skills that have been linked to academic success inside the classroom and intellectual curiosity outside the classroom. It includes such assets as academic motivation, engaging in learning activities, and having a sense of belonging at school and caring about the school. Although some youth enjoy the advantage of a genetic endowment that contributes to intellectual ability (Bouchard, 2004), attitudes toward learning and school are also influenced by experiences in the home and school (e.g., rewarding experiences in the classroom and positive relationships with teachers) and the peers with whom adolescents identify and affiliate (Harris, 1995).

Positive Identity

Positive identity includes the asset of personal power—youths' belief that they have some control over what happens to them; it is conceptually similar to an *internal locus of control* orientation (Rotter, 1966) or self-efficacy

(Bandura, 1997). It also includes high self-esteem, a sense that one's life has a purpose, and an optimistic outlook on the future. In other words, youth with these assets have positive beliefs about themselves and their ability to influence the course of their lives, and they have positive expectations about the future and what they can accomplish.

Social Competence

According to Scales and Leffert (1999, p. 173), "Social competence involve the *personal skills* that children and adolescents use to deal with the many choices, challenges, and opportunities they face." It involves planning and decision-making skills, as well as the interpersonal skills necessary to interact effectively with peers and adults, including people who differ in terms of culture, race, and ethnicity. Dealing with challenges includes resistance skills to deal with peer pressure and to avoid dangerous situations, and conflict-resolution skills to find peaceful ways to resolve disputes.

Positive Values

Positive values include prosocial values and values involving personal character that are generally supported and promoted by adults in the United States (Benson, Leffert, Scales, & Blyth, 1998). The values include caring or helping other people, promoting equality and social justice, showing integrity by acting on convictions and standing up for one's beliefs, being honest, and taking responsibility for one's actions. It also includes the belief that it is important not to engage in risky behaviors, such as using drugs and alcohol or being sexually active at an early age. Adolescents are better able to chart a positive developmental course and avoid potential hazards if they internalize these values and use them to guide their behavior.

In the book *Developmental Assets*, Scales and Leffert (1999) reviewed hundreds of studies with relatively large samples examining the relation between their 40 developmental assets (or similar constructs) and outcomes among adolescents. Their review provides support for the importance of the various asset categories, but there was more extensive research and empirical support for some assets, such as commitment to learning and positive identity, than for others, such as positive values and social competencies. They also acknowledged that their list of 40 assets does not include everything that adolescents need for healthy development, noting such basic necessities as food, shelter, and medical care. However, it does provide parents, professionals, and policy makers with a framework for thinking about ways of promoting positive youth development and addressing gaps in the infrastructure of communities.

Data from Search Institute surveys of communities have also shown that youth with many assets are less likely to engage in risk behaviors than youth with fewer assets. For example, data collected by Roehlkepartain, Benson, and Sesma (2003) from 150,000 students in grades 6–12 showed that the percentage of youth who used illicit drugs three or more times in the past year was 38% (0–10 assets), 18% (11–20 assets), 6% (21–30 assets), and 1% (31–40 assets). Similar findings were reported for using alcohol and tobacco, engaging in violence and antisocial behavior, and being sexually active. Those with fewer assets were also more likely to report being frequently depressed or to attempt suicide.

Individual Attributes Consistently Identified as Protective Factors

The list of individual attributes in the second column of Table 4.1 was compiled by Masten and Powell (2003) and includes characteristics of individuals that have been linked consistently to competence in diverse studies of youth who have experienced significant adversity. This section examines why these attributes may be important for youth exposed to risks.

Cognitive Ability

Intelligence and a commitment to learning are important attributes for school success, a key developmental task from the elementary years through young adulthood. Academic success opens up opportunities, leads to positive responses from others, and contributes to a positive sense of self-worth. In homes where youths' self-esteem is undermined, children may benefit from discovering and developing their talents in other settings, such as in the classroom and extracurricular activities, and having those abilities affirmed by other important adults. However, the cognitive abilities associated with resilience include more than academic skills. Decision-making skills and "street smarts" are particularly important for youth growing up in environments with many hazards; good judgment is required for avoiding risks and dealing with the challenges that youth encounter in those settings. Problem-solving skills and resourcefulness are also important for youth who encounter many obstacles as they negotiate age-related developmental tasks in communities with limited resources for youth. *Executive functioning skills* are important for all children but may be particularly important for youth who have limited resources in their homes and communities. This includes setting goals, planning, prioritizing, and organizing the steps that need to be taken to achieve the goal, executing the plan, keeping track of the results, and making modifications as needed based on the results.

Another cognitive skill that is useful to youth who experience considerable adversity is processing and achieving insight regarding their adverse experiences. Clinical studies of adults who grew up in abusive homes show that those who are resilient managed to process their experiences in the home and understand that the problems they experienced were due to their "crazy" families rather than because of their shortcomings (Higgins, 1994; Rubin 1996). Children who have these insights are better able to psychologically distance themselves from their troubled families than those who accept their abusive parents' message that they deserve what they get.

Self-Esteem and Self-Efficacy

According to Harter (1999), self-esteem depends both on youths' accomplishments in areas of importance to them and the affirmation they receive from people who are important to them. Werner and Smith (2001) found that resilient adolescents typically developed talents that led to success and recognition in some area and almost always had some adults who conveyed to them the message "You count."

Self-efficacy refers to the youth's belief that he or she is capable of performing the behaviors need to accomplish a task or achieve a desired outcome (Bandura, 1997). This belief help explains why resilient people show persistence and determination when they are faced with difficult tasks and encounter obstacles. Youth who doubt that they have what it takes to succeed are likely to expend little effort and may struggle with depressive symptoms or feelings of helplessness. As Rutter (2006b) has pointed out, self-efficacy can be enhanced by successfully dealing with challenging tasks. He used the term *steeling effect* to describe the phenomenon of youth getting stronger and more confident and successfully negotiating stressors, much as steel is made stronger by exposure to heat.

Temperament and Personality

Temperament and personality influence how we respond to other people and events and how others respond to us. Wachs (2006) described five ways in which temperament may contribute to resilience, and Wachs's conclusions regarding those five processes are summarized next. First, youth with difficult temperaments may be exposed to more risk if parents, teachers, and prosocial peers respond negatively to these characteristics. In contrast, some youth have appealing characteristics that lead to favorable responses from others. These appealing characteristics are particularly important for youth who experience abuse or neglect at home and need to develop positive relationships with adults outside the home. Resilient youth from troubled families were found to have characteristics referred to as "adoptability" (Higgins, 1994); sometimes these youth were figuratively adopted by the family of a friend, which helped affirm that they were likeable individuals and also provided role models of positive family functioning.

Second, to some extent children select environments and temperament that may influence the selection process. Highly active, impulsive, and uninhibited children may put themselves in more risky situations than their peers. Children who are good at regulating their attention, emotions, and behavior may be more likely to select academic pursuits than children with the opposite profile.

The third way in which temperament may influence resilience involves goodness of fit. Children are more likely to receive support from parents and teachers if there is a good fit between the child's characteristics and the adult's values, interaction style, and expectations for the child. While an intuitively pleasing idea, Wachs (2006) notes that the empirical evidence in support of this concept is limited and inconsistent.

Fourth, children who differ temperamentally may be more or less reactive to the stressors they experience and to environmental supports. Resilient children may be less reactive to environmental stressors. Finally, children with different temperamental characteristics may also differ in the strategies they use to cope with stress. Based on his review of prior research, Wachs (2006) reported that children who are high on the temperament dimensions of positive emotionality, approach, and activity level were more likely to use *active coping strategies* while children with the opposite profile were more likely to use *avoidant coping strategies*. Children who used more active, flexible coping strategies are likely to deal more effectively with stressors and thus are more likely to be judged to be resilient.

Self-Regulation

Self-regulation refers to a person's ability to control his or her attention, emotions, and behavior. Being able to control attention and stay focused is important in many settings, but particularly in the classroom. Achievement is related to children's ability to stay on task, tune out distractions, and persist when tasks are difficult; teachers tend to respond favorably to children who have these characteristics (Sanson, Hemphill, & Smart, 2004). Finding ways to control emotions may be particularly important and difficult for youth who experience trauma and have to cope with strong emotions (e.g., anger, depression, guilt) following the trauma. Self-regulation can also contribute to whether youth are accepted or rejected by peers. Children who can control their emotions and behavior tend to be more popular with peers than children with self-regulation problems (Asher & Coie, 1990). Self-regulation may also be viewed as a moderator variable that influences how adolescents respond to peer deviance; peer deviance was less likely to predict antisocial outcomes in youth who were high on self-regulation than for youth who had difficulty with self-regulation (Dishion & Connell, 2006). Similarly, there was a stronger relation between stressful experiences and depressed mood among adolescents who were low in self-regulation than for adolescents who were high in self-regulation.

Positive Outlook on Life

A positive outlook on life includes hopefulness and optimism, which are viewed as being critical for persevering in challenging circumstances (Seligman, 1995). According to Gilham and Reivich (2004, p. 147), "Hope is often defined as a wish for something with some expectation that it will happen, while optimism is typically defined as a tendency or disposition to expect the best." So hope tends to be situation specific and optimism is a general expectation or outlook on life. Optimism has been linked to many positive outcomes including success in school and on the job, less depression and anxiety, better physical health, and even longer life (Gilham & Reivich). Optimism is also related to self-efficacy, with some individuals generally confident about their ability to succeed and others generally pessimistic. Attributions, or our explanations for why we succeed or fail, play an important role in whether we have an optimistic or pessimistic outlook (Gilham & Reivich). If we attribute an outcome, such as failure on a test, to an internal characteristic that is stable (I am stupid), there would be little reason to work harder and be optimistic about the next test. If we attribute failure to an external factor (an unfair or unusually difficult test) or an unstable factor (not studying enough), we can maintain our optimism and even increase the likelihood of greater success on the next test by working harder. Similarly, negative attributions that are global (I am a terrible student) have a more pervasive effect than negative attributions that are specific (I struggle with algebra but do well in other subjects).

People who overcome adversity often have an outlook on life that includes a belief that life has meaning (Frankl, 1962) and a sense of mission that involves helping others, possibly others who are experiencing similar hardships (Rubin, 1996). This outlook of making meaning and sense of mission may be tied to their religious or spiritual beliefs. Religious beliefs may influence an individual's cognitive appraisal of stressful situations (God has a reason why this is happening), foster hope that things will work out well in the end, and provide coping strategies for dealing with stress (e.g., prayer, mediation, and support from fellow members). Religious faith has been linked to positive physical health, mental health, and happiness in several studies (Wessells & Strang, 2006). Moral views based on religion may also reduce adolescents' involvement in risky behaviors such as early sexual intercourse or use of drugs and alcohol (Dryfoos & Barkin, 2006).

However, many resilient individuals arrive at their philosophy of life and commitment to helping others without having strong ties to organized religions (Higgins,1994; Rubin, 1996).

Risk and Vulnerability

Risk Factors

A factor that is associated with or predictive of a problem outcome is called a risk factor. Like assets, risk factors are often divided into characteristics of the individual (internal) and contextual factors (external). Individual risk factors include such things as attention-deficit/hyperactivity disorder (ADHD) and learning disabilities. Contextual risk factors are found in the key environments where adolescents spend most of their time including the home (abuse and neglect), peer group (friends who engage in risky behavior), school (unsafe, disengaged students), neighborhoods (violence), and the larger cultural and historical context (availability of guns, war). Another way to classify risk factors is to divide them into chronic stressors or traumatic events. *Chronic stressors* include such things as parental neglect or chronic poverty that occur over a long period of time. *Traumatic events* are extreme experiences including living in a community that is attacked during a war or devastated by an earthquake, being kidnapped or raped, or witnessing terrible events such as the murder of friends in a school shooting. Most adolescents who develop problems are exposed to multiple risk factors, and the term *cumulative risk* has been used to describe this phenomenon. Moreover, the risk factors that are important are likely to depend on the outcome of interest, although some risk factors are associated with a host of problem outcomes. Dryfoos and Barkin (2006, p. 217) identified the following risk factors that are associated with many high-risk behaviors among adolescents: (1) early use of drugs and alcohol; (2) alienation, out of the mainstream; (3) high-risk friends; (4) poverty; (5) lack of support, lack of attachment to adult; (6) low achievement; and (7) learning disabilities.

Other risk factors identified by Dryfoos and Barkin (2006, p. 218) that are classified as individual characteristics are low expectations for the future, depression, hyperactivity, low birth weight, and aggressive as a young child. Some risk factors are related to the individual's developmental history and include such things as a history of physical and sexual abuse, malnutrition, or lead poisoning; these experiences during childhood are likely to influence attributes of the adolescents such as personality and cognitive abilities.

In general, risk factors have the potential to undermine optimal development and interfere with children's ability to successfully negotiate age-salient developmental tasks (Masten & Powell, 2003). As a result, children may be disadvantaged relative to their peers in terms of their cognitive, language, social, and self-regulation skills; lagging behind their peers in these competencies may influence their relationships and interactions with teachers, peers, and others. Peers may be especially hard on youth who are viewed as "different" and not fitting in (Harris, 1995). Skill deficits and lack of acceptance by others are likely to influence how youth view themselves (self-esteem), their ability to succeed (self-efficacy), and their outlook on the future. Even bright, talented, and socially competent youth may perceive limited prospects for the future in very high-risk environments where the adults they know struggle to make it. (For additional information on risk factors see also Fraser, 2004, and Coleman & Hagell, 2007.)

Vulnerability

The risks that adolescents are exposed to are important for their development, but adolescents are also likely to differ in terms of their vulnerability to the risks they face. By comparing monozygotic (identical) and dizygotic (fraternal) twins, behavioral geneticists have been able to demonstrate that some adults are at greater risk genetically for problem outcomes such as schizophrenia, depression, alcoholism, criminality, and bulimia (twin studies of children have also demonstrated a genetic risk for ADHD and reading disorders) (Bouchard, 2004; McGue & Bouchard, 1998). Although we often think of genetic factors as contributing to vulnerability, inheritance also plays a role in the development of individual characteristics viewed as protective factors such as intelligence, sociability, positive emotionality, and optimism (Bouchard, 2004; Seligman, 1995).

Behavioral genetic studies also suggest that those who are genetically vulnerable for developing disorders are most likely to actually develop the disorder if they are reared in a high-risk environment (Mednick, Gabrielli, & Hutchings, 1984). Mednick and colleagues compared adoptees who had biological fathers with a history of criminal convictions (high risk) and adoptees whose biological fathers did not have criminal records (low risk). Although high-risk adoptees were more likely than low-risk adoptees to have a criminal record, the group that was most likely to have a criminal record had both biological and adoptive fathers with criminal records. Similarly, youth with a genetic risk for alcoholism should be much more likely to become an alcoholic if they live where drinking is a big part of the culture than if they live in a culture where drinking is not accepted, such as in some Islamic countries (Long, 2008).

Caspi and his colleagues (2002) used longitudinal data to show that the effect of a significant risk factor (severe maltreatment) on antisocial behavior among male youth depended on the *monoamine oxidase A* (MAOA) gene. The effect of severe maltreatment was much greater for youth who were low in MAOA activity than for those who were high in MAOA activity. Caspi and colleagues noted that although only 12% of the male birth cohort had the combination of low-activity MAOA and maltreatment, they accounted for 44% of the cohort's violent convictions.

In addition to *genetic vulnerability*, prior experience may also make some adolescents more or less vulnerable to the risks in their current environment. As noted above, a history of success in overcoming obstacles is likely to make youth more confident when confronted with a new stressor. A lack of success in dealing with obstacles is likely to undermine confidence and motivation for youth facing new challenges. Youth make predictions about the likely outcomes of their actions based on prior experience.

A Summary of Protective and Risk Factors

Assessing internal protective and risk factors must be part of a general look at the range and balance of protective and risk factors affecting the adolescent. The ecological model provides a foundation for understanding how the internal factors work within the border context of the adolescent's life. It guides the practitioner toward problem definitions and interventions that aim to strengthen the adolescent within his or her context. A brief summary of internal protective and risk factors drawn from the discussion so far is provided in Table 4.2.

TABLE 4.2. Internal Protective and Risk Factors

Internal factors that promote positive development and resilience	Internal risk factors that deter positive development and resilience
• Commitment to learning	• Learning disability
• Cognitive abilities (IQ scores, attentional skills, executive functioning skills)	• Mental health diagnosis
	• Low expectations for the future
• Positive identity	• Low academic achievement
• Self-perceptions of competence, worth, confidence (self-efficacy, self-esteem)	• Low birth weight
• Social competencies	• Aggression toward peers and adults
	• Alienation from peers and adults
• Self-regulation skills (impulse control, affect, arousal regulations)	• Substance abuse
• Positive values	• Physical or sexual abuse
• Temperament and personality (adaptability, sociability)	• Eating disorders
	• Criminal activity
• Positive outlook on life (hopefulness, belief that life has meaning, faith)	

Interventions to Enhance Assets
and Assessments of Outcomes

Having identified characteristics associated with positive outcomes in youth, a logical follow-up question is What can be done to enhance these individual assets in youth? Evaluation research has shown that a number of intervention programs have successfully contributed to increasing assets and decreasing problem outcomes among youth (Dryfoos & Barkin, 2006; Fraser, 2004; Gillham & Reivich, 2004; Greenberg et al., 2003). Based on a review of the literature, Greenberg and colleagues concluded that "school-based prevention programming—based on coordinated social, emotional, and academic learning—should be fundamental to preschool through high school education" (p. 467). Comprehensive school-based programs that focus on social and emotional learning (SEL) enhance many of the individual assets described above while simultaneously improving academic performance, the classroom environment, and relationships youth have with significant others (Greenberg et al.; see also *www.casel.org*).

Because it has been implemented successfully in two states and takes advantage of existing infrastructure, such as schools, universities, and Cooperative Extension Service, the PROSPER model will be used as an example of a successful approach to increasing assets and decreasing problem behaviors among adolescents (for an overview of the model see Spoth et al., 2007). PROSPER stands for promoting school–community–university partnerships to enhance resilience. It is a universal program, rather than one that focuses only on youth considered to be at risk, which may be important for sustaining parental and community support. Other things that are appealing about the model is that it allows local communities to select intervention components from a menu of effective, evidence-based programs and pays particular attention to implementing these successful programs with fidelity. Local leadership is provided by a team consisting of County Cooperative Extension agents, school personnel, local community service providers, and parent and youth representatives. Extension agents serve as links between the local communities and universities that provide training, technical assistance, and evaluation resources.

PROSPER includes a component that aims at strengthening family through improving parenting skills, such as nurturing, setting limits, and communication (Spoth et al., 2007). It also enhances the skills of the youth including peer resistance, self-management, and social skills; in addition, it focuses on the student's knowledge and beliefs about risk-taking behaviors such as knowledge of alcohol and drug use.

An evaluation of PROSPER, focusing on substance use outcomes, showed positive effects on substance initiation and use of marijuana and inhalants during the past year. Differences between the experimental and comparison groups also approached significance for drunkenness and cigarette use during the past year (Spoth et al., 2007). Because local communities take leadership in selecting and implementing the program components that fit the needs of their community, hopefully the PROS-PER program will be sustained over time, unlike many previous model programs initiated by researchers with external funding.

The evaluation of PROSPER described above focused on reducing risky behaviors that are of concern in most communities. However, there is also interest in knowing whether intervention programs contribute to positive youth development or thriving, and how to measure these positive outcomes. An examination of available measures is beyond the scope of this chapter, but interested readers can consult a book on this topic edited by Moore and Lippman (2005). Also, some schools and communities collect data about their youths' assets, thriving, and risk-taking behaviors by using surveys created by the Search Institute; information about these surveys can be found at their website (*www.search-institute.org/home*).

The Lost Boys of Sudan: Resilience in Conditions of Extreme Adversity

The last section of the chapter provides an example of the role that individual attributes played in the resilient outcomes of youth who experienced extreme adversity. The source of this information was first-person accounts given to the author by several Sudanese youth in the hope that their experiences could help others. In the late 1980s, Sudanese children, typically between the ages of 4 and 12, were separated from their parents when their villages were attacked during a civil war. In the chaos of the attack, the children lost track of other family members and fled not knowing whether their parents and siblings were dead or alive—a situation known as *ambiguous loss* (Boss, 2006). They joined with other survivors of the attack and began an arduous journey to refugee camps in Ethiopia that lasted weeks or even months; along the way they encountered many hazards—lack of food, water, and blankets, and attacks by wild animals and government militias. The separated children grappled with fear and sadness, as they witnessed peers and adults perish on the journey.

Once in the Ethiopian camps, the children lived in peer groups with a few caretakers assigned to look after them—approximately 12 per 1,000 children in the camp at Panyido (Derib, 1998). Sanitation problems in the camp resulted in unsafe drinking water and disease. Older children had to bury younger peers who died. Lacking basic necessities, the children longed to be reunited with their parents, and children could be heard calling out the names of their parents during the night.

In May 1991, the refugees were violently expelled from the camps when there was a regime change in Ethiopia and had to flee back into Sudan. At the Gilo River on the border of Ethiopia and Sudan, thousands of children were trapped between a flood-swollen river and a pursuing army; many of the children could not swim and had to make a choice between jumping into the roiling river or being gunned down on the riverbank.

Back in Sudan, survivors were bombed by government forces who viewed them as future rebel soldiers. Thus, the youth had to make another long trek to the Kakuma refugee camp in Kenya. In Kakuma, they continued to live with peers in homes they helped construct, and attended class under the few trees in the area until relief agencies could construct school buildings. From the mid-1990s onward, food rations were so limited that the youth ate one meal per day and had to go some days without any food until the next ration arrived. They lived in Kakuma from 1992 to 2000–2001, when 3,800 Lost Boys (including 89 girls) were resettled in the United States.

Before being resettled, the youth had to go through a "best-interest determination" interview to determine whether they were eligible for resettlement and that it would be in their best interest to be resettled given that reunification with their families was unlikely. Julianne Duncan (January, 2000), who conducted 174 of these interviews, noted that "virtually every child is suffering from symptoms of *unresolved trauma*" (p. 4). She reported that youth were still experiencing disturbed sleep, nightmares, startle reactions, and other trauma symptoms 7 years after arriving at the Kakuma camp. But Duncan (May, 2001, p. 10) also reported, "Strength and resilience are the overwhelming characteristics of this group of children." She also described them as "really nice kids." Our research team was also struck by their remarkable resilience when we started working with these youth shortly after their resettlement.

How was it possible that these youth could endure so much hardship and adversity without the support of their biological parents and still have characteristics that most parents would be very pleased to see in their offspring? In the 8 years that we have conducted research with the group, we have attempted to answer this question. We have identified protective factors that include individual attributes, relationships, community resources and opportunities, and cultural factors. The individual attributes are listed in Table 4.1.

One of the key attributes of the youth was their strong commitment to education. Although it was not true of everyone, many of the youth dutifully marched off to school each day in the refugee camps without their parents there to prod them. There were a number of reasons for that. First, many of the children realized that their parents were not there to support them, and they would eventually have to support themselves, which required getting an education. In fact, they had a saying: "Education is my mother and my father." Second, they were strongly committed to rebuilding Sudan once the war was over and helping those left behind. Throughout their stay in the camps, the adult caretakers sounded the same drumbeat—Sudan needs educated people to rebuild after the war. The youth were from a culture that values the wisdom of elders, so the youth were primed to heed the advice of their elders. Moreover, the decision to attend school was supported by a peer culture that shared the views of the elders on education. Finally, the youth held onto the hope that they would be reunited with their parents, and they wanted their parents to be proud of the people they had become. As one youth put it, "I said, I will find my parents one day, and if they find me as a person they don't like, that would not be good."

We wondered if those who were most intelligent were most likely to survive, so we asked the youth about this. Generally, the youth thought that achievement in the classroom was not strongly related to who survived, but decision-making skills and resourcefulness were important. The decisions they made on their treks and the decision to stay in the camp, rather than try to return to their villages, had implications for whether they survived or perished. Similarly, they had to be resourceful in a context where inadequate resources were a chronic problem.

Having cared for themselves without their parents and having managed to overcome a long litany of obstacles, the Sudanese youth developed a *strong sense of self-efficacy*. Rutter's (2006b) notion of a "steeling effect" was evident in the words of this youth who had been complimented for adjusting rapidly to a new culture following resettlement: "This is the easy part. If I could do all of those things when I was only a child, I should be able to manage living in the United States as an adult." Their sense of efficacy was evident in their determination and persistence in the wake of setbacks. As we shall see later, their determination and sense of efficacy were also tied to their *religious beliefs* that God had kept them alive for a reason and there was something important they needed to accomplish.

Moreover, although resilience has been linked to an internal locus of control orientation (a belief that adolescents have some control over their destiny) (Werner & Smith, 2001), the Sudanese youth needed to accept that some things were beyond their control (the war, separation from their parents) and have a tempered sense of mastery (Boss, 2006). This meant focusing their effort on things they could control (e.g., going to school) and adapting to what was beyond their control.

Although this chapter focuses on individual attributes, an important part of the story of the survival of the Sudanese youth involves their relationships with adults and peers. One should not get the impression that their impressive personal strengths were all that they needed in this situation. It was important that they have temperamental and personality characteristics that were appealing to others and elicited positive reactions and support from others. The term *adoptability* has been used to describe children who have the ability to elicit help from other adults when their own families cannot or will not provide the support they need (Higgins, 1994; Rubin, 1996). Many of the Sudanese youth found adult mentors among the older adults and families living in the refugee camp. Caretakers and teachers assigned to look after the youth also played an important role in their lives even though they were burdened with large numbers of children.

Peer relationships were also an important part of their story. One of the U.S. officials who did "best-interest determination" interviews with the youth in Kakuma concluded that *sociability* was important to their survival; in an interview with us, he noted that it would have been very difficult for a person with a "lone wolf" mentality to have survived his or her ordeal. The youth needed to pool their resources and help each other through difficult times in order to survive. Peers provided protection and mutual support, and talking or playing with friends was a welcome distraction from their daily stresses. After years of being together, the peer group functioned like a surrogate family for the youth. As one youth said, "We decided to come together, older boys and younger boys and those in the middle and stay together as a family." These *second families*, as the youth referred to them, looked out for the welfare of the group, unlike the fictional youth in *The Lord of the Flies*. They were guided by two important cultural values: (1) it is important to share whatever you have with others, and (2) it is important to maintain your reputation and the reputation of your family. A person who would steal food from another hungry person would not be viewed as a suitable marital partner when he reached adulthood in their culture.

It is also important to remember the relationships the youth had with their parents prior to separation. The youth who were old enough at the time of separation to remember their parents noted the psychological presence of their parents despite their physical absence. When confronted with a difficult decision, they tried to think about what their parents would want them to do in this situation or how their parents handled similar situations. Older youth could remember specific advice their parents had given them and stories that their parents told them that included lessons about right and wrong.

Two of the most significant stressors that the youth had to contend with were separation from their parents and *ambiguous loss*, not knowing whether their parents were dead or alive. Thus, especially in the early years after separation, the youth had to deal with some very strong negative emotions and find ways to regulate those emotions using coping strategies. The coping strategies they used can be divided into *emotion-focused coping strategies* and *problem-focused coping strategies*. The emotion-focused coping strategies included avoidance (pushing thoughts of their families out of their minds), distraction (keeping busy with peers or schoolwork), and mental disengagement (sleeping more than usual). Problem-focused coping strategies including trying to contact their families by sending letters to their villages with Red Cross workers and asking new arrivals to the refugee camps from their area if they had seen their parents. For most youth, attempts to find out information about their families were unsuccessful, and eventually they reached a point of acceptance regarding their situation. As one youth put it, "Life is something that you get used to."

In addition to regulating their emotions, the youth had to regulate their behavior. While playing soccer all day was an option, the youth willed themselves off to school, even though hunger made it difficult to focus on schoolwork. Despite their hunger, most of them managed to control impulses to acquire food by any means. On the long treks to Ethiopia and Kenya, they resisted the strong urge to lie down on the trail and sleep; if the group moved on without them, they were easy prey for lions and hyenas. Thus, self-regulation was important for educational advancement, relationships with peers, and even survival in a hazardous environment.

Despite their bleak circumstances, the youth managed to maintain a positive outlook on life and find meaning in their experiences. Religion was an important part of how they made meaning of their experience. Noting the many times on the journey that he eluded death, one youth reflected, "If God had wanted me dead, I would be dead now, but I am not. So He must have other plans for me." When we first met him in 2001, he trusted that God had a plan for him but he was not certain what it was. Three years later when he reconnected with his surviving siblings, he concluded that God had made him suffer through this ordeal so that he eventually had a job in the United States that allowed him to provide for his siblings; his parents had not survived the war.

The youth also noted the importance of *hope*; as one youth put it: "If I did not have hope of something, I would have not made it." Viktor Frankl described how he survived in a concentration camp using this quote from Friedrich Nietzsche, "He who has a *why* to live for can bear almost any *how*." For the Sudanese youth, the "why" seemed to be their hope of being reunited with their families and their desire to help rebuild southern Sudan when the war ended. Several of the youth we interviewed noted that the hope of being reunited with their parents helped them get through the darkest days of their ordeal. Once they learned that they would be resettled in the United States, they also had hope of a better future.

Although the Sudanese youth were doing remarkably well given what they had endured, it is important to note that they did not come out of the experience unscathed. Many of the youth struggled with post-traumatic stress disorder (PTSD) symptoms after resettlement, although there was wide variation in reported symptoms (Bates et al., 2005; Geltman et al.,

2005). Some of the youth have also experienced depressive symptoms, and a few of the youth have been disappointed since resettlement because it has been very difficult to pursue educational goals given the need to work long hours to support themselves and family members still in Africa. Some of the foster parents of the minors have expressed concerns about alcohol consumption in group members, and view alcohol use as a way to temporarily forget painful memories.

The experience of the Sudanese youth confirms the importance of personal assets and attributes in understanding resilient outcomes in youth. However, their experiences also demonstrate the importance of *context* in understanding resilience. One important lesson from the Sudanese is that when parents are not able to carry out their parenting responsibilities, other adults need to step up and provide guidance and support. Adult caretakers and mentors encouraged the youth to remain hopeful about finding their parents, suggested coping strategies for dealing with their separation, and stressed the importance of focusing on the present and the future (education) rather than the past and what they had lost. The Sudanese youths' experience also points to the potential of *peer groups* to contribute to positive developmental outcomes. Much of the prior research on adolescent peers has focused on the ways their behavior contribute to problem outcomes, but clearly peer relationships can be important sources of support; in this case, supportive peers helped each other to survive. Moreover, even in a bleak refugee camp, community resources, such as schools, churches, and recreational activities, helped restore some normality to the lives of the youth and provided additional adults to support their development. Finally, Sudanese culture also influenced the relationship between the youth and the adults in the camp; many Sudanese adults followed the *cultural dictum* that "Any child is everybody's child" and the youth had been socialized to respect their more knowledgeable elders "Because they saw the sun first." In subsequent chapters, a more extensive discussion of contextual influences on positive youth development is provided.

QUESTIONS FOR THE REFLECTIVE PRACTITIONER

1. Which of the 20 internal assets listed in Table 4.1 do you have?
2. When you consider your personal strengths, what do you consider to be your most valuable individual assets?
3. Have you had these assets for as long as you can remember or have you developed some of these assets more recently?
4. In what ways did your relationships with others contribute to the development of these assets?

5. Do you view your school and your community as environments that help youth develop the individual assets they need? Why or why not?

6. Are there any assets listed in Table 4.1 that you would like to acquire or improve upon?

7. Put yourself in the place of the Sudanese Lost Boys. How do you think you would have reacted if you were separated from your parents by war sometime between the ages of 4 and 12?

8. What would you need to do to make it through that situation?

9. How are war experiences likely to affect children?

10. The Sudanese youth depended a great deal on their peers to survive. What are some of the ways in which peers have had a positive influence on your life?

11. The Sudanese youth also needed adults outside their families to serve as surrogate parents and mentors. Who do you consider to be the most important adult in your life outside of your immediate family members?

12. The Sudanese youths' experiences also highlighted the role that culture can play in the development of individual assets. How has your culture helped shape your characteristics (e.g., beliefs, values, and norms of behavior) that would help get you through difficult times?

Chapter Summary

Through the lens of the Sudanese Lost Boys, we can better understand the many attributes and assets youth possess to be resilient in times of trouble. Though most of our clients will never experience the difficulties the Lost Boys endured, the knowledge that is gained of how these youth survived helps us all better understand youths' reaction to more common-place stresses and difficulties. In the next chapter, the youth in the family context is discussed.

CHAPTER 5

The Family Environment

Douglas Davies

Chapter Overview

As adolescents are challenged by developmental imperatives and cultural expectations to achieve higher and more integrated levels of functioning, they do best when they have a strong family in the background supporting their transition to adulthood. A history of secure attachment, parental warmth, responsiveness and support, and functional family communication patterns provide a strong foundation for adolescent development. The quality of parenting and family relationships are critically important to adolescent growth and development (Allen, 2008). This chapter addresses these concerns and offers options for assessment and intervention with adolescents and their families, which readers can apply to a case example.

CASE EXAMPLE:
Who Are the Youth Represented in This Chapter?

The following case example represents some of the concerns related to adolescents and the family environment. Considering the implications for this case within the context of the risk factors, theory, assessment, and intervention strategies presented in the following pages will prepare you to assess and suggest interventions for the more developed case study at the end of the chapter.

Melissa's single-parent mother, Debbie, was aware that she had given Melissa too much freedom and that she had little control over her now. Melissa had not gotten into trouble in the neighborhood, but this self-reliant and opinionated 15-year-old refused to work in school and was hostile and provocative toward some of her teach-ers. Her mother was very concerned that Melissa's poor grades and oppositional behavior toward teachers would compromise her future. But she also seemed to identify with Melissa's adamant independence, saying, "She's so bright and strong willed—I just wish teachers would reach out to her." Debbie seemed to believe that by being independent Melissa would be less likely to become a teen parent as she did 17 years ago.

Melissa's history suggested that her current refusal to be influenced by her mother or allow her activities to be monitored was just the adolescent iteration of a pattern of self-reliance and independence that had begun in early childhood after her mother was diagnosed with multiple sclerosis, and her father, in response, abandoned the family. As the illness slowly progressed through Melissa's school-age years, Debbie became less physically capable and increasingly self-involved in her health issues.

Debbie seemed to alternate between an indulgent style of parenting, giving Melissa a great deal of personal freedom and failing to convey clear disapproval of her behavior at school, and the indifferent style of parenting, not intentionally, but because she was frequently depressed and preoccupied with her progressive illness. Melissa was intelligent and appeared to cope well until adolescence, when she took the stance that she was able to look out for herself and insisted not only that she did not need adult supervision but also that adults, such as teachers, had to "prove" they were worthy of being involved with her. Melissa's early loss of her father and progressive loss of her mother had promoted excessive self-reliance and a prevail-ing mistrust of adult intentions. When she was 13, Melissa "abandoned" her father, refusing to go to visit him in a distant state (as she had done once a year up to that point) explaining that "If he really wants to see me, he'll have to come to me."

*   *   *

The adolescent's gradual progression to autonomy and increased identity development impacts the parent–child relationship. Based on the development of formal operational and abstract thinking, the adolescent becomes more analytical, more capable of self-reflection, and able to see his or her parents more objectively. Because of these cognitive changes, the adolescent differentiates him- or herself more sharply from parents than was possible in childhood. Parents are de-idealized and seen in terms of both positive and negative qualities. For adolescents with a history of secure family relationships, these cognitive changes do not predict a rejec-tion of parents; nevertheless, the adolescent is more likely than a younger child to view his or her parents with a critical eye.

These changes in the adolescent's view of parents are elements of a major developmental reorganization of the sense of self, that Blos (1979) named the "second separation-individuation" (p. 10). Recall that the separation-individuation of toddlers, as described by Mahler, involves the young child's developing awareness that he or she is *actually* separate from his or her mother and that the child and the mother are individuals, with their own separate thoughts and feelings (Mahler, Pine, & Bergman, 1975). Blos argued that the second separation-individuation involves an equally fundamental shift in the early adolescent's view of self in relation to parents. The young adolescent gradually gives up the view of him- or herself as a dependent child and his or her parents as being all-knowing and in charge. This view is replaced by an awareness that "I'm responsible for what happens to me," and that "My choices will determine who I become."

Across adolescence, feelings of closeness and interdependence with parents decline, as does time spent together. As adolescents increasingly pursue their own agendas, and interact preferentially with peers, parents become less central. However, the quality of early relationships tends to persist. An adolescent with a history of good relationships with his or her parents continues to feel close to them and to rely on them, even though he or she is more independent and more involved with peers (Collins & Steinberg, 2006).

As adolescents make more decisions independently from parents, parents attempt to influence, guide, and sometimes control the adolescent's choices. In this process, both teen and parents find themselves in different roles than in childhood. The adolescent is doing more asserting, while the parent may find him- or herself in a reactive stance, trying to get the adolescent to slow down or change course. From the perspectives of both, this transactional process requires a lot of negotiation and, in many cases, conflict and confrontation (Steinberg & Silk, 2002). In the abstract, parents want to support the adolescent's assertiveness and self-reliance because these capacities are essential for adult functioning. Similarly, adolescents want to remain connected to parents as they move toward independence. Relationship renegotiation revolves around these themes and both parents and adolescents implicitly hope for the successful outcome of autonomy while still maintaining connection (Beveridge & Berg, 2007). In this healthy pattern, adolescents and parents increasingly engage in give-and-take, and gradually a more egalitarian relationship emerges (Steinberg & Silk). However, until the egalitarian relationship evolves, there may be periods of disagreement, distrust, or hostility.

Perspectives on Parent–Adolescent Relationships

This section introduces several conceptual frameworks that inform a discussion of the family context of adolescent development and clinical work with teens and parents: attachment theory, family systems theory, and models of parenting styles. Although there are many parallels and points of convergence in these frameworks, they are described separately.

Attachment Theory

The attachment system that develops between caregiver and infant serves the functions of providing protection, a sense of security, mutual regulation of affect and arousal, and a scaffolding for the infant's development. In the second year of life, the attachment relationship expands to include a "secure base" from which the toddler can explore the world. Over the first few years, based on how the young child has been responded to and cared for within the attachment relationship, the child internalizes working models of what can be expected in relationships and a view of the self within relationships. These working models tend to "organize" the individual's perception of future relationships (Bowlby, 1969, 1973).

Studies of adults' assumptions about attachment demonstrate that adults have attachment styles that tend to parallel their infant's attachment patterns. *Secure* adults tend to value attachment, feel their attachments shaped their personalities, and are able to take a realistic view of their relationships. *Dismissive* adults tend to deny the importance of attachment and often report distant or cut-off relationships with their own parents. *Preoccupied* adults tend to be focused on their dependency on their own parents, to feel responsible for difficulties in relationships with parents, and to worry about how others see them. *Unresolved* adults tend to have histories of childhood trauma and loss, and express ongoing anxiety about loss. Their descriptions of attachment experiences tend to be incoherent and disorganized. There are strong correlations between parents' adult attachment classification and their children's attachment types (Main, Kaplan, & Cassidy, 1985).

Attachment History and Adolescent Development

Secure attachment in infancy and early childhood predicts the capacity of adolescents to function with increasing autonomy *and* remain strongly connected to parents (Sroufe, Egeland, Carlson, & Collins, 2005). Adolescents benefit developmentally when they continue to feel close to parents, even as they are striving to become autonomous. Adolescents with histories of secure attachment tend to be able to balance attachment and autonomy. Although overt attachment-seeking behavior declines in adolescence, when an adolescent with a history of secure attachment is under extreme stress, the attachment relationship becomes a source of resilience, as he or she turns to a parent for help and support (Boutelle, Eisenberg, Gregory, & Neumark-Sztainer, 2009).

Adolescents increasingly meet attachment needs through friendships and romantic relationships with peers; but adolescents and even young adults continue to see parents as fulfilling a main function of attachment, providing a secure base (Nickerson & Nagle, 2005). As securely attached adolescents explore new experiences, particularly through interactions with peers, they still consider a parent as the person they can depend on. In one study, 90% of adolescents with secure attachments named a parent as their primary attachment figure; by contrast a significant majority of insecurely attached adolescents named a peer (Freeman & Brown, 2001). An important aspect of the secure base is the parent's ability to acknowledge and empathize with the adolescent's full range of emotions, including negative ones. Adolescents feel supported when parents are willing to talk about negative experiences and emotions and to explore how to cope with them (Stocker, Richmond, Rhoades, & Kiang, 2007).

In contrast, insecure attachment history confers developmental risk. For example, an adolescent with an avoidant attachment will have low expectations about his or her parent's ability to give support in times of developmental stress; in fact, his or her working models will suggest that the parent will be dismissive, critical, or rejecting (Feeney & Cassidy, 2003). Avoidantly attached teens are more likely to turn to peers with similar negative views and to maladaptive coping strategies such as substance abuse.

Family Systems Theory

Families function as a system, and assessment of adolescents must understand whole-family functioning, as opposed to focusing exclusively on the referred adolescent's relationship with parents. Change in one member of the family ripples through the system, affecting all other members as well as the overall stability of the family. *Family cohesion* is a term describing the degree of closeness and contact among family members (Foster & Robin, 1989). Families that are optimally *cohesive* provide clear expectations about how family members will be involved with each other and what their responsibilities to each other will be, while allowing a degree of autonomy for individual members that is consistent with their culture. Families at either end of the cohesion continuum (with *enmeshed* at one end and *disengaged* at the other) may face conflicts when children reach adolescence.

Enmeshed families tend to have inadequate boundaries between parents and adolescents. Emotional overdependency has been encouraged, privacy may have been discounted, and interference in each other's affairs is the norm. Enmeshment may take different patterns but essentially parents require the adolescent to curtail striving toward independence and instead serve the parents' needs (Mayseless & Scharf, 2009). Enmeshed adolescents may avoid self-assertion in deference to their parents' views in order to maintain the relationship with the parent, in some cases continuing in a parentified, caretaking role with a parent and younger siblings, or keeping their autonomy seeking secret. In *triangulation*, the parents require the adolescent to take an inappropriate mediating role in the family, as when one parent enlists the adolescent in a quasi-spousal relationship to deal with alienation or divorce from the other parent. Girls are at higher risk for enmeshment because they tend to be socialized to become caregivers (Brody, 1996). Enmeshed adolescents may argue a lot with parents, but without resolution, and the arguing seems to function as a means of remaining engaged (Allen, 2008; Beveridge & Berg, 2007).

Disengaged families are at the other end of the cohesion continuum. In these families, everyone is pretty much on his or her own. The adolescent's independence may be fostered to an extreme degree, often because his or her behavior is ignored or unmonitored by parents. Parents may show little concern about serious problems (such as substance abuse or delinquency), and fail to establish consistent and effective rules for in-family and community behavior. Disengaged families do not provide enough structure to support the transition through adolescence. Expressions of anger and conflict are common within the family, yet the family tends to be able to "absorb" conflict and keep functioning. An adolescent who has been emotionally abandoned in this way during a time of stress is at high risk for increased substance abuse or delinquency (Dodge & Pettit, 2003). Disengaged adolescents tend to dismiss their parents' perspectives and operate self-reliantly, and their parents may stop trying to influence their choices, or only sporadically assert themselves.

Parents' "Working Models" of Adolescence

In addition to enmeshment and disengagement, parenting is influenced by each parent's unique family history including how they were parented and how they experienced their own adolescence. Family systems theory, like attachment theory, maintains that family styles tend to persist across generations, with parents setting up interaction schemas and roles for children that reproduce patterns in their families of origin. In assessment, a three-generational genogram often reveals these continuities. Parents may have "working models" about adolescence based on their own teenage experiences. A mother who became pregnant at 17 may be frightened that the same thing will happen to her daughter and place rigid restrictions on dating. This leads to conflict and, with some youth, open rebellion—including becoming sexually active in defiance of her mother. Another example is the father who minimizes his adolescent's antisocial behavior as normal, based on his own history of delinquency in adolescence. A father whose son had been suspended from school and charged with assault for attacking another kid might say, "All kids get in trouble at this age. I know I did. I think everyone is overreacting." Parents' own histories can create problematic assumptions that blind them to the actual needs of their teens.

Parenting Styles

Knowledge of parenting styles helps the practitioner think about how particular parent–adolescent relationships function. There are four different types of parenting styles that focus on dimensions of responsiveness and demandingness (Baumrind, 1991).

1. *Authoritative*. This type of parenting is most supportive of adolescent development (Collins & Steinberg, 2006, p. 1018). Authoritative parents are involved with their teens, convey warmth, set firm expectations and limits, and maintain family routines, while supporting the adolescent's individuality and autonomy.

2. *Authoritarian*. These parents tend to be harsh and demanding, and absolute and punitive in discipline, practices that interfere with the adolescent's autonomy and promote passivity, dependency, and, sometimes, rebellion. Their children may keep their behavior and friends' identities secret, to avoid their parents' criticism. As a result, authoritarian parents often know very little about their adolescent's life outside the home.

3. *Indulgent*. In this pattern, parents demand little of their adolescents and allow the adolescent a lot of freedom, yet are warm and responsive. Adolescents from indulgent families tend to have less sense of direction, are immature, and tend to be followers. They receive little positive guidance and parents' indulgence may extend to failing to monitor the adolescent's activities or friendships.

4. *Indifferent*. These parents are basically neglectful, investing little interest or time in interacting with the adolescent, monitoring his or her behavior, or supporting his or her development. Their children tend to have poor self-regulation, and are most likely to experience a range of adolescent problems, including delinquency, substance abuse, and precocious sexuality (Collins & Steinberg, 2006).

However, in real families these parenting styles may be on a continuum, especially when components such as degree of warmth or monitoring are considered. A parent may be firm in expecting and supporting high achievement (authoritative), yet indulgent in allowing the adolescent more use of a car than most parents would. Further, just as it is possible to have different attachment relationships with each parent, in two-parent families the parents may embody different parenting styles, and these may be exacerbated if the parents are divorced. This will likely be a source of tension for the parents and for the adolescent, as the teen attempts to adapt to parents' different levels of responsiveness and demandingness.

Protective and Risk Factors: A Family Perspective

Family Disruption and Stress

Disruptions in the family, such as illness, divorce, mental health issues, death of a parent, parental incarceration, or in the wider environment, such as economic conditions that shift a family into poverty, may threaten to derail adolescent development. Single-parent families and stepfamilies are more vulnerable to disruptions (Collins & Steinberg, 2006). Consistent with resiliency research showing that the child's relationships with nonparental adults promote development (Werner & Smith, 1982), recent studies show that involvement with nonparental relatives, particularly grandparents, support prosocial behavior and good mental health, especially in single-parent families, divorced families, and stepfamilies. A supportive grandparent can be a source of continuity for an adolescent whose family system is under stress or in flux (Attar-Schwartz, Tan, Buchanan, Flouri, & Griggs, 2009; Ruiz & Silverstein, 2007).

There is also evidence that the *timing* of adolescence in many families interacts with parents' midlife developmental issues and may enhance family conflict. For example, midlife, from the late 30s to early 50s, is often a time of increased stress for parents. Career pressures may be intense during this period, and in two-parent families marital satisfaction tends to decline and the possibility of divorce heightens (Gottman & Notarius, 2000). Parents may experience adolescents' growing autonomy as a loss of personal importance. They may feel less competent in their role as parent, adding to midlife stress (Paley, Conger, & Harold, 2000).

Monitoring and Knowledge

Because adolescents spend so much time outside the family, knowledge and monitoring practices are important to assess when adolescents are referred for evaluation. Adolescents whose parents know their "whereabouts, companions, and activities" are less likely to engage in problematic behavior or identify with antisocial peers (Laird, Criss, Pettit, Dodge, & Bates, 2008, p. 299). While age-appropriate parental monitoring is a protective factor throughout development, it is particularly important during early adolescence, when developmental imperatives push the adolescent toward autonomy and personal freedom at a time when good judgmental and decision-making abilities are not yet firmly established.

Adolescents whose parents know about their lives—and are ready to set necessary limits—are much less likely to join, or be influenced by, antisocial peer groups. Parents who establish rules and expectations and engage adolescents in talking about what they do in their free time convey to the adolescent an expectation of self-control (Laird et al., 2008). Moderate strictness and high but reasonable expectations for the adolescent's behavior, especially when combined with parental warmth, is a protective factor, while both coercive and lax discipline predict more behavior problems (Coley, Morris, & Hernandez, 2004; Hair, Moore, Garrett, Ling, & Cleveland, 2008). This risk is particularly acute in authoritarian families where coercive discipline becomes physical or abusive (Dodge & Pettit, 2003; Patterson, 1995).

In turn, adolescents' acceptance of parental monitoring is strongly related to the history of parent–child attachment. Adolescents who have experienced a secure attachment over time are likely to feel valued and respected by their parents and therefore to be more motivated to find a balance between efforts toward independence and meeting parental expectations (Allen, McElhaney, Kupermine, & Jodl, 2004; Vitaro, Brendgen, & Tremblay, 2000).

Parent–Adolescent Conflict: Risk Factor or Normative?

The extensive research literature on parent–adolescent conflict tends to debunk the image of adolescence as a rebellious period when parents are rejected, suggesting instead a more nuanced view, in which parent–adolescent conflicts are frequent and sometimes disturbing, but in most families tend to occur in the context of warm and involved relationships.

Parent–adolescent conflicts are more frequent and more intense in early and midadolescence (McGue, Elkins, Walden, & Iacono, 2005). The parent–adolescent relationship tends to stabilize again in late adolescence, as power and decision making become more egalitarian (De Goede, Branje, & Meeus, 2009). Young adolescents, however, tend to think the quality of their relationship with parents decreases (McGue et al., 2005). From a psychodynamic perspective, it is likely that young adolescents project onto their parents their own struggles to differentiate and distance themselves from parents; yet parents of young adolescents often agree that relationship quality decreases in early adolescence. Some research has found that young adolescents' conflicts are more intense with mothers compared to fathers and that girls engage in more conflict. Girls' greater conflict has been explained as a function of "gender intensification," as parents try to enforce traditional gender expectations on girls; however, this has not been consistently found in research (Allison & Schultz, 2004; McGue et al., 2005).

Most studies of nonclinical early adolescents find that conflicts are in the mild to moderate range and revolve around disputes about homework, chores, personal appearance, time management and use of free time, messiness, choice of friends, early dating, and substance use (Collins & Steinberg, 2006). Any of these areas can become a theater of conflict, as adolescents assert themselves and parents try to maintain control and authority. In a mundane example, an adolescent client might say: "My parents were always yelling at me to turn my music down. Then after I got my iPod, they told me I was hypnotized in my own world, and why couldn't I be part of the *family*? They have no clue what they want. I finally just stopped arguing with them." Even though many conflicts are over "little things," as this example suggests, both adolescents and parents may become frustrated when conflict is poorly resolved. Rather than reaching a mutually agreed-upon compromise, many conflicts are settled (or perhaps "unsettled") by one party either giving in or disengaging (Collins & Steinberg). Parents often regard common issues of conflict (such as failure to do chores) as moral issues, while teens think of them as personal choices. Parents may view an adolescent who does not pick up his or her room as violating the values they have taught the adolescent, while the adolescent feels (and may say), "It's no big deal." This perspective recasts adolescent "storm and stress" as an artifact of *parents'* distress and disappointment when teens resist or contradict their expectations (Collins, 1997). In many families, the changes and day-to-day conflicts accompanying early adolescence are harder on parents than on teens (Smetana, 1989; Steinberg & Steinberg, 1994).

In most families conflicts are more than counterbalanced by interactions that reflect mutual respect and admiration, warmth, and love. Relationships are maintained even in the face of frequent disagreements in early adolescence. A parent who tolerates conflict, hears the adolescent's perspective, and sees disagreement as a chance to resolve problems and guide the adolescent protects his or her development. Even though parents and adolescents disagree on the "small stuff," like curfew or appearance, they tend to agree about the larger issues such as ethical, political, or religious values. Adolescents who are supported emotionally by their parents, identify with them, and adopt similar views of the world are also most likely to turn to parents for help in making major life decisions (Collins & Laursen, 2006).

At the other extreme, parents who denigrate the adolescent's ideas, take authoritarian and judgmental stances, and provoke anger and alienation impede adolescent development. Attempts at psychological control through derogation and rejection may seriously undercut the adolescent's identity formation.

Conflict is normative in early adolescence, so the issue is not conflict in itself, but rather how developmentally influenced conflict intersects with familial protective and risk factors. Families with major conflict during adolescence tend to have had a long history of parent–child difficulties that are intensified by—not created by—the adolescent's developmental changes. They lack adaptive strategies for dealing with conflict and do worse handling conflict as it increases in adolescence (Collins & Laursen, 2006). Steinberg estimates, however, that "only a very small proportion—somewhere between 5 and 10%—experience a dramatic deterioration in the quality of child–parent relationships during adolescence" (1990, p. 260).

A Summary of Protective and Risk Factors

Assessing family protective and risk processes must be part of a general look at the range and balance of protective and risk factors affecting the adolescent. However, analyzing past and current family processes guides the practitioner toward family-based problem definitions and interventions that aim to strengthen parent–adolescent relationships. A brief summary of family protective and risk factors drawn from the discussion so far is provided in Table 5.1.

TABLE 5.1. Internal Protective and Risk Factors

Parent and family factors that promote positive development and resilience	Parent and family factors that deter positive development and resilience
• Parental knowledge and monitoring of the adolescent's activities • Parental warmth • Parental ability to tolerate conflicts and still remain engaged • Parental encouragement, support, and flexibility as the adolescent becomes more autonomous • Open communication between parents and adolescent • Moderately strict discipline, clear boundaries • Authoritative parenting • History of secure attachment • The adolescent's use of parents as a secure base • Cohesive family structure and boundaries, past and present • Availability of supportive nonparental adults	• Parents' critical, negative, dismissive views of the adolescent • Low knowledge and parental monitoring of the adolescent's activities • Chronic high levels of conflict in the family predating adolescence • Poor communication between parents and adolescent • High levels of psychological control: coercion, criticism, shaming • Lax, inconsistent, or highly punitive discipline, including harsh physical punishment and abuse • Authoritarian, indifferent, or indulgent parenting style • History of insecure attachment • High level of marital conflict or alienation, with adolescent assigned role of mediator or supporter of one parent • Family disruption or crises • Isolation of family from supports

Assessment and Engagement with Adolescents
and Their Families

Assessment of family issues is essential to any evaluation of an adolescent. The above review of family protective and risk factors points to areas of assessment with regard to family processes. Central questions from a family perspective are

> Do parent–adolescent relationships and family processes support or interfere with adolescent development?
> What needs to be changed to allow development to proceed more healthfully?

However, some adolescents struggle with problems that are primarily internally generated, or based on trauma experienced outside the family, or derived from biological risks. Obvious examples are teens with adolescent-onset bipolar disorder. Even in those cases where the family is not central to the problem, it is nevertheless valuable to assess the family's strengths and challenges, because mobilizing the family's support can create a context for ameliorating individual problems.

Within any family there are likely to be areas of strength and adequacy. Most parents have tried to do their best, within the constraints of individual and family history. Most parents want their children to succeed. Nevertheless, dysfunctional family processes maintain symptomatic behavior and compromise development (Olson, 1996). Evaluation should develop hypotheses about how family interactions create risk, as well as identifying parent strengths that can support teens' development.

Meeting the Family for the First Time

Early accounts of family systems therapy argued that the family should be seen together from the outset. However, there are strong reasons, especially during the evaluation, to first see the parents and adolescent separately. One option is to have a brief meeting (5–10 minutes) with adolescent and parents together to get their respective views of the problems, then spend the rest of the first session with the adolescent alone. This is important because many adolescents are defensive about being evaluated and they worry, when parents are seen first, that the practitioner, on hearing parents' negative views will prejudge them and form a coalition with the parents. This is followed by one or two meetings with the parents alone, possibly another session with the adolescent, and then a family session. The major goal of these separate meetings, in addition to gathering information and developing hypotheses, is to make a connection with each family member that will hopefully evolve into a therapeutic alliance. Seeing parents and adolescent together for the first session risks "fireworks" before family members know the practitioner and before the practitioner understands the family well enough to intervene. It is not sufficient to rationalize that one has at least seen an enactment of dysfunction if family members leave the session aroused, distressed, or hopeless. If parent–adolescent conflict is the reason for referral, it is useful to first hear how parents and adolescent frame the conflict before bringing them together. In these separate sessions, information gathering and engagement go hand-in-hand, as the practitioner listens carefully, attends to the family members' perspectives and affects, elicits interpretations of the sources of the conflict, and, in parent sessions, conveys interest in the parents as individuals and as a couple by asking about their current issues as well as taking a brief history of their families of origin. Engaging parents also involves eliciting their hopes for therapy. Most parents, even those with dismissive or authoritarian styles, wish to repair the relationship with their adolescent. The practitioner tries to help them articulate that wish, to establish relationship change as a goal of treatment, and to convey a sense of hope that change is possible. When parents have been heard, respected for their individual histories, and helped to formulate "relational goals" for therapy they are more likely to develop a therapeutic alliance (Diamond, Diamond, & Liddle, 2000). Consequently, as noted above, the first task, which should inform the practitioner's responses from the first minutes of the first interview, is to make empathic connections with all family members. Since motivation of parents is central to changing family processes, the assessment period must be seen as a time to engage the parents and help them develop an attachment to the practitioner so that they will be able to enter a therapeutic alliance on the adolescent's behalf. Early development of an alliance with parents contributes to better outcomes for adolescent clients (Hogue, Dauber, Stambaugh, Cecero, & Liddle, 2006).

First, let the family know that it is most helpful to learn how they communicate and relate with another. Also caution them that they should not expect a quick solution to a conflict that has been ongoing, but that the practitioner can best serve their needs by understanding how the family functions, as a basis for collaborating on reducing conflict. It is fairly common for both parents and adolescent to come to the family session ready to tell their side of the story and to express intense affects during the session. The practitioner can feel more balanced in this session if he or she has made a beginning connection with parents and adolescent. Similarly, family members may be able to better tolerate the fact that the practitioner will not intervene decisively in the conflict if they have been prepared for the family session and if they also, as individuals, feel a beginning bond with the practitioner. Within these caveats, the family session (or at least a parent–adolescent session) is central to the assessment process. In adolescent cases where family dysfunctions play a large role, parents and adolescents are likely to present views of one another and interactions that allow the evaluator to observe how their transactional dysfunction "works." Although parents and teens have separately reported these interactions, there is no substitute for seeing them enacted.

Observing Family Interactions

Identifying interaction patterns that interfere with the adolescent's development helps clarify what needs to be targeted in intervention. The changes a family is able to make in reshaping communication patterns, dampening conflicts, reducing insecurity in attachment, or understanding one another's perspectives will have the most impact in helping an adolescent shift to a more positive developmental trajectory. Consequently, assessment must focus not only on general impressions of family processes, but specifically on those areas of parenting that may be amenable to change. Change in "the caregiver is viewed as the key to long-term positive outcomes for the youth" (Henggeler & Lee, 2003).

At the outset, however, it is necessary to respect the reality that dysfunctional interactions, even those that distress family members, may be resistant to change and may also be adaptive. For example, some parents, for reasons that are not clear, are leery of allowing their teenager to test him- or herself outside the family, and may feel that their limitations on him or her are somehow protective. Clients often have an unstated or unconscious rationale that informs or supports the continuance of their symptomatic behavior. This line of reasoning helps us understand why advice giving, telling someone what they need to do to change, or making the "big interpretation" about what seems self-evident to us, rarely works.

Intervention Approaches

Family approaches have dual goals of improving parent–adolescent relationships and increasing adolescents' developmental competence.[1] The two goals are realized in tandem, as positive systems change supports individual change. On the adolescent's side, goals include reducing symptoms,

---

[1] Space limitations do not allow for full description of the many family-based treatment models. For reviews, see Malone (2001) and Cottrell and Boston (2002). The discussion of treatment approaches illustrates many themes and treatment activities common to contemporary family therapy approaches.

restricting self-harming or risk behaviors, and helping him or her become more engaged in the development of competence. On the family's side, goals often include strengthening boundaries, increasing monitoring and expectations for the adolescent, improving parent–teen communication patterns, developing problem-solving strategies, and restoring damaged attachments.

In almost all cases, then, except perhaps for some older, well-individuated adolescents, parents will be an integral part of treatment. Recent research shows that the best treatment results are gained when there are strong components of *both* family/parent treatment and individual adolescent treatment (Hogue, Dauber, Samuolis, & Liddle, 2006). Within this dictum, treatment can take many forms, including whole-family systems interventions; sessions with parents alone focusing on psychoeducation, guidance, and the understanding of the parent's relational emphases; sessions with family subsystems (e.g., father and adolescent) focusing on perspective sharing and relationship enhancement; planned parent–adolescent meetings focusing on problem solving; and regular individual therapy with the adolescent that includes, as one theme, understanding the adolescent's interactions with other family members (Mackey, 2003). Certain situations, especially divorce, may preclude working with parents together; however, in most cases of divorce, even though parents may be unwilling to meet jointly, both should be engaged in separate sessions. Stepfamilies are at higher risk for conflict in adolescence, especially when the stepfamily is established when children are teenagers. Consequently, the practitioner should attempt to engage stepparents, and be alert to certain dynamics that often create conflict, such as the stepfather who takes over disciplining teens before he has a solid relationship with them, or the stepmother who is given the job of being the primary caretaker for children before she knows them.

Framing the Problems

In the first phase of treatment the goal is to help family members describe presenting problems and family dynamics from their individual perspectives. Although problematic interactions will often be enacted in early sessions, family members are asked to step out of the dynamics in order to analyze them and see how they operate. *Narrative therapy* provides techniques for helping family members think about the effects of problems more objectively. White and Epston (1990) ask family members to describe how the problems influence them individually and as a family. This encourages them to consider the costs of the problems. A related question asks each individual to describe how he or she personally influences the problem and keeps it going. This question implicitly shifts consideration from blaming others to personal responsibility, and can become a basis later for exploring what individuals can do to change the dynamics of the problem.

As problems are described in more neutral, objective, and interactional terms, family members are encouraged to contemplate them from the outside. One implication of a detailed, multiperspective problem description, as emphasized by narrative therapies (White & Epston, 1990), is that problems are externalized. Even though parent–adolescent relationship patterns are central to the problem, the problem is temporarily taken out of the enacted relationship realm, as family members view its circularity of cause and effect "objectively." Of course, objectification makes family members uncomfortable by challenging either/or views they have previously embraced, and they are likely to try to revert to familiar patterns through accusations and blaming, or by challenging the therapeutic process, as in "Just talking about it isn't solving the problem." This is often a first test of the alliance. If the practitioner has been able to develop an alliance with each family member, he or she can respond by asserting that he or she is asking them to try out a new way of thinking that has the promise of changing how the family deals with conflict. The practitioner can also explicitly state that falling back into the established script will not lead to solutions, since it clearly has not up to now.

A related useful technique is to ask parents to describe *the adolescent's perspectives and needs*, with the adolescent listening and elaborating or correcting the parents' impressions. Then roles are reversed and the adolescent is asked to speak from the parents' perspectives. During this exercise, the practitioner is active in keeping the current speaker focused on attempts to understand the other's viewpoint. Further, the practitioner asks for confirmation that the representations of other's perspectives are generally accurate. The goal is to help polarized family members realize they are capable of understanding one another's viewpoints. The practitioner can point out commonalities in the family members' views of the conflict and, especially important, note instances of empathy shown by either parents or adolescent. Parents and adolescent are encouraged by the practitioner to construct an overview description of the problems and their interactional correlates that they can tentatively agree on. Since the perspectives of both must be included in the problem description, it is likely that the problem will be redefined as interactional and systemic. At the outset, the adolescent's view of the problem might have been "My parents are totally unreasonable," and the parents' might have been "Our daughter has no control over her anger." By contrast, the new problem definition is likely to describe chains of action, reaction, and mutual negative reinforcement. This may open the way to a "relational reframe" (Moran, Diamond,

& Diamond, 2005) in which problems previously described as deficits in individuals are now framed in interpersonal, process terms.

Behavior Problem and Relational Problem: A Brief Clinical Example

Tiana, just turned 15, and her single-parent mother, Ms. Jamison, were seen because of intense conflict that seemed to have originated when Tiana was caught shoplifting a bathing suit a few months earlier. This was the only known incident, and the family conflicts had been minor prior to it. Tiana complained that her mother blamed her over and over and now got angry at her for much smaller problems, a recent explosion coming when she'd forgotten to return some library books. Her mother agreed that she was still very upset because she'd never expected a child of hers to steal. After observing the mother's disappointment and the daughter's wounded sense of her mother's unfairness, the practitioner tried to understand the context of the shoplifting. She asked Tiana if she had shoplifted before, and Tiana responded indignantly that she had not. The practitioner said, "You got almost all the way to 15 before the first and only time. Usually kids begin much earlier. That makes me wonder what was going on that one time." Tiana pointed to her mother and said, "She knew I was going to go to camp in a week, and she wouldn't buy me one." Ms. Jamison was completely taken aback, and said that Tiana had not asked her for a bathing suit. Tiana said, "Yes, I did, a few weeks before, and you were too busy to pay attention, like you always are, so I had to get it myself. I wasn't going to go to that camp with that old, little girl bathing suit. Then when I got caught you didn't let me go to camp anyway." Ms. Jamison began to cry, then rallied and said, "Honey, if I didn't hear you . . ., (*to practitioner*) Lord knows, I am often really tired working two jobs . . . you should have asked me again." The practitioner said, "Tiana tried to get your attention about this, but you were very tired that day, and it seems like she gave up and went out on her own. It sounds like neither of you wanted it to turn out the way it did, but you didn't know what she needed, and she didn't want to bother you by asking again." What had been defined as a behavioral infraction was now recast as a relational issue. This ushered in a period of targeted work on how this teen and parent could communicate more clearly. It emerged later that underlying this relational issue was an insecure attachment history based on Ms. Jamison's drug addiction during Tiana's early years. Although Ms. Jamison had remained drug-free for over 10 years, her daughter's vulnerability to a perception of parental inconsistency, no doubt intensified by her young adolescent developmental status, caused her to act out. In the later part of therapy, Tiana and Ms. Jamison were helped to talk directly about this early history, with the result that their current attachment was strengthened (Diamond, 2005).

Problem Solving and Communication

As the problems are framed, treatment in family sessions can shift to concrete problem solving and improving communication. Even though one is aware that "deep" patterns of insecure attachment history and problems related to cohesion underlie family conflict, it is usually more effective to begin with present-oriented work. Relationship changes are likely to follow when parents and teens have experiences of understanding one another and working together.

Problem Solving

Problem solving focuses on specific and well-defined conflict situations, usually involving the push–pull of adolescent exploration and limit testing, and parental granting of independence and limit setting. One option, following Taffel (2005), is to use separate sessions to establish an issue to negotiate in a family session. In separate meetings with parents and adolescent, goals and format of the family session can be defined in advance and the practitioner can clarify his or her role as facilitator and mediator. The issue taken up in the first problem-solving session should be one that adolescent and parents are motivated to negotiate, but since this is the first foray into problem solving, it should not be the most *difficult* issue. Further, it must in fact be an issue the parents agree *is* negotiable. (For a structured approach to problem solving, see Barkley, Edwards, & Robin, 1997, part II, steps 10–12.)

From Communication to Relationship

Clearly, effective problem solving leads to better communication. However, it is also important to focus explicitly on changing communication patterns. From the outset, the practitioner has already tried to model good communication by striving to understand the perspectives of parents and teen. He or she has listened carefully, tried to be attuned to emotions behind words, asked for clarification and explanation, and has tried to summarize what family members have said.

The practitioner takes the role as a communications "broker" between the adolescent and parents. From his or her stance as an observing helper whose alliance with each family member supports his or her credibility, the practitioner can intervene in poor communication. It is helpful for the practitioner to state his or her belief that better communication will improve family relationships. When rote patterns of arguing or suppression of ideas dominate the family's communication patterns, the practitioner may frequently call a time out and initiate a dialogue that requires participants to shift from rolling along with scripted arguments rife with miscommunication to a focus on content, affect, and intention. For example, a practitioner observes that parents and adolescent interrupt, talk over one another, and do not seem to listen well. After listening to an argument that drags on without resolution, a practitioner can say, "I want to stop you and tell you what I'm hearing. This feels to me like a conversation that goes in circles. A big reason is that you're talking at the same time rather than listening to each other." The practitioner can summarize the argument that has just occurred and note possible points of mutual agreement. Then the practitioner can ask them to have the same discussion using some familiar strategies for improving communication, such as confining themselves to "I" rather than "You" statements, and restating the other's point before making their own.

The practitioner should pay particular attention to affects in conflictual interactions. Communication can become more functional if family members reduce the intensity of expressed affect. Intense affect raises the level of arousal in listeners, and in conflictual families intensity in one person potentiates arousal in others. As arousal increases, capacity for reflection decreases. The practitioner can point this out, summarize the conflict with neutral affect, and directly suggest that family communication will improve if they can bring down the "emotional tone" (Mackey, 2003). Essentially, the practitioner (temporarily) takes on the role of family affect regulator.

The practitioner's attunement to affects puts him or her in a position to find pathways around overt anger and hostility that often dominate in conflictual families. By attending to family members' expressions and body language, as well as to his or her own affects in response to the family, the practitioner can begin to call attention to their "underneath" feelings such as sadness, disappointment, frustration, loneliness, insecurity, and worry about rejection or loss of love. Shifting attention to these more vulnerable feelings can remind family members that they care about each other. An example of a "shift intervention" (Liddle & Schwartz, 2002) addressed to the whole family might be "While you were arguing just now, I had the sense that maybe it was because of the pain, not just anger, I could see in your eyes that there was a lot hurt and sadness in the room, because the family feels stuck in all this anger. It feels painful because you care about each other." A statement like this has the potential to focus the family away from defensive anger and toward the insecure attachments that overt anger obscures.

While such interventions have the potential to reframe communication difficulties as reflecting insecure attachments, it is necessary to approach them carefully (Moran et al., 2005). If the practitioner's shift from conflict to painful feelings about relationships is dismissed by some family members, the family is likely to retreat to an entrenched defensive position. While some therapists would consider this grist for the mill, a better option is to explore tender feelings and wishes for acceptance and love first in separate adolescent and parent sessions. This provides a better gauge of the teen's and parents' readiness to focus on relationship issues. Further, in separate sessions the practitioner can state his or her conviction that addressing such feelings will be helpful and solicit family members' buy-in. Then the practitioner and the family can explicitly make plans to focus on vulnerable feelings in upcoming whole-family sessions. In therapy with conflictual adolescents and parents, an implicit goal is to increase mutual trust. A practitioner who states his or her intentions in advance, as opposed to springing on the family a powerful and potentially threatening shift in focus, is embodying and modeling trustworthiness.

Separate Parent and Adolescent Sessions

Even when the primary goal of treatment is to improve relationships, there are many advantages, as noted above, to flexibly combining separate parent sessions with parent–adolescent sessions. These sessions can focus on direct guidance and advice on limit setting and monitoring, helping parents think about their child's needs and behavior from a developmental perspective, and how to communicate clearly.

When parents disagree about parenting style and practices, the adolescent is exposed to differing, and therefore inconsistent, expectations and discipline. Sometimes parenting disagreements reflect more pervasive marital conflicts. At other times, they may reflect polarized reactions to the adolescent developmental transition, with one or both parents struggling with anxiety about how to parent an adolescent. For many parents, anxiety may be stimulated by memories of their own adolescent difficulties.

Work on resolving parenting conflicts is an important focus of parent sessions. The major goals of this work should be to limit the conflict parents act out with the adolescent in the middle, to control tendencies to undercut one another, and to reduce competition to be the "better" parent. If parents can set limits on their own conflicts, the adolescent will not have to focus so much on attending to, or distancing him- or herself from, parental struggles over him or her and will be freer to pursue adolescent tasks.

Parents' differences may be based on different assumptions about attachment. Consequently, it is important to take a history of the attachment and parenting styles each parent grew up with. Based on this information, the practitioner can help parents articulate their working models of parenting. When these assumptions are put into words, parents can view their differences more objectively.

Some parents face a personal developmental crisis as they become aware that their adolescent needs them less. Parents with histories of ambivalent attachment become anxious as their adolescent becomes involved with peers and the pursuit of autonomy. Such parents will benefit from the practitioner's empathizing with and defining the reasons for their anxiety, providing developmental information that normalizes adolescent autonomy seeking and reframes the current task of parenting as providing a secure base for exploration, and, often, helps the parent reflect on his or her hopes for the next stage of his or her life. The parent's impending loss must be acknowledged, but particular emphasis should be put on helping him or her reframe the role of parenting in terms of supporting his or her adolescent's development.

Case Study: Treatment of an Adolescent Coping with Family Disruption

Alex Cernak was referred by his mother, with his father's assent, at age 16½. He was entering his junior year of high school. His grades had been poor during his first 2 years of high school, in contrast to his history of having been a very good student in elementary school. His mother viewed him as unhappy and possibly depressed, and felt he had not recovered from his parents' divorce 2 years earlier. Alex was spending alternating weeks at his mother's and father's houses, and his mother said that this was difficult for him. For example, he sometimes left homework assignments at her house, and then did not have them when he was at his dad's. She recognized that she was less available to Alex now, because she was feeling a new sense of freedom herself.

In a separate interview, Alex's father expressed concerns about his grades and tendency to procrastinate. Mr. Cernak said that he had recently told Alex that if his grades did not rise in the first quarter of his junior year, he would take away his music lessons. Alex's father did not think he was depressed, but said, "I'm not sure what he's feeling a lot of the time. He's quieter than he used to be." Regarding the divorce, which was initiated by Alex's mother, Mr. Cernak said, "I realize it's been rough for him. He was surprised as I was when she said it was over. If that's what she wanted, OK, but I think she should have waited until Alex was off to college."

Alex's two older siblings, Mark, age 22, and Chad, age 20, had not lived at home since the parents' divorce. Mark was seen by both parents as well adjusted and high achieving. He was beginning a graduate school program in a field related to Mr. Cernak's. Chad had begun college, but had dropped out and now is a keyboard player in a rock band. Chad and Mr. Cernak had fought often during Chad's adolescent years, and Alex had observed many of these arguments. At issue were Chad's disinterest in school and mediocre academic performance, his devotion to music, and physical expressions of "alternative" identity that now included multiple tattoos and body piercings. The parents' marital conflicts had coincided with and been exacerbated by the father's anger with Chad, whose side Ms. Cernak frequently took. Chad's and Mr. Cernak's relationship remained tenuous.

Prior to the parents' divorce Alex had been a good student who was not seen as having behavior problems. According to his mother, he had been a "wonderful kid," who had been "well loved" by both his father and mother. Like his older brother, he had developed a strong interest in music and had become a talented saxophonist. At the time of the parents' separation, which also coincided with his brother's leaving for college, Alex was troubled by the divorce and became depressed. When he entered high school, his grades fell and he seemed apathetic about school, with one exception— he was accepted to the school's prestigious popular music band.

In the first few individual sessions Alex spoke very articulately about the feeling of having the rug pulled out from under him. His parents had not fought a lot, but he realized they had deep differences and hadn't been close in their relationship for a long time. But the divorce took him by surprise. He talked about how difficult it was to be in a joint custody arrangement spending alternate weeks at each parent's house. He had to adjust to new relationships with both parents and had been really struck by the differences between them that were not so obvious before, now seeing his father as demanding and strict, and his mother as more laid back and nurturant. When the parents were together, his mother had served as a buffer against the father's strictness. At the same time, his mom made it clear that during the weeks he was at his dad's, she expected him to make his dad's house his home base and not to drop in unexpectedly at her house. Alex spoke about how disorganized he felt going back and forth between houses and, more profoundly, between different parental styles and values. He also missed not having any siblings at home.

QUESTIONS FOR THE REFLECTIVE PRACTITIONER

1. What risk factors does Alex have?
2. What protective factors does Alex have?
3. As a family practitioner, how do you improve Alex's relationship with his mother?
4. As a family practitioner, how do you improve Alex's relationship with his father?
5. What issues would you address in individual sessions with Alex?
6. What issues would you address in family sessions?

Chapter Summary

In this chapter the reader was presented with family contexts and dynamics that can promote or hinder growth and development. The complicated nature of the parent–adolescent relationship was discussed through attachment theory, family systems theory, and parenting styles. In the next chapter, we discuss the important environment of the school.

CHAPTER 6

The School Environment

Chapter Overview

This chapter explores the unique characteristics of the school microsystem and its influence on the adolescent. Particularly, we present the protective and risk factors in the school microsystem, and the effect of bullying on youth academic performance and emotional health. Additionally, ADHD and interventions that are appropriate in the school setting are discussed. Also discussed are issues relating to experiencing trauma in the school. Throughout the chapter, we provide suggestions for clinical interventions for individuals working with adolescents in a school context. A case study is presented and questions for discussion about that case are offered. We begin here with a brief case to introduce some of the adolescent concerns the reader will meet in this chapter.

CASE EXAMPLE:
Who Are the Youth Represented in This Chapter?

The following case example represents some of the concerns related to adolescents and the school environment. Considering the implications for this case within the context of the risk factors, theory, assessment, and intervention strategies presented in the following pages will prepare you to assess and suggest interventions for the more developed case study at the end of the chapter.

Janine is 15 years old, bi-racial, and attends a large public high school with some of the same peers she has known since middle school. Her academic abilities in middle school were considered above average. She was active in sports in middle school and viewed as one of the best basketball players on the girl's team. However, once she entered high school all of that changed. Janine's friends from middle school stopped wanting to spend time with her and refused to sit with her at lunch. Feeling left out, Janine tried to find a way to make new friends, but most of the girls told her she was too old for being a tomboy and that none of the boys would like such a smart girl. Her parents were shocked when the first report card came out and Janine had all C grades. They were more shocked when the basketball coach called them because Janine showed up for practice and appeared to be high. They wondered why there had been no calls from the school before now.

The School Microsystem and the Adolescent

The school microsystem is a venue that is dynamic and continually changing. Because youth spend at least 6 hours a day at the school, and much longer if involved in clubs or sports, it is a focal point in their lives. It is the venue where they meet people of their own age and interests, where they may be admired, despised, emulated, or shunned by their peers. It is also the place where they may gain notoriety for their academic ability, their athletic or artistic prowess, their ability to make and keep friends, or for less positive behaviors but just as noteworthy: their ability to be disruptive or angry, their ability to use drugs and alcohol, and their sexual escapades.

For some youth, the school can be a refuge from the problems that they are facing outside of school. They might be able to forget about the fight between their parents the night before, or their brother's drug use, or their younger sister's health issues while they are at school. Because of the level of activity and energy the school engenders, some youth can frequently live in the present and push nonschool issues aside. However, other students may not be able to disengage from their outside lives.

Some students may feel that the school is a place of humiliation, frustration, or isolation. School is not a happy place for them. They hate the place that makes them feel demeaned, stupid, different, or disliked because of bullying. Many youth vacillate between feelings of warmth toward their alma mater to feelings of distrust or contempt. So what can help youth in the school microsystem feel supported? The short answer is to increase the protective factors that exist in the school microsystem.

Protective Factors Associated with Healthy Adolescent Outcomes in the School Context

Sense of Belonging

A sense of belonging reduces feelings of disengagement and alienation (Bogenschneider, 1998; Garcia-Coll et al., 1996; Maughan, 1992; Roth & Brooks-Gunn, 2000; Wang et al., 1994). It is the proverbial "Cheers" effect.

People want to go where people know their name and feel a connection to them. Students who feel that they are connected to their teachers, class-mates, school, instructional programs, and school functions are better equipped to handle adverse circumstances (McMillan & Reed, 1994; Wang et al.). If the student feels he or she belongs, then he or she feels a desire and a commitment to be in school during the good times or the bad times. If youth feel that it matters whether they go to school or not, they will make a commitment to be in school. Therefore, creating this sense of belonging in youth for school goes a long way to reduce truancy and absenteeism. A strategy that has been successful is for administration, teaching staff, and support staff to know the students' names (not just those of the really, really good or really bad kids), and to say hello to everyone on a daily basis as they arrive at school or throughout the day. Additionally, if a student was absent it helps if school personnel inquire about him or her, to let the youth know that he or she was missed when he or she was not there. This is very valuable for youth because it ties into their cognitive understandings of feeling unique and also helps them establish an identity that is authentic, an identity of being a student at his or her school.

Size of School

Schools that are smaller have a greater need for all to participate, which then reinforces the sense of belonging to the school (Gump, 1981). If the school is smaller, the individual's absence is sorely felt. Also, it means that all members are needed to be part of a sports team, music event, club, or play. Schools that are very large have only a small percentage of the students involved in activities and have to be very selective about who is chosen. Small schools need everyone to function and therefore allow all to join.

Being Involved in a School Activity or Club

Involvement in a school activity, sport team, musical activity, or club helps the youth feel connected to a particular group of students. They share a common purpose and common goals and thereby create their own micro-system for growth. This microsystem is then a reference group for the other activities in their life and provides a circle of friends with common interests. Activities also give the youth an opportunity to "shine" in a particular venue. This is especially important when he or she does not receive positive notoriety in other spheres of his or her life.

Activities also help the youth establish an identity of who he or she is in the school microsystem. Since identity development is so very important for youth, it gives them the parameters of an emerging identity. For example, if a female youth is a member of a swim team, she has a ready group of friends who also enjoy swimming, receive positive encouragement for their swimming, and share similar beliefs: namely, that practice is important, that one needs to give maximum effort to improve, eat well and be healthy for continued success, and that it is important to support each other on the team. She has "bought into" these basic beliefs. Who she is, what she does, and where she spends her time are influenced by this. Certainly, her identity is more than just as a swimmer, but this identity helps to set the groundwork of who she is and who she will become.

Therefore, it is important for practitioners to support the youth they are seeing in counseling to join activities or clubs. Encourage them to take the "plunge" to try out for a sport or a musical, or show up at a club meeting. It may be quite anxiety producing for them at first since they are entering into a new microsystem where they may not know very many people. But it is a very important venue for social and emotional support and a great opportunity for identity development.

Teaching Techniques That Foster Group Processes

It has been found that how youth are taught effects their functioning. Teaching techniques that facilitate group cohesion impact resilience in youth (Hawkins, Catalano, & Miller, 1992; Novick, 1998). As it is important to create a group in school activities, it is also important to create a group in learning activities. O'Donnell, Hawkins, Catalano, Abbott, and Day (1995) found that children who were at high risk for academic failure, who were taught learning methods in a cooperative team, were significantly more academically successful than children who had not been taught in this manner. Therefore, belonging to a smaller group helped them succeed academically where they were being unsuccessful on their own. Interestingly, a cooperative learning style was most significant for at-risk girls.

Feelings of Accomplishment and Praise

Rutter's (1987) research of institutionally reared girls found that "the experience of pleasure, success, and accomplishment at school had helped the girls to acquire a sense of their own worth and of their ability to control what happened to them" (p. 324). Furthermore, Rutter's earlier work (1981) found that the use of rewards, praise, and appreciation were associated with better pupil outcomes. It is a self-fulfilling prophecy that if they believe they are bright and capable, they will act and behave in bright and capable ways. If youth believe that they can be successful, they will more likely be successful. This is the essence of self-efficacy, which we have spoken of earlier.

O'Donnell and colleagues (1995) similarly found that opportunities for rewards was an important factor contributing to at-risk girls staying in school. If they believe they are "getting something out of their being in school" they will stay the course and persevere, even when school is difficult or there are other issues that interfere with academic life. Therefore, incentives for good attendance do work, if they need an incentive.

The sense of accomplishment at school has positive effects on the other microsystems that the youth inhabits. Maughan (1992) found that a sense of accomplishment at school compensated for the lack of opportunities for positive growth in their home environment. Therefore, difficulties at home were not so keenly felt if they were being successful in the school environment. Practitioners who are aware of difficulties in the student's home must help the youth get the support he or she needs to be successful at school.

Furthermore, it is noteworthy to realize that positive experiences at school have residual effects throughout life. Werner and Smith (2001) found that positive attitudes about school at age 18 predicted satisfaction with interpersonal relationships at age 40. Nearly two decades later, those who experienced positive experiences at school were able to transfer those experiences to other spheres of their life.

When practitioners who work with youth show a sincere interest in his or her studies, and positively encourage his or her academic progress, there is a beneficial outcome, even when the practitioner is not affiliated with a school. Asking how the youth did on a test or papers and praising his or her accomplishment or progress helps the youth stay the course and feel that he or she is important and special.

Teaching with an Explanatory Style

Seligman (1995) found that youths' success or failure at school was "enormously influenced" by the explanatory style that teachers and coaches used with children at school even at an early grade level. Therefore, how lessons are framed makes a huge difference for students on whether they will be successful or not. Those students who were criticized for insufficient effort were less adversely influenced than those who were criticized for poor ability. Seligman hypothesized that effort is a temporary issue and can be easily remedied; however, ability is a more permanent attribute and therefore more detrimental to the individual if this criticism continues over time.

Schools with High Expectations for Their Students

Attending effective schools increased resilience (Emery & Forehand, 1996; Garbarino, Dubrow, Kostelny, & Pardo, 1992; Garmezy, 1993; Hawkins et al., 1992; Jessor et al., 1995; Masten & Coatsworth, 1998; Maughan, 1992; Novick, 1998; Sandefur, 1998; Wang et al., 1994). Howard, Dryden, and Johnson (1999) and Maughan found that schools that encouraged caring relationships, high expectations, and opportunities for participation had students who succeeded. If school personnel believe that their students can achieve, overcome obstacles, and surpass their expectations, their students will do exactly that.

School as an Oasis

For some resilient students, the school became a home away from home (Wang et al., 1994). If positive growth and development was not occurring in the microsystem of the home, the student could flourish at the school. Some resilient students have seen the school as an oasis or a refuge (Wang et al.). Therefore, if the home microsystem is difficult, the school mirosystem may be a venue where the youth can blossom.

Physical Environment of the School

A positive atmosphere for growth is not merely limited to the ambiance of the school. The actual physical environment of the school is also associated with improved student outcomes (Garmezy, 1993; Wang et al., 1994). A school that is physically attractive and well cared for improved students' behaviors and attainment. School practitioners can create or support opportunities for beautifying the school through cleanup days, painting, mural painting, or creating school gardens. This also increases pride in the school and connection to the school for the students.

School Mentor

Garmezy (1985, 1993) believes that the presence of an external support person is fundamental to resilient outcomes. This individual may act as a parent substitute for the adolescent. Gottlieb and Sylvestre (1994) discuss that mentors through acceptance, sustained interaction, and a willingness to ease authority and age disparities create strong, healthy relationships between adolescents and adults. Luthar and colleagues (2000), in their review of resilience research, discuss the recurring theme of the importance of "connections with competent, pro-social adults in the wider community" (p. 545). A supportive teacher or school social worker can play a major role in reducing stress (Larson, 2000; McLoyd, 1998; McMillan & Reed, 1994; Nettles & Pleck, 1996; Roth & Brooks-Gunn, 2000; Wang et al., 1994; Werner & Smith, 2001). The school mentor can encourage the youth to persevere.

Teachers Who Take a Particular Interest

Howard and colleagues (1999) reported that the most frequently encountered individual outside of the family system who had a positive effect on a resilient child were teachers who took a personal interest in the child. These teachers were able to transcend their role as an academic and became a positive model for personal identification. Rutter (1981), Wang and colleagues (1994), and McMillan and Reed (1994) found that the models of behavior their teachers exhibited influenced students far beyond the years in school. Students felt that someone was on their side and gave them confidence to continue in school, many years after the actual school year when they met their special teacher. A student who is noticed for something special that he or she said or did by a teacher had a positive impact on how the youth felt about him- or herself and who he or she understands he or she is.

With each of these protective factors the youth receives a sense of individual identity and value, which is paramount for healthy development. It is important for school practitioners to remind teachers and school administrators about the pivotal role that they play in the lives of youth. Frequently they are so overwhelmed with teaching content that they forget how the little kindnesses that they can confer to students make a huge difference in the students' lives.

The school social worker or school-based practitioner holds a very important role of helping the teachers and administrators understand the emotional and social components of the students in their classes and school. The school social worker can act as a bridge between these groups. Frequently, the school social worker is able to uniquely contribute to the school microsystem by his or her knowledge of the workings of the school and the particular needs of his or her students.

Clinical Interventions for Individuals Working with Adolescents in a School Context

The school social worker is often responsible for working with students who are experiencing social or emotional issues that are affecting their academic performance. The school-based practitioner is often involved in a myriad of activities at the school. These may include special education evaluations, running small groups, classroom groups, or organizing schoolwide programs.

Special Education Evaluations

Before the special education process is initiated, the school practitioner may have worked with the student for some time and may have insight into the student's behavior. Frequently the school social worker is responsible for completing a portion of the special education evaluations. Most often, the school practitioner is required to write the developmental history of the student being evaluated, including a review of the developmental milestones of the student's life. A family history given by the parent and the youth is often included. Additionally, classroom observations, home visits, and contacts with other agencies, organizations, or health professionals that may have worked with the youth are often included. Of course, any collateral conversations about the student need parental permission.

The *individualized educational plan* (IEP) is the formal meeting between the parents, youth, and school professionals who report about the outcomes of the special education evaluation. Each member of the school team—the school social worker, school psychologist, classroom teachers, and reading and/or math specialists—give their reports. Often, the school social worker serves in the invaluable role of helping the family understand the results and advocating for the youth. Frequently, the IEP can be very intimidating for parents and youth when so many school professionals come together. The school social worker can be a great support to the family and help interpret the reports in "real" language. Sometimes, the school reports are peppered with school acronyms and jargon that are unintelligible to the outsider. Once the reports are given the parents need to decide whether they agree with the recommendations of the IEP, which may be to certify the student for special education services or decline services.

Small Groups

The school practitioner may see general education and special education students in small groups. Small groups may have a special purpose such as grief/loss, anger management, ADHD, positive self-image, positive body image, understanding feelings, or may be just a weekly group to offer support. The groups may be short term or ongoing. Students in small groups may play therapeutic board games, role play difficult situations so that they gain a way of using words to cope with a particular situation, do art therapy, be involved in active outside activities, or initiate a behavior modification program.

Classroom Groups

The school social worker or counselor may run classroom groups that are psychoeducational and focused on supporting positive peer relations, reducing risk behaviors, or understanding one's emotions. Frequently these groups are co-led by the school practitioner and the classroom teacher.

School-Wide Programming

Schoolwide groups may be organized by the school social worker or counselor to change the climate of the school. Such programs include peer mediation, violence reduction, gay–straight alliance, or bullying programs. These programs often tackle large issues that are affecting the school environment or morale. Often the school social worker, with the help of the administration and the support of the teaching staff, is instrumental in creating these large-scale programs.

Bullying within the School Microsystem

Since social interaction is such an important component to healthy youth development, being demeaned, humiliated, or ostracized by one's peers decreases one's sense of self and undermines one's ability to have friendships at school. Having been bullied as a child impacts the self-esteem of the adolescent, which may affect social interactions and optimal functioning in adults (Cleary, 2000; Duncan, 1999; Laser, 2006; Olweus, 2001a, 2001b). Bullying harassment by peers has a continuing affect on the victim. Duncan reports that 46% of young adults, who were bullied as children, still think about having been bullied. In addition, Laser and Olweus found that several years after the bullying incidents, adolescents who had been bullied in late elementary school were still being affected by higher levels of physical and mental distress than their nonbullied peers.

A 2001 study by the *Journal of the American Medical Association* (JAMA) of nearly 16,000 students found that 16.9% of the respondents had been bullied (Nansel et al., 2001). Likewise, the National Center for Education Statistics polled 6,500 sixth- through twelfth-grade students. It was found that 56% of the students reported that bullying behavior happened in their school, 42% had witnessed bullying, 18% worried about being bullied, and 8% had been bullied (Nolin, Davies, & Chandler, 1996). Similarly, the school personnel were also cognizant of violence perpetrated in the school environment. Twenty-five percent of public school teachers rated physical conflict between students to be a serious to a moderately serious problem in their schools (Nolin & Davies).

Gender Differences in Bullying Victimization

The gender of victims of bullying has also been examined in a number of studies. Duncan (1999) found that American children of both genders were nearly equal in becoming victims, unlike European and Asian children who were predominately male victims (Morita, Soeda, Soeda, & Taki, 1998; Olweus, 1993; Smith, 1997).

Borg (1998) investigated the emotional reaction of being bullied for boys and girls and found that sixth-grade boys who were bullied most often felt vengeful after the victimization. Girls of the same age who had been bullied most frequently had feelings of self-pity. Following the bullying event, sixth-grade girls and younger students of both genders were more likely to confide in their parents regarding the event. Similarly, girls were more likely to share their feelings with their friends than were boys. The lack of reaching out to others after the bullying event puts boys at greater risk for becoming further isolated and for harboring residual feelings of vengeance.

The Developmental Context of Bullying

The late elementary and early middle school years are the pinnacle of bullying behavior (Duncan, 1999; Oliver, Hoover, & Hazler, 1994; Olweus, 2001b; Rigby, Cox, & Black, 1997). The middle school years are also the developmental period where peer influences are most strongly felt and peer conformity is most valued (Brown, Clasen, & Eicher, 1986; Brown, Eicher, & Petrie, 1986). Therefore, this combination of desiring group affiliation and conformity to group norms and being singled out for victimization is very devastating for the developing youth. In early adolescence, youth do not yet have a strong sense of identity and therefore the victimization is particularly hurtful since they are not fully certain of who they are and who they are not.

The Impact of Bullying Victimization on Adolescents

Olweus (2001a) studied the mental and physical health implications of being bullied. He found that children bullied in late elementary school were still being affected by higher levels of physical and mental distress in comparison to their nonbullied peers several years later. The enduring effects of bullying victimization reached far beyond the middle school years. Laser (2006) found that schoolwork was three times more likely to be poor in female youth who had been bullied. Females who had been bullied were also twice as likely to suffer from sleep problems, feel sad or depressed, or admit that they lie or cheat on a regular basis than their nonbullied peers. Males who had been bullied were twice as likely to have trouble concentrating and three times more likely to be sad or depressed than their nonbullied peers. For both genders, those who had been bullied were twice as likely to feel unsafe at school, feel that they were not being graded fairly at school, and that the discipline was not fair at school than their nonbullied peers (Laser). The differences associated with being bullied undermined the youth's emotional stability, academic performance at school, feelings of safety at school, and acceptance at school.

In extreme cases, negative feelings due to bullying victimization can manifest itself in suicidal or aggressive behavior. Cleary (2000) investigated the correlation between bullying victimization and suicidal or aggressive behavior. His research focused solely on high school students in the New York City public schools. He found that violent or suicidal behavior occurred 1.4 to 2.6 times more frequently among students who had been victimized by bullying than in students who had not been bullied (Cleary). Similar findings by Olweus (2001a) acknowledged that there was a relationship between bullying behavior and suicidal ideation.

Factors Related to Bullying Victimization in the School Microsystem

Youth who become the victims of bullies are classified into two distinct groups: provocative victims and passive victims (Olweus, 1993, 2001a, 2001b). The provocative victims are often described as needling and inciting the bully into action. The provocative victims are often blamed for the actions that beset them. Students and teachers alike often feel that these provocative victims "deserved the rough treatment that they got" (Olweus, 2001a, p. 12). Interestingly, it was found that sometimes an entire class colluded or conspired against these provocative victims. Perhaps there were only a few students who actively bullied the victim, but the other students either by their passivity, or their tacit approval, allowed the victimization to occur (Olweus, 2001a).

Oliver and colleagues (1994) investigated student beliefs regarding bullying and found that the majority of their sample believed that bullying victims played a role in their own victimization. The respondents also believed that being bullied made the victim stronger and could be instructive for the victim. In that, by being bullied they would learn that their behavior was inappropriate and needed to be changed. These findings suggest that many students may not realize the harm that is done to these bullied individuals.

Although this sort of victim blaming has been implicated as part of the trivialization of bullying incidents, it is estimated that provocative victims make up only 10 to 20% of the total number of bullied victims (Olweus, 2001b). The overwhelming majority of bullied children are passive victims who have done nothing to call attention to themselves, other than simply coexisting in the same environment where the bully resides.

Frequently, the youth who is being bullied is different than his or her peers in appearance: he or she may wear clothes that are not in fashion, or have hair that is not well cut or kept. He or she may be gay or transgender. The youth may have emotional issues that makes him or her prone to cry or quick to anger. He or she may not be as financially well off as his or her peers. Therefore, perceptions that these bullied youth are somehow responsible for their own fate are untrue and further prejudice the already injured youth. Such perceptions also undermine the ability of school personnel to stop the occurrence of bullying as valuable time is needlessly spent on investigating the rationale for why these youth were bullied instead of simply eradicating the bullying behavior (Franson, 2000).

Bullyproofing in the School Microsystem

Since we are aware of the long-term repercussions for bullying behavior, how can we stop bullying from occurring in schools? Olweus (2001a, 2001b) has found a number of particular characteristics of successful bullying programs that make bullying behaviors desist.

Inclusion

Bullying behavior negatively changes the environment of the school for everyone: those who are being bullied, those who are aware of the bullying behavior and not speaking up, and those who are the bullies. Including everyone in the trainings and requiring all to be responsible to call out bullying behavior supports those being bullied, gives power to those who have been afraid to say something before, and calls attention to the bullies that their behavior is unacceptable. It also means that everyone from the lunch lady to the principal needs to be trained and aware of the program and how to report bullying behavior.

Ongoing and Continuous Programs

Programs need to be ongoing and continuous. This means programs designed to teach bullying behavior for only a week or a month do not work. The students, teachers, and parents need to be reminded about bullying behavior and how to stop it, so that it becomes second nature.

Teacher and Parent Accountability

Both teachers and parents need to be accountable for enforcing a moratorium on bullying behaviors. Teachers can no longer pretend that they did not see or hear the bullying behavior and sit idly on the sidelines. Neither can teachers criticize or intimidate students allowing others to copy their behavior. This also means that parents who teach their children that bullying is OK or a normal rite of passage need to be educated, as well. Parents who allow their youth to solve problems through violence need to be made aware that this is against school policy and will create school problems for their child.

Student Accountability

Regardless of whether the bully is a star athlete or the diva in the school play, he or she will receive the same punishment for bullying behavior. There are not special rules for privileged students. This social hierarchy unfortunately operates in many high schools and is often part of the problem. Once the hierarchy is dismantled there can be greater reduction of bullying behaviors.

Zero Tolerance of Bullies

There is zero tolerance for bullying behaviors. This means that students who previously believed they were allowed to taunt others because they exhibited unusual behavior are no longer given an opportunity to explain away their behavior. If they bully, they will receive the punishment the school has created for this behavior. This punishment may include after-school study hall time, restitution to the school in the form of service, Saturday cleanup help, and so forth.

Swift, Consistent Discipline for Bullying

Principals and teachers cannot push off decisions about discipline to the next week or even the next day. The follow-through needs to be swift for bullying behavior so that the two events—the bullying and the punishment—are remembered together.

Attention-Deficit/Hyperactivity Disorder

ADHD is probably the most discussed health concern in the school microsystem. Practitioners working in the schools must have a good working knowledge of ADHD.

What Is ADHD?

ADHD behaviors are seen as problems with attention span, problems with impulsivity, problems with excitability, problems with hyperactivity, problems with organization, problems with poor judgment, problems with following directions, and problems with making and keeping friends. Inside the brain there are biochemical abnormalities in the neurotransmitters that actually slow down processing (Carver, 2009). This is why giving stimulant medication actually improves functioning. This, however, does not mean that the intelligence of the ADHD youth is compromised or that the brain is somehow unhealthy. Often, there is a genetic component to ADHD. When practitioners construct a genogram this helps the family understand this genetic component and helps them to discuss how other family members dealt (or did not deal very well) with ADHD in the past. They may not have been diagnosed, but the family probably remembers how Uncle Jimmy had problems in school or Grandpa had boundless energy.

Prevalence of ADHD

ADHD has a prevalence rate of 3–5% in the United States (Parker, 1992). However, ADHD is being seen in community samples up to a rate of 18% (Centers for Disease Control [CDC], 2005). This disparity points to difficulties in diagnosing ADHD and misdiagnosing ADHD. If other issues such as child abuse, inconsistent parenting, child neglect, PTSD, anxiety disorder, or perinatal drug exposure have not been ruled out, the youth may be receiving a diagnosis that does not address his or her problems and perhaps is receiving medication that will not affect his or her symptoms. Because ADHD is a biological condition, medication is often helpful when ADHD has been properly diagnosed.

Additionally, 83% of children with ADHD become adolescents with ADHD and 70% of children with ADHD are adults with ADHD (Barkley, 1990). This means that the majority of youth with ADHD experience this as a lifelong issue.

Interventions for Youth with ADHD and Their Families

The majority of problem behaviors come from the inability to do a task and *not* from purposeful noncompliance. However, others may interpret the youth's behaviors differently. Frequently, parents or teachers believe that the youth is purposeful in his or her inability to complete a task and are frustrated with the youth. This misconception needs to be addressed by the practitioner. There are two groups that the practitioner needs to work with: parents of youth with ADHD, and youth with ADHD. Both groups, youth and parents, need to understand that ADHD behaviors can be managed but not cured. There will be days that the youth will be able to follow directions better and stay on task and other days that he or she will be less successful. The most effective manner of working with both groups should be a mixture of education about ADHD and social support.

Particularly for Parents

It is important for the practitioner to explain to parents that consistency is extremely important. Consistency should be attempted in routines, in expectations, and in household rules. Parents should practice how to give instructions as simply and clearly as possible. The most important house rules should be explained, written down, and placed in a prominent location in the home (e.g., on the refrigerator). Parents should praise the youth's accomplishments (even the small ones). This may seem awkward at first, especially if in the past the parent has spent a lot of time yelling at the youth for his or her transgressions (which sadly is often the case), but the youth will be very pleased when the parent says something nice to him or her and realizes his or her progress. Once the parent learns to see the behaviors as related to ADHD and not ornery adolescent behavior, the parent and youth can move forward in their relationship.

Frequently, ADHD youth misplace their possessions on a regular basis, which can be very difficult and frustrating for parents who must continually pay for lost items. The parent can help the youth become better organized with homework and possessions. The parent should be instructed by the practitioner to work with the youth to organize his or her room, backpack, and desk. Parents should be encouraged to use a family calendar to plan upcoming events and have the calendar placed in an area of the house that is highly visible. The practitioner should also help the parent reduce the stimulation at home while the youth is doing homework.

Particularly for Youth

The practitioner should encourage the youth to write notes to self, or text notes to self, to remind him or her of things that need to be done, deadlines, and appointments. The practitioner should encourage youth to see their own successes, and the progress that they are making. This promotes the development of healthy self-esteem in these youth.

The practitioner in small groups of ADHD students can help them to reinforce learning positive social skills by role playing "What would you do" scenarios. This can help youth explain and understand social situations and ethical dilemmas. Frequently, ADHD youth have trouble making or keeping friends because they have not clued into many of the nonverbal or nonovert behaviors of social interactions, or students stay away from the ADHD youth due to their frequent misbehavior. Therefore, ADHD youth need to learn how to make and keep friends. The practitioner can lead discussions about behaviors that promote or deter friendships. Additionally, the practitioner can give examples of behaviors that can be modeled to support prosocial behavior in the small ADHD group.

The ADHD small group can actually act as a method of supporting friendships and alliances between ADHD youth. It can also promote connections to other youth with ADHD as a support network outside of the group. The practitioner can encourage group members to praise accomplishments of fellow group members, which also supports group cohesion and positive regard for each other.

Additionally, it can be extremely effective to have ADHD youth create note cards to be put in their assignment notebooks and their wallets that promote slowing down to think. An example of this would be 1 = Think about situation, 2 = Think about what would happen if . . . , and 3 = Active decision. It is important for the practitioner to stress that in the end the choice is theirs to make. The youth can either make a good choice and positive outcomes will be created, or a negative choice for which he or she will be the recipient of negative consequences.

Even if the youth is taking stimulant medication, this is not a cure for ADHD. The youth needs to learn how to slow down and think about the decision that needs to be made. The medication will give him or her the time to think. However, he or she still needs to do the thinking about an appropriate solution.

Finally, the practitioner can help promote a positive energy outlet for ADHD youth such as involvement with a school sports team or individual sports such as running or biking. Since ADHD youth often have boundless energy, it is always a good idea for them to have a physical activity that can provide an energy release and some camaraderie.

Trauma in the School

Unfortunately, schools have been the location of frequent violence. This violence can occur between students, between students and staff, between parents and staff, or brought in from outside of the school through an outside individual or through technology in the case of texting or online communications (MySpace, Facebook, YouTube, or Twitter). Additionally, it is not uncommon for students during the adolescent years to die in an accident, overdose, or by suicide. Similarly, a beloved staff member may die an untimely death. Due to the many and diverse possibilities for experiencing trauma at school, a school crisis counseling plan needs to be established prior to any incident.

Crisis Counseling

The first components to creating a working plan is to designate who will be involved in offering counseling services, when counseling services will begin, for what duration, and where the services will be located. If the trauma has closed the school, the school practitioner will have to find an off-campus location in which to hold counseling sessions. If many have been affected by the trauma, the school practitioner should have community practitioners who can offer their services as well. Planning for crisis counseling should be organized in advance as part of any school preparedness plan. Additionally, helping families access support services may also be a responsibility of the school practitioner.

Debriefing Groups

Debriefing groups are effective with adolescents and with staff. These groups can be organized by proximity to the trauma for the individual or by the connection of the individual to the bereaved. Debriefing groups can help students and staff cope with the loss of the individual(s) they are grieving and/or help students and staff grieve the loss of feeling safe in their school and community. Students and staff should attend separate groups. Sometimes, students will connect deeply to a student who died, even if they had no particular relationship to the deceased student. The practitioner should assess students' and staff's feelings of suicidality (see Chapter 12) in both those who knew the student or staff well and do not believe that they can live without the deceased student or staff, and in those who did not know the student or staff well but feel a keen connection to the deceased student or staff. These debriefing groups may need to be ongoing throughout the school year. The anniversary of the trauma may require additional supportive services for students and staff.

Case Study

Ivan is a 15-year-old Russian immigrant freshman at a suburban high school. The school has over 800 freshmen. Ivan has had a difficult transition from middle school to high school. He rarely sees kids he knows at high school. His middle school was one of the five schools that filtered into the high school. He has never had a lot of friends, but he feels more isolated at high school. At his middle school, people knew who he was, though sometimes it was for the wrong reasons. Sometimes Ivan had trouble following the school rules. He has also had problems sitting in his seat. He sometimes daydreamed in class. When he was caught daydreaming by the teacher he always had a funny comment, which would make the entire class laugh. However, the laughter was often accompanied by a visit to the principal's office.

Ivan excelled at sports. He was one of the fastest runners at his middle school. However, because of his frequent visits to the principal's office, he often was in after-school detention and not at track practice. Since he missed so many practices, he was not allowed to compete in track meets. He is considering trying out for high school track this spring. However, the competition is fierce.

Ivan does very well on tests but often loses a lot of points in class because he frequently forgets his homework. Therefore, his grades are mixed; in classes where he mainly takes tests he does better. His penmanship is atrocious; often the teachers have trouble deciphering his writing. He is quite bright, but often seems very scattered. He is very gifted at seeing multiple vantage points.

Ivan has an older sister who has been a model student. She has been on the honor role throughout high school. His parents often compare his lackluster performance to hers. She just found out that she would be attending a prestigious university in the fall. Both his mother and father are very proud of her. Ivan is tired of always being told that he is inferior to his sister.

Ivan's mom was fed up with receiving the calls from the principal last year. She has threatened to send him to boarding school if he does not "shape up" in high school. She has taken away his Wii and his iPod to punish his "being smart to the teacher." However, that didn't really seem to change his behavior. Regardless of what is being taken away, it does not keep Ivan from blurting out in class. Ivan is frustrated with himself and he does not know how to curtail his behavior.

QUESTIONS FOR THE REFLECTIVE PRACTITIONER

1. What risk factors does Ivan have?
2. What protective factors does Ivan have?
3. If you were a school social worker, how would you begin working with Ivan?
4. How could you help Ivan to perform better in school?
5. How could you work with Ivan's teacher's to improve his school success?
6. How could you work with Ivan's family to improve better functioning?

Chapter Summary

This chapter presented the ups and downs of school life for the adolescent. The protective and risk factors across the ecological levels that influence a teen's challenges or successes in school were discussed. School-specific concerns such as ADHD and bullying were addressed. Interventions aimed at individual adolescents, such as treatment for ADHD, response to trauma, as well as at the school structure itself (bullyproofing) were also presented. A case study at the end of the chapter challenged the reader to apply the protective and risk factors in an assessment and to consider which of the suggested interventions would be most useful for a specific adolescent and his family. In the next chapter, we discuss the neighborhood environment.

CHAPTER 7

The Neighborhood Environment

Chapter Overview

We present a clinical orientation to the role of neighborhood in adolescents' lives. We define three major factors—neighborhood social cohesion, neighborhood collective socialization, and neighborhood disorganization—and present questions for assessing these factors in clinical practice. We discuss theory and research that demonstrate how these factors affect youth and the application of intervention modalities such as cognitive-behavioral, existential, narrative, and multisystemic approaches. The chapter ends with a case example.

CASE EXAMPLE:
Who Are the Youth Represented in This Chapter?

The following case example represents some of the concerns related to adolescents and neighborhood. Considering the implications for this case within the context of the risk factors, theory, assessment, and intervention strategies presented in the following pages will prepare you to assess and suggest interventions for the more developed case study at the end of the chapter.

James, bi-racial, age 14, whose parents recently got divorced, has moved from a small town in Vermont to New York City because his father's work is there. He did not have the choice to stay in Vermont because his mother refused to raise a teenage boy on her own. He now lives with his father in a 10th-floor apartment in Manhattan and attends high school at a magnet school with a focus on the performing and visual arts. His mother, an artist, encouraged him to make this choice. James's father comes home from work because he is ill and is surprised to find James at home in the middle of a school day. Upon further inquiry, his father finds out that

113

James has skipped 17 days of school in the last month. James tells him he is tired of being harassed and getting off at the wrong stop on the subway that he takes to and from school. He breaks down in tears, telling his father he just wants to go back home to Vermont where he doesn't have to deal with violence and people who look so down and out, like the woman who asks him for money every day.

A Clinical Orientation To Neighborhood

Clinically oriented practitioners do not commonly consider the influence of neighborhood in their work with adolescents. However, the M-E approach impels us to account for how neighborhoods influence clients. Neighborhoods influence teenagers' experiences of protection and risk and should be considered in assessing overall behavior adjustment. Neighborhoods are both physical and social environments that effect the development of personal identity, competence, cognitive, social, and motor skills, and security and trust. For example, cognitive, social, and motor skills as well as competence develop from neighborhood opportunities to explore physical environments that allow for mastery and control (David & Weinstein, 1987). Moore (1986) points out that achieving competence is limited when the physical environment of a neighborhood prohibits one's capacity for play and exploration unless the young person has opportunities for these activities in other environments.

Negative perceptions of one's neighborhood result in behaviors that isolate young people and their families from neighbors and neighborhood services that might serve as important resources (Brodsky, 1996; Furstenberg, 1993). For example, when vandalism, litter, and deteriorated or vacant homes characterize a neighborhood, residents tend to view it as having more crime and other problems such as the presence of homeless people, drug dealers, and prostitutes (Perkins, Meeks, & Taylor, 1992). Neighborhood residents who perceive their neighborhoods as dangerous places are more likely to avoid being out and about in them and tend to isolate themselves from neighbors and neighborhood services (Coulton, 1996). For example, residents in some neighborhoods only go out at certain times of the day when they know that the streets are free of gangs and drug dealers (Brodsky, 1996).

Danger and violence in a neighborhood prohibit the development of trust among neighborhood residents. Trust among neighbors and in local services make a neighborhood beneficial for parenting (Furstenberg, 1993). Neighborhood social processes, such as the development of trust, can either positively or negatively influence parents' power to help their adolescents in "school completion and the attainment of economic security, staying out of trouble with the law, the postponement of childbearing, and avoidance of excessive use of drugs and alcohol" (p. 236). The question is How do practitioners in community mental health agencies, private practice offices, or schools think about and assess the role of neighborhood risk and protection in the lives of the teens?

Some teens live in neighborhoods that promote easy access to safe physical and social environments and some live in places where this access is limited or nonexistent (e.g., see Kotlowitz, 1991). Therefore, practitioners need to understand that neighborhoods have varying influences. Neighborhoods are complex, multidimensional ecosystems. Events that occur among people who reside and work within them (proximal influences) and events that occur in systems outside of them (distal influences) shape neighborhoods.

We address the proximal neighborhood influences on adolescents. However, it is important to acknowledge that neighborhood conditions develop from interactions between local residents' micro and meso relationships as well as distal processes in exosystems and macrosystems. Therefore, accounting for neighborhood includes recognizing that broader social processes of prejudice and discrimination influence neighborhood protective and risk factors. For example, stigma is attributed to certain neighborhoods such that when job applicants list particular addresses in neighborhoods known to be dangerous and/or poor, potential employers do not consider them for the position because they perceive that they will not be "productive and will introduce problems to the work place" (Holloway & Mulherin, 2004, p. 433). Outsiders label residents of lower-status neighborhoods as lazy, irresponsible, and gullible even when there is no evidence to prove the accuracy of those assumptions (Cherulnik & Souders, 1984). Issues such as these are confirmed when young people who reside in poor neighborhoods tell researchers about their experiences at school. For example, one 12-year-old boy told a researcher, "You never tell teachers your address if your momma live in a bad neighborhood 'cause they think you be like all the knuckleheads where your momma live even if you don't be there all the time . . . even if you live somewhere else most of the time . . . they still trying to make you like them knuckleheads just cause they think that's where you be most of the time" (Burton & Price-Spratlen, 1999, p. 87).

Ecological theory compels us to account for the multiple systems that shape neighborhood conditions and outsiders' responses to those conditions. Hence, assessment of and intervention in neighborhood risk factors in clinical practice requires a social justice orientation because the helping professional must avoid blaming clients who reside in troubled neighborhoods for the troubles that exist in that neighborhood.

An Overview of Neighborhood Protective and Risk Factors

The protective and risk factors associated with neighborhood include social composition, economic composition, social processes, and physical composition/resources (see Table 7.1). Neighborhood-level risk factors include high crime rates, access to drugs and weapons, crowding, high rates of residential mobility, deteriorated properties, absence of social cohesion, and diminished attachment to the neighborhood. On the other hand, neighborhood-level protective factors include collective efficacy and social cohesion, low crime rates, and higher rates of affluent residents (Jensen & Fraser, 2006). It is important to assess for both protective and risk neighborhood factors regardless of the practitioner's intuition about how positive or negative a teen's neighborhood is, because the presence of protective factors or the presence of risk factors in a neighborhood is not always associated with a client's income or education level (Nicotera, 2003, 2008).

Practitioners are not likely to use U.S. census data or crime data to gather information about a client's neighborhood. Census and crime data provide useful information about a neighborhood, however; they represent geographical areas that tend to be different than the geographical

TABLE 7.1. Four General Categories of Neighborhood

1. Social composition	3. Social processes
• Age	• Organizational participation
• Race/ethnicity	• Unsupervised teens
• Residential mobility	• Neighboring
• Density of children and adolescents	• Crime
• Percentage of elderly	• Value consensus
• Percentage of single parents	• Community monitoring
	• Social capital/social networks
2. Economic composition	4. Physical composition/resourses
• Percentage of affluent neighbors	• Condition of housing
• Poverty	• Trash/litter and graffiti
• Employment	• Traffic and street conditions
• Percentage of white-collar workers	• Playgrounds/parks
• Percentage of managerial/ professional workers	• Proximity to employment
• Education levels of residents	• Community centers
• Public housing	• Schools and libraries
• Home ownership	• Bars
	• Abandoned homes and vacant lots

Note. Adapted with permission of the author from Nicotera (2003, pp. 102–103).

area an adolescent and his or her family might consider their proximal neighborhood. Additionally, these structural measures of a neighborhood omit the social processes in a neighborhood that might be risk factors, but also might be protective factors, depending on how the teen and his or her family perceive them. Hence, for purposes of clinical practice, the teen and his or her family provide the best information about their neighborhood.

Neighborhood Protective and Risk Factors Associated with Adolescent Strengths and Problems

The research and theory on neighborhood influences tends to concentrate on deficit-type neighborhoods. As a result, there is little research or theory to suggest the qualities of strength-based neighborhoods. However, pluralistic neighborhood theory (Aber & Nieto, 2000) suggests that all neighborhoods, regardless of their socioeconomic status, have strengths and deficits.

The three broad areas for assessment in clinical practice are (1) neighborhood social cohesion, (2) collective socialization, and (3) neighborhood social organization and disorganization (see Figure 7.1).

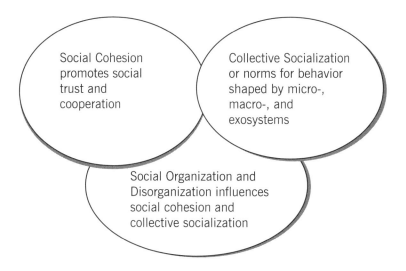

FIGURE 7.1. Neighborhood factors that influence adolescents.

Neighborhood Social Cohesion

Neighborhood social cohesion includes the social ties or micro- and meso-level relationships between residents in a neighborhood. These ties vary from neighborhood to neighborhood and even from neighbor to neighbor within the same neighborhood. They are the social ties that make a person feel comfortable when out of town because there is a sense that the neighbors will look out for one's home. Neighborhood cohesion is also trusting that there are neighbors who will help out, such as helping a child who has fallen off his or her bike or making dinner for a neighbor's family while one of the parents is in the hospital. Neighborhood social cohesion serves as a protective factor because it provides a sense of comfort and safety that residents will (1) recognize strangers in the neighborhood and monitor their actions if necessary for neighborhood safety, (2) contribute to a friendly neighborhood climate where people know each other and help each other, and (3) promote an experience of general satisfaction related to residing in the neighborhood (Sampson, Raudenbush, & Earls, 1997).

Youth who perceive more social cohesion in their neighborhoods report better health regardless of their race and ethnicity and regardless of the type of neighborhood where they live (Abada, Hou, & Ram, 2007). Additionally, adolescent females who perceived their neighborhood as being more socially cohesive report lower rates of depression (Nebbitt & Lombe, 2007). Other researchers (Plybon, Edwards, Butler, Belgrave, & Allison, 2003) found that teen perception of neighborhood cohesion influences a stronger sense of school self-efficacy and higher grades.

Collective Socialization

Collective socialization is a neighborhood protective and risk factor for teens. Just like families, neighborhoods develop and communicate norms about positive and negative behavior and aspirations that influence teens. William Julius Wilson (1987, 1996) developed foundational theories about how collective socialization works as a risk factor. The following quote reflects his theories: "Adult neighbors provide important models of behavior for local adolescents so that youth living in neighborhoods in which many residents experience school failure, joblessness, poverty, and family instability, will themselves be less likely to complete school, gain employment" (Crowder & South, 2003, p. 661). Collective socialization also works as a protective factor. For example, when neighborhood residents tend to have completed school and hold jobs neighborhood youth learn that the future will be brighter if they stay in school (Crowder & South).

Teens in neighborhoods with the risk type of collective socialization are more likely to drop out of school, especially when they have greater association with neighbors who experience high rates of unemployment and poverty (Crowder & South, 2003). Hence, when we assess for neighborhood collective socialization it is imperative to ask about protective- and risk-oriented neighborhood norms and about the level of contact a teen has with neighbors whose life experiences resonate with those norms.

Collective socialization is also a factor in behaviors beyond educational and employment aspirations. Novak, Reardon, and Buka (2002) studied adolescents' beliefs about drug use and its relationship to the norms in their neighborhoods. They discovered that in neighborhoods where there is a collective view that the use of hard drugs is low risk then teen residents also viewed hard drugs as low risk. This relationship between the collective neighborhood norm and youth's views was persistent even after the researchers accounted for how individual proclivities and experiences of teens effect their perceptions of the risk of hard drugs. Interestingly, this collective socialization risk did not apply to the teens' sense of risk for alcohol and marijuana use. Their views on these substances were dependent on individual inclinations and personal experiences. The evidence from this research assists in clinical assessment decision making. On the one hand, assessments for substance use and/or abuse typically explore an adolescent's internal processes and experiences such as exposure to media that glamorizes alcohol. On the other hand, these assessments also need to include information about a teen's neighborhood collective socialization.

One caveat about collective socialization is that practitioners need to be nonjudgmental about a client's neighbors and neighborhood. For example, a teen might state that none of the adults in his or her neighborhood have jobs and that they hang out in the park all day. It is imperative for practitioners to remember that unemployed neighbors are not like a contagious disease from which we must protect youth any more than employed neighbors represent upstanding or "germ-free" citizens. We would not suggest that our adolescent clients blindly seek association with employed neighbors without further assessment of those neighbors' abilities to be safe mentors.

Neighborhood Social Organization or Disorganization

Neighborhood social organization or disorganization includes a combination of neighborhood social cohesion and collective socialization. It is the third neighborhood factor important for clinical practice. We refer to this concept as "disorganization" because the prominent literature applies that label even though there is a continuum that moves between social organization and disorganization. Bowen, Bowen, and Ware (2002) describe the concept on the disorganization end of the continuum as including (1) lack of neighborhood support (e.g., how interested adult neighbors are in teens, neighbors helping each other out, access to youth activities in the neighborhood, satisfaction with the neighborhood, how safe the teen feels in the neighborhood), (2) the perception of prosocial and negative behaviors of neighborhood peers (e.g., youth get good grades, graduate from high school, work or go to college after high school versus youth get in trouble with the police, use drugs, join gangs, consume alcohol), and (3) resident exposure to neighborhood crime (e.g., being threatened with a weapon, hearing gun shots, witnessing a drug deal). Bowen and his colleagues found that residing in neighborhoods with more disorganization negatively impacted teen school experiences, even after they accounted for the influence of families.

Neighborhood social disorganization influences teen proclivity for violent behavior. Vowell (2007) found that residence in a disorganized neighborhood had a direct effect on the violent behavior of teens. For example, the greater the levels of disorganization the more likely that teens perpetrated some of the following violent actions: use of force to get something, hurting someone enough to need bandages, physically assaulting someone or hitting a member of their family, using force or trying to use force to get someone to have sex, setting fire to someone's property, and using a weapon to make someone give away personal items (Vowell). Hence, witnessing violence, along with other neighborhood dangers, has an impact not only on academic achievement, but on behavior as well.

Law and Barber (2006) explore how neighborhood social disorganization influences adolescents' sense of loneliness, sense of community integration, and antisocial behaviors. Their assessment of neighborhood social disorganization includes a combination of strengths and deficits. This combination includes (1) youth perceptions of adult control in the neighborhood (e.g., if an adult neighbor saw a youth doing something wrong, like spray painting or skipping school, would that person say or do something about it?); (2) youth views on how they feel about living in the neighborhood, how many neighborhood youth they know, and how often they feel lonely in the neighborhood; (3) how often youth had contact with neighbors, local church, and community leaders; and (4) youth perceptions of the presence of litter, trash, graffiti, and unsavory characters such as drunks in a park. They found that youth who perceived fewer of the neighborhood strengths noted in numbers one, two, and three, and more of the deficits noted in number four, were more likely to engage in antisocial behaviors such as spending time with peers who cheat, lie, steal, or get into trouble. The youth who perceived more of the strengths in the neighborhood tended to spend less time with antisocial peers.

Neighborhood social disorganization also influences depression in adolescents. Researchers Nebbitt and Lombe (2007) studied teens to assess whether family encouragement, association with delinquent peers, and personal beliefs would outweigh the influences of neighborhood social disorganization on youth's depressive symptoms. The teens in their study completed the Center for Epidemiological Studies Depression Scale (CES-D). They were also asked to rate the level of neighborhood disorganization (e.g., violent crimes, drug use and dealing, and the presence of police who harass people who are not doing anything wrong) and neighborhood cohesion (e.g., people are friendly, youths know each other, adults know each other). The study's results demonstrate the role of neighborhood social disorganization in depressive symptoms in spite of family, peer, and individual factors. Thus, witnessing violence and a lack of safety in one's neighborhood is concomitant with depression.

In addition to depressive symptoms, neighborhood factors can also influence a teen's experiences of feeling hassled or stressed, which over time could lead to sadness and depressive symptoms. In a different study, Anthony and Nicotera (2008) explored elements of neighborhood social disorganization through youth perceptions of neighborhood hassles. These hassles include drug dealers approaching neighborhood residents, not having places in the neighborhood to hang out with peers, and feeling scared in one's neighborhood. The results demonstrate that the presence of neighborhood resources such as grocery stores, libraries, recreation facilities, fast-food stores, and banks help youth to feel less hassled or safer.

Thus far we have considered how youth's experiences of neighborhood social cohesion, collective socialization, and social disorganization influence their internal struggles (e.g., depression) and external actions (e.g., antisocial behavior). In addition, lack of physical activity or exercise can exacerbate emotional-psychological and behavioral problems. Therefore, it is important for practitioners to understand how neighborhoods influence teen access to exercise. Mota, Almeida, Santos, and Ribeiro (2005) studied how neighborhoods of residence influenced adolescents' participation in organized and nonorganized sports outside of school. Teens who were more active lived in neighborhoods that (1) provided easy access to resources such as stores and recreation facilities, (2) had a social environment in which locals were seen being physically active, and (3) had sidewalks, less traffic, lower crime rates, and enjoyable sights such as gardens. Practitioners often find themselves working with teens who experience (1) depression, (2) antisocial behavior, and/or (3) pressure from antisocial peers. We also work with teens to increase their commitment to stay in school and to seek higher education or positive employment as well as increasing levels of physical activity. Yet many practitioners do not recognize that a youth's neighborhood conditions might play a role in these concerns.

Considerations for Assessment

The research suggests that we should assess for neighborhood protective and risk factors from four perspectives: (1) youth experiences with neighbors who may assist in the development of competence and who provide support, (2) sentiments (positive and negative) about the people and places within a youth's neighborhood, (3) neighborhood-based activities in which the youth engages, and (4) the resources available within the neighborhood (Nicotera, 2005). These four perspectives are contained in assessments of neighborhood social cohesion, collective socialization, social disorganization, and physical-resource neighborhood factors such as access to resources.

Begin your assessment with general open-ended questions about the teen's neighborhood and neighbors. These general questions may lead to information that helps the practitioner assess the more specific neighborhood protective and risk factors for a particular client. However, before beginning the neighborhood assessment practitioners need to explain the reason for inquiring about this part of a client's life. It is important to refrain from jargon words like *collective socialization, neighborhood social disorganization*, and *neighborhood social cohesion*. For example, the practitioner might say:

> "Sometimes when a person is having a problem it's easy to look inside him- or herself and wonder, what is wrong with me? I take the view that whatever is going on inside someone is also connected to things that are going on around him or her, even things in the neighborhood. So I am not only going to ask you about yourself, family, and friends, but also about the neighborhood where you live."

Practitioners may want to begin with a discussion about places a client likes and does not like in his or her neighborhood. The next step is to have the teen describe what he or she would change in his or her neighborhood and how that would make the neighborhood different from its current state. Additionally, practitioners can ask the teen to think about a neighbor he or she likes and to describe why he or she likes that neighbor and some of the things that neighbor does for or with him or her. Once the teen is chatting about his or her neighborhood, practitioners can draw on the following list of questions to gather more information (see Table 7.2). In addition to posing questions like the ones noted in Table 7.2, the practitioner may want to conduct a home and neighborhood visit, if their practice setting provides for this type of assessment process.

TABLE 7.2. Questions to Ask Adolescent Clients about Their Neighborhoods

"Tell me about your neighborhood."

"Tell me about what goes on in your neighborhood."

"Where do you spend time with friends? How far from your home is it? How do you get there?"

"Do you go shopping for food or other things for or with your mom or dad? How do you get there?"

"Where do you go to school? How far from your home is it? How do you get there?"

"Where do your friends live? How far from your home are they? How do you get there?"

"Tell me about a favorite place in your neighborhood. Why is it your favorite place? How often do you get to go there? Does your mom or dad know about this place?"

"Tell me about a place you don't like in your neighborhood. Why is it a place you don't like? Do you ever go there? Does your mom or dad know about this place?"

"Do you know other teens in your neighborhood? Do you spend time with them? What do you do for fun?"

"Do you know adults in your neighborhood who don't live with you? Do you spend time with them? What do you do when you are together?"

"Do you see neighbors talking with each other, children playing together, and teens and adults interacting?"

"Tell me about the places you can go by yourself in your neighborhood. Tell me about the places you cannot go by yourself."

"What types of businesses are in your neighborhood—for example, laundries, banks, grocers, schools, community centers, churches? Can you walk to these or take a bus there?"

"What types of green spaces are in your neighborhood? Are they parks? Do they have swings and other play equipment? Do they have athletic equipment? Are there streets near the green spaces? How busy are they?"

"How busy are the streets? How fast does traffic move on them? What types of vehicles are driving on them?"

"Does your neighborhood have sidewalks? What, if any, kinds of activities do you see on the sidewalks?"

"Do you see litter, vandalism, vacant housing, dilapidated housing, abandoned cars, and unkempt lots?"

"Do you see people drinking alcohol, doing drugs? Do you see homeless people?"

Note. Based on Nicotera (2005).

Case Study

Max is a 16-year-old African American teen who lives with his parents (Ruth, age 43, and Ben, 44 age) and younger sister (Sasha, age 14) in a middle-class urban neighborhood in a midsize metropolitan area in California about 100 miles west of Lake Tahoe. Typical of this part of California, their neighborhood is culturally and ethnically diverse and Max has friends who are also African American as well as white, Asian, and Latino.

He attends a private Catholic high school in another neighborhood near his home and it is close enough that he walks to and from school when the weather is not too cold. He tends to make A's and B's in his classes and also has good friends who he has been in school with since kindergarten. He is a member of the school's ski team and they practice at the Heavenly ski area near Lake Tahoe.

The new school year began 8 weeks ago and Max's parents were astonished when the midsemester grade report sent home by the school showed that his usually good grades had dropped to B-minuses and C-pluses. They were also surprised when he told them he has decided to quit the ski team because they know it is one of his favorite activities. At first his parents figured it was typical teenage rebellion and while they made it clear that they expected his usual good grades; it was his choice to leave the ski team. However, over the next couple of weeks they noticed that Max was spending more and more time alone in his room avoiding them and his sister. Whenever they asked him to join the family for pizza out or to choose the DVD they would watch he would either act irritated and/or say he didn't feel well. Around this time, one of the neighbors, a parent of one of Max's friends, called Ruth because she caught her son and Max wandering out of one of the homes on the street that had been abandoned because of a bank foreclosure 6 months earlier. When she questioned the boys they confessed that they had skipped school. Then later when she pressed her own son, he told her they had skipped school several days over the past couple of weeks because their work hours conflicted with it. She shared with Ruth that her son said they had gotten jobs at the local grocery store because "times are rough for everyone and Max and I are just looking out for our futures and yours."

Both Ruth and her husband, Ben, are alarmed and talk with Max, who defends his behavior the same way that his friend did. "All the kids are making some kind of plan like this mom," he said, "look at all the neighbors who have had to move and lose their homes!" When his parents reassure him that the family finances are strong he says, "Well that's what all the families in Florida thought until everything went south." He tells them he saw photos about this on the Internet and all of his friends have been scheming about it since they are not old enough to work at regular jobs. Then he confesses that he wanted to quit the ski team to save his parents money, but he also wanted to do more.

The family reports that about 35% of the homes in their neighborhood have been empty for the past 6–8 months. Ruth and Ben say they had not been close to those families since they had only moved there over the last couple of years. However, Max and Sasha pipe up that they miss the kids who lived there and still get e-mails from them about how unhappy they are in their new neighborhoods now that their parents are "broke." Sasha shares that "all those houses look haunted now with the grass dried up and dead and two or three of them have broken windows, too!"

Clinical Interventions with Adolescents in a Neighborhood Context

Keep Max in mind while reading this section and be prepared to decide which of the suggested interventions are applicable to him. Clinically oriented practitioners are uniquely prepared to assist adolescents and their families in unpacking the clinical effects of the neighborhood risk factors presented in this chapter. Practitioners are also adept at creative strategies for helping teens become aware of the ways in which they can capitalize on neighborhood protective factors as they work toward emotional and behavioral changes. These types of interventions are the focus of this section. It is also possible that as we become aware of neighborhood-level conditions that are deleterious to our teenage clients we may want to create neighborhood- or community-level interventions aimed at working with residents to increase neighborhood social cohesion or to decrease the elements of neighborhood social disorganization. However, neighborhood- and community-level interventions to change the risk factors identified in this chapter are beyond the scope of the clinical interventions and also beyond the scope of this book. We encourage those who want to create neighborhood interventions to collaborate with colleagues who are trained to practice community social work or community psychology in order to practice ethically within their level of competence.

Few interventions aim specifically to reduce the effects of deleterious neighborhood influences on clinical concerns. Therefore, it is incumbent on the practitioner to apply interventions, such as cognitive-behavioral therapy (CBT; Beck, 1995; Ellis & Wilde, 2001), in a way that assists clients in having control over the effects of neighborhood social disorganization, negative collective socialization, or limited neighborhood social cohesion. Practitioners should uncover any automatic thoughts or irrational beliefs (Cooper & Lesser, 2008) that their adolescent clients have in relation to their neighborhood experiences such as "All the kids are painting graffiti," or "No cool kids in this neighborhood ever use the community center or the library." Then the practitioner continues to pose questions that help the teen to provide evidence that disputes the automatic thoughts as well as developing a plan for not letting these thoughts interfere with his or her own positive behavior. This type of intervention is similar to assisting teens in coping with peer pressure. The difference is that the level of pressure is not always as apparent as it is with peers, since neighborhood factors exist outside the tangible sphere of the teen himself or herself.

Existential approaches (Frankl, 1969; Walsh & Lantz, 2007) to clinical practice are also useful for helping teens to deflect the effects of neighborhood risk factors because they allow the teen to make sense of the meanings he or she makes as a result of living within negative neighborhood conditions. This approach also allows the practitioner and the teen to focus on the neighborhood protective factors as a way to build meanings that create positive behavior choices. Narrative therapy (Epstein & White, 1990; Kelley, Blankenburg, & McRoberts, 2002; Zimmerman & Dickerson, 1996) is another useful strategy in clinical work that accounts for neighborhood influences and the meanings teenagers make out of them. The approach allows a teen to externalize negative neighborhood stories that affect the narratives with which he or she identifies and uses when making choices.

Finally, multisystemic therapy (MST; Henggeler, 1999; Henggeler, Clingempeel, Brondino, & Pickrel, 2002; Randall & Henggeler, 1999) is an overall approach that practitioners can use in the development of strategies for intervention. Unlike the intervention approaches just discussed, MST does not prescribe any particular strategy for making change. Instead, it serves as a framework for working with the teen and his or her family so that individual, family, school, and neighborhood factors play a role in assessment and intervention. The following ideas will be useful regardless of the theoretical approach used in intervention (see Table 7.3).

TABLE 7.3. General Intervention Ideas

Youth and family	Youth and family and neighbors
• Assist youth to draw positive meanings about self and future in spite of neighborhood problems witnessed.	• Work with families to connect with neighbors to discuss and seek solutions to troubling neighborhood events.
• Facilitate family discussions related to troubling neighborhood events.	• Facilitate the family in assessing neighborhood troubles and the strengths that may be useful in alleviating the troubles.
• Support child, youth, and family in recognizing the role macro structures play in neighborhood conditions.	
• Support positive social contacts between youth, family, and appropriate neighbors.	• Facilitate the family's development of skills for work with local power players to change troubling physical and social conditions.

1. Describe all of the psychological and behavioral factors that might be playing a role in Max's current issues. What information from the case example provides clues to these factors?

2. Describe all of the neighborhood factors that might be playing a role in Max's behavior and choices. What key words, used by Ben, Ruth, Max, and Sasha, suggest some of the neighborhood factors at play for this family and for Max's presenting issues?

3. Describe how you will explain the neighborhood factors and their relationship to Max's psychological and behavioral presenting concerns to the family without using jargon.

4. What questions (see Table 7.2 for a summary) should the practitioner ask the family in order to assess which of the neighborhood processes (collective socialization, social cohesion, social disorganization) might be influencing Max? What questions do you ask to assess whether they might also be influencing Sasha?

5. We discussed several intervention strategies in this chapter. Based on the issues confronting Max, which are most useful and why?

6. Recall the neighborhood where you lived as a teenager. How would you rate that neighborhood in terms of collective socialization, social cohesion, and social organization?

7. Recall the neighborhood where you lived as a teenager. Describe the macro- and exosystem factors that may have played a role in collective socialization.

8. How might your experiences of the neighborhood where you grew up influence the way you think about your clients' neighborhoods?

9. How would you apply the concepts of social cohesion, social organization, and collective socialization to teen clients who live in rural areas or smaller towns? How might these be different than in urban neighborhoods?

Chapter Summary

This chapter challenged you to consider the ways in which neighborhoods influence adolescent clients. We discussed three general neighborhood factors: collective socialization, social cohesion, and social disorganization. We presented research evidence to help you understand how these factors play a role in clinical issues. We covered general areas for assessment and several approaches to intervention. A case example helped you to think about applying the ideas to practice with teens and their families. We posed questions for general discussion and self-reflection so that you could think about how your own experiences of neighborhood might influence the way you view the neighborhoods of clients. In the next chapter we discuss the media's influences on youth.

CHAPTER 8

Media Influences

Chapter Overview

Teenagers in the United States spend about 6 to 7 hours each day interacting with various media sources (Roberts, Foehr, & Ridout, 2004, as cited in L'Engle, Brown, & Kenneavy, 2006). This chapter addresses how the media, as a "significant other" (Cooley, 1902; G. Mead, 1934; M. Mead, 1965) in a teenager's world, filters through the ecological levels to impact him or her. Theoretical foundations that provide evidence for the need to assess media influences are presented together with evidence from research on media effects on body image and sex/sexuality in adolescents. The section on assessment provides information on how to talk with adolescents about their use of the media. Interventions that arise from behavioral theory, existential theory, and public health theory with a focus on peer opinion leaders are discussed. A clinical case example allows you to apply the knowledge gained from the chapter.

CASE EXAMPLE:
Who Are the Youth Represented in this Chapter?

The following case example represents some of the concerns related to adolescents and the media. Considering the implications for this case within the context of the risk factors, theory, assessment, and intervention strategies presented in the following pages will prepare you to assess and suggest interventions for the more developed case study at the end of the chapter.

Joanne, European American, age 16, is considered an outcast in her high school. Peers have teased her since middle school where she was viewed as a teacher's pet and bookworm. Joanne does not fit in with any of the student groups, not the athletes, not the student council, and not the debate team. Over the years she seemed to weather this treatment with outside interests such as taking classes at the local community college and tutoring elementary school kids in reading and math. When she begged her parents to get connected to the Internet so she could communicate with her community college classmates about homework, they agreed and willingly spent the extra money to pay for her Internet access at home. However, since then Joanne's father noticed that she appears depressed and tired. He also noted that she was refusing to sit down to dinner with the family and would eat only raw fruits and vegetables. While he did not want to snoop into Joanne's life, he was shocked when he went into her room and found printed material from websites about how to commit suicide without leaving any evidence.

A Clinical Orientation to the Media

New technologies have increased adolescent access to media. Socially interactive media such as text messaging, Facebook, and MySpace have brought teens into closer contact with both known and unknown peers and adults. While traditional media represent macro- and exosystems and are delivered *to* the adolescent, the interactive nature of more current sources bring media into the meso- and microsystems of the young people. Stokols (1999) points out that these interactive media opportunities "blur" the "boundaries among one's micro-, meso-, and exosystems" (p. 343).

The theories and research that support our understanding of media influences cut across several disciplines, including mass communication, psychology, social psychology, and sociology. Over the past several decades various studies have made contrasting claims to the effects of the media on behavior (Bandura, Ross, & Ross, 1963; Bushman & Anderson, 2001; Donnerstein & Smith, 1997; Drabman & Thomas, 1975). Current scholars (Lloyd, 2002) suggest that noninteractive media, such as television, serve as a practice arena for adolescents through which they may or may not decide how to behave in a real-life situation. As Lloyd notes, while "the potential for imitation of aggressive behaviors [experienced through various media technologies] exists, it is more likely that adolescent viewers use these viewing opportunities as times to rehearse (cognitively) interactions with peers and selectively apply them as appropriate situations arise" (p. 75). Lloyd suggests that cognitive rehearsal is a chance to try out different ways of acting "without risking peer rejection" (p. 75). When teens use interactive media sources where communication is direct and immediate (e.g., e-mail, MySpace), then rehearsal of options for how to behave in real life disappears. The result of this can range from small mistakes to tragedies that cannot be undone. Similar to words spoken out loud, once an e-mail is sent or a blog is posted it cannot be taken back.

Each teenager has his or her own unique responses to the varying media sources in his or her life. These responses result from variations in gender, race/ethnicity, social class, and sexual orientation as well as from the level of access a teen has to different types of media. The theory of symbolic interaction (Blumer, 1969; G. Mead, 1934; M. Mead, 1965; Spencer, 1999) provides a foundation for understanding how the media filters through to influence adolescents in varying ways. Symbolic-interaction scholars point out the importance of language and other forms of communication through which "culture, socially structured situations, interpersonal relationships, and social identities are created and maintained" (Heise & Weir, 1999, p. 139). For example, two teenagers viewing the same Internet site do not develop the exact same perspective of that site; each comes to his or her own personal meaning about it. Their families and other social contexts also shape this meaning. However, a new shared meaning develops as the two teens discuss the site with each other and their peers. Over time, this meaning can turn into expectations for behavior within the teen peer group and have more influence than the teens' families (Heise & Weir). In fact, Lloyd (2002) suggests that "within the context of media influence, it is postulated that the features of mass media entertainment (e.g., language, clothing, and cultural settings in television programming) take on a primary role in the transmission of implicit social knowledge within the adolescent peer culture" (p. 83).

Prior to the advent of current technologies, teen interactions about the media occurred only in face-to-face settings or via the telephone in the home of one's family. However, with cell phones, text messaging, and sites like MySpace, these interactions occur in a continuous fashion, among a broader range of peers and out of earshot of adults. While teens require a sense of privacy, they also need opportunities to discuss the ideas they gather from the media with trusted adults. For example, teens can form "parasocial relationships" with celebrities via the Internet or other media (Giles, 2002). These parasocial relationships influence an adolescent's choices for acting, thinking, and feeling (Larson, 1995). They "also provide cultural materials for developing gender role identity, forming values and beliefs, and learning sexual and romantic scripts (Arnett, 1995, as cited in Giles & Maltby, 2004, pp. 814–815). If adolescents discuss the ideas they get from the media and parasocial relationships with parents and trusted adults, then they are more likely to use that media to grow. On the other hand, the media can be a risk factor when parental or adult input on media messages is absent.

Virtual Identity and the Media

In face-to-face interactions, "performance of identity" or self-expression involves physical cues about gender, height, weight, age, skin color, and "fashion sense, hair style, and other bodily markings . . . [which] are assessed by others as they determine whether we might make a good friend, partner, or employee" (Thomas, 2007, p. 5). Performance of identity in face-to-face settings is distinguished from the virtual performance of identity in cyberspace (Thomas). A teen who was interviewed by Thomas describes it like this: "I'm not sure if anybody here [in cyberspace] totally gets to know me—I'm sort of a persona. It's a lot like me, but minus the things I don't like about myself" (p. 5). Agger (2004) suggests that virtual communication has ushered in opportunities to present or invent the self in ever-changing ways that were not possible prior to its development. He notes that "the internet opens up a new world of self-creation, storytelling, global communities, interactive instantaneity, and possibly even political organizing quite unknown in a slower paced stage of modernity" (Agger, 2004, p. 146). The most recent presidential election cycle in which President Obama and his campaign capitalized on the Internet as a tool for fundraising and getting out the vote are a testament to Agger's statement.

When Erikson (1968) developed his theory on the adolescent developmental crisis of identity versus role confusion and when Marcia (1966) expanded those ideas, neither of them imagined the number of selves or identities the 21st-century teenager could play with via cyberspace (Lloyd, 2002). We might consider cyberspace as the adolescent version of the preschool dress-up corner or closet without the physical constraints of the body. This is not to suggest that the teen's experience of Internet communication and communities is disembodied since the emotions of these experiences are clearly felt in the physical body. Thomas (2007) states, "real emotions and bodily reactions are intimately connected with communication, whether online or offline. Real people, experiencing real reactions are involved in cybercommunities and online interactions" (pp. 9–10). Given this, cyberrelationships may be considered an important area for assessment in clinical practice with teens. One example of this importance is taken from a tragic incident in which a young girl committed suicide after experiencing unrelenting cyberbullying (Maag, 2007). This tragedy and other Internet exploitations that wreak havoc on the lives of youth and their families paint a dangerous picture of this media form. However, it is imperative that practitioners develop awareness about the positive influences of cyberspace. Positive influences of the media are not common, but examples can be found in the literature.

Loader (2007) discusses the positive ramifications of the Internet on the political, civic, and community engagement of young people. Thomas (2007) interviews teens about their cyber experiences and provides examples of how they build cyberspace communities and learn social-emotional skills as a result. She describes a role-playing cybercommunity created by an international group of 13- and 14-year-old teens. Role playing via the Internet requires writing and Thomas notes the support the teens give each other by commenting and being open about their emotional reactions to their peers' writing. The youth also work out conflicts that develop as a result of the role playing. For example, a conflict was aptly handled when one cyber-community member wanted to review all poetry to ensure it was "G-rated before [the poem] went public" (Thomas, p. 108). Other members were upset with him for not trusting that his peers could self-censor the content of their poems. Another teen discussed the tears he shed and community mourning (virtual hugging) that occurred when another teen was thought to have died in a car accident and the subsequent cybercommunity relief when the teen's brother announced he had only suffered a broken arm and ribs (Thomas). Thomas's interviews also indicate that teens are well aware of the fact they are changing their identities online as one teen noted, "You *have* to change the way you are depending on which space you're in at any given moment. Although I am always 'me' underneath, I present my words and actions very differently depending on what space or place or window or whatever you like to call it, that I am in" (p. 43). In this sense, teens are regulating their "presentation of self" (Goffman, 1959) in ways that they often do in the nonvirtual world such as the way they might talk with their teachers and parents as compared to their friends.

Body Image and the Media

Media messages play a role in the body image of adolescents. Messages about what constitutes the ideal body are culture bound such that teens from different ethnic and racial backgrounds may experience the impact of the media differently. The research on media influences on body image tends toward a European American focus. However, some studies demonstrate differences such as Adams and colleagues (2000) who found that African American girls espoused a larger ideal body for women than European American girls. Another scholar (Botta, 2000) who studied racial differences in girls' pressure for an ideal body type found that African American girls were less pressured by media images of thin women than European American girls. In another study, Gentles and Harrison (2006) begin to sort out these differences noting that larger African American teens who watched Eurocentric television shows such as *Sex and the City*, *Seventh Heaven*, and *That 70s Show*, were more likely to think that their peers expected them to *conform* to a media standard of feminine thinness. In contrast, African American teens with more petite body sizes who watched similar television shows felt that their peers expected them to *exceed* the same media standard for the thin female. These researchers note that more research on racial and ethnic differences in media influence on body image needs to be conducted and that future studies need to examine exposure to television shows that are geared toward people of color, such as the programming on Black Entertainment Network, Latino/Latina-oriented networks, and Asian-oriented networks (Gentles & Harrison).

Concerns about body image have long been considered a female issue (Ricciardelli & McCabe, 2003), but current research indicates that media and other social factors also influence adolescent males' body image (Baird & Grieve, 2006; Leit, Gray, & Pope, 2002; Pope, Philips, & Olivardia, 2000). There is, however, a gender difference in response to media images of the ideal body. In general, teenage girls tend to be influenced toward making their bodies thinner and boys tend to wish for larger muscles. Teenage boys are more likely to have concerns about living up to stereotypical media images of the muscular male while girls are prey to media stereotypes of thinness (Ricciardelli & McCabe, 2003). In fact, McCabe and Ricciardelli point out that "pressure to attain the ideal body weight has been used to explain the emergence and maintenance of body dissatisfaction among boys and girls" (p. 655). Other researchers note the specific influence of the media on adolescent boys' body image. Their results demonstrate that advertisements portraying muscular males tend to decrease teenage boys' sense of body satisfaction (Baird & Grieve, 2006; Leit et al., 2002). Body dissatisfaction has been noted as a catalyst for future eating disorders that require mental and physical health treatment, making assessment of body image and satisfaction an important element in clinical work with teenage boys (Gentles & Harrison, 2006). Peterson, Paulson, and Williams (2007) support this notion with their research, which demonstrates that teenage boys were more apt to diet to attain a male body ideal when they were regular viewers of media images about dieting. Research on media influence on boys' development of body dissatisfaction is limited. However, it is incumbent upon practitioners to seek out future studies that provide evidence on the effects of the media on boys' body image.

Teenage boys and girls who aspire to resemble a media figure they admired also worry more about their weight (Field et al., 2001). However, even though media messages influence male and female teens, research shows that girls tend to be more affected by the messages. Numerous studies demonstrate a connection between media images promoting thinness in women and the development of body dissatisfaction among teenage girls (Harrison 2000). For example, teenage girls indicate that images of women in magazines influence their views of their own body. Sixty-nine percent report that the images cause them to view thinness as an ideal female body and 47% said that the images affect their plans to lose weight (Field et al., 2001). In contrast, 50% of teenage boys report that images of males in the media have no influence on their eating habits and body image (Ricciardelli, McCabe, & Banfield, 2000). Nevertheless, research does show that adolescent boys' and girls' body images are affected by media pressures to attain and maintain stereotypical body types; thinness for young women and muscular for young men (Ata, Ludden, & Lally, 2007). In fact, a longitudinal study indicates that both teen boys and teens girls are susceptible to body-image messages from the media and that the effects of these messages increase over time as the youth move through adolescence. However, these influences are more potent for girls than boys over time because boys' concern with body image fades as they age while girls' does not fade (McCabe & Ricciardelli, 2005). Regardless, assessment of media influence on both male and female teens is important.

Sexuality and the Media

Teens report being more influenced by friends and the media than they are by their parents (Ballard & Morris, 1998; Stodghill, 1998). Media aimed at teens provides an abundance of sex- and sexuality-related material. For example, 83% of teenage-focused programs contain portrayals of sex and sexuality (Kunkel et al., 2003, as cited in Epstein & Ward, 2008). Additionally, 44 to 76% of music videos and DVDs contain similar content (Ward, 2003). One important point is that media content about sex and sexuality is aimed at heterosexual messages as Brown and Keller (2000) point out: "Homosexual and transgendered youth rarely find themselves represented in the mainstream media. Although a few youth-targeted programs, such as *Dawson's Creek*, have recently included gay characters, what some have called 'compulsory heterosexuality' prevails" (p. 255).

Teens *are* curious about sex, and age-appropriate images related to sexuality do not have to be a negative element in their lives. The caution lays in teen claims that their peers and the media have a greater impact than parents on their understanding of sex. When teens and parents view media with sexual content together and are able to talk about the content, then parents can mediate these messages and transmit the values about sex they deem appropriate for their adolescents. In fact, mass-communications scholars demonstrate that parents and other adults have a role in mediating teens' exposure to media (Austin, 1993). About 30% of teens between the ages of 15 and 17 years indicate that they approach their parents about sexuality as a result of television exposure to sexual content (Kaiser Family Foundation, 2002, as cited in Collins, Elliott, Berry, Kanouse, Kunkel, & Hunter, 2003). Another study examined teens' reactions and parental influence on teens' reactions to an episode of the television program *Friends* about pregnancy and condom failure (Collins, Elliott, Berry, Kanouse, & Hunter, 2003). The results support the mediating influence of parents. Hence, parents are not powerless over the media messages that their teenagers receive. However, in order to be part of the conversation about these messages, parents need to be viewed as approachable and open to their teens' questions about sex and sexuality.

While 51% of late-adolescent boys report that they learned information about birth control, AIDS, and sexually transmitted diseases (STDs)
from their parents and friends, 96% of them indicated that they learned
about these from the media (Bradner & Lindberg, 2000). Other notions
about sexuality are also influenced by the media, including boys' attitudes
condoning sex outside of ongoing relationships as well as their perception
of the age-old view of women as sexual objects (Ward & Friedman, 2006;
Zurbriggen & Morgan, 2006). Adolescent boys described the top messages
about sex from the media as including "Sex is fine anytime, anywhere, for
any purpose"; "Sex from one night stands is kind of common"; "Everybody
is having sex"; and "Sex is popular/cool" (Epstein & Ward, 2008, p. 121).
Other ideas about sex and sexuality were also gleaned from the media, but
with less frequency than those just listed. Some of these other attitudes
range from the notion that "finding and being in a relationship is the best
way to fit in" to "Women who have sex are sluts" to "Be safe about sex" and
"AIDS kills" (p. 121).

Teenage girls have different reactions to media than the boys. Currie
(1997) assessed teen girls' reactions to advertisements in teen-oriented and
beauty-oriented magazines. She reports that the girls in her study judged
some ads in terms of realism and logic. For example, when discussing a
fragrance ad in which a man is painting a woman's toenails, one girl, whose
view was similar to the other girls in the study, stated, "I would think why
is he painting her toenails—How would he know how to do it?" (p. 465).
Another typical statement of the study respondents was made by a 15-year-
old girl who responded to a car advertisement, stating, "This is strange,
weird, like just a girl, a drink, and a car. If I looked at it, I wouldn't know
what they're trying to do—It's confusing" (p. 465). Still another reaction
to an ad for comfortable jeans further indicates this critical thinking when
a 14-year-old girl notes, "that she simply did not understand an ad that
associates the comfort of jeans, rather than the discomfort of high-heeled
shoes and false nails, with women" (pp. 465–466).

Currie's (1997) study indicates that this use of logic and critical thinking goes out the window when the ads move from images that girls can
compare to their own lives to images with ideological components beyond
their adolescent development. Perception of messages change when the ads
"portray three icons of traditional adult (hetero) femininity: a diamond
ring, a bride, and an infant child" (p. 467). A 17-year-old girl in Currie's
study reacts this way to an ad for diamond rings: "I like this one . . . it seems
really, he seems really like he's *really* in love with her and it kind of shows, I
guess, that guys care about girls and they're the ones that are kind of taking care of them and buying them stuff . . . which is good—plus it's also just
kind of cute" (p. 467). Another 17-year-old girl reacted to a perfume ad that
depicted a woman holding a toddler noting that the ad was realistic because

even though the woman in the ad is a model, she could also be a mother and in fact the image "is how mommies and little kids interact—It's real" (p. 467). Currie points out that when the girls did not have personal experience with an image then "ideological appeals of romantic love and motherhood were so strong that they overrode the criterion of logic" (p. 468).

The notion that ideological norms for the role of romance and motherhood in women's lives influences female teens' noncritical reactions to advertisements helps us to understand male teens' easy acceptance of media messages. They portray traditional, ideological roles for men such as those that equate manhood with gaining as much sexual experience as possible or having muscular bodies. In fact, the studies discussed thus far indicate the age-old gender schism that equates women with romantic love and motherhood and men as the sexual aggressors of women, who become sluts when they say yes, is alive and well in the 21st century. Some teens may have more enlightened, 21st-century attitudes about working and parenting roles for men and women. However, their relationships are still influenced by this age-old dual standard for heterosexuality with males as sex seekers and girls as sexual gatekeepers as perpetuated in the media.

Researchers have also studied responses to media messages about abstinence and the potential for sexual experiences to end in negative consequences (Epstein & Ward, 2008). However, study participants recall messages about responsible sex far less often than messages about sex without consequences. For example, nearly 21% of male participants noted media messages condoning casual sex, but only 6% of them recalled messages about abstinence and 5% recalled messages that sex can lead to negative consequences (Epstein & Ward). Brown and Keller (2000) note that only a small percentage (9%) of television programs that provide portrayals of sex depict situations that cover the potential risks of unprotected and early-initiated sex. In contrast, other studies demonstrate that more than 50% of teens studied report that they learned about saying no to sex and about 40% learned to talk about safer sex from the content of television programs (Kaiser Family Foundation, 2002, as cited in Collins et al., 2004).

Given the messages teens get from the media, it's fair to ask whether the messages have an affect on their behavior. Several scholars explored this by examining the relative influence of peers, family, school, religion, and the media on adolescents' sexual intentions and behavior (Brown et al., 2006; Collins et al., 2004; L'Engle et al., 2006). Collins and colleagues (2004) assessed differences between teens who watch television shows with greater amounts of sexual content and teens who watch shows with less sexual content. The results indicate that adolescents who view television programs containing greater amounts of sexual content are more likely to adopt sexually advanced behaviors, including sexual intercourse, than the teens who watch television shows with less sexual content. Viewing television programs with more sexual content still stood out as a major influence on teen behavior, even when Collins and colleagues accounted for other factors that influence teens' choices about sexual activity such as parental monitoring, being religious, and having parents who would disapprove.

L'Engle and her colleagues (2006) provide a few more details on how the media influences the intentions and actions of adolescents. They compared the relative influence of parents, school, religion, and the media on the sexual intentions (how likely it is that the teen would engage in sex in the next year and how likely he or she would do this while in high school) and current sexual behavior (light sexual activity and heavy sexual activity) of 3,261 teens in 7th and 8th grades. L'Engle and her colleagues found that over time, viewing media with sexual content and messages suggesting that sexual activity in teens is acceptable and had a greater influence on teens' intended and actual sexual behavior than religion (attendance at services, beliefs, and perception of clergy's view of sex) and school (being happy at school, perception of teachers' view of sex, and grades on a recent report card). When it came to peers, their study indicated that the media had greater effects than peers on teens engaging in light sexual activity: "(1) having a crush, (2) dating at least once, (3) being in a private place, (4) light kissing, and (5) 'French' kissing" (p. 189). However, peers had a greater effect than the media on influencing intentions to have sex and heavy sexual activity: "(1) breast touching, (2) vagina or penis touching, (3) oral sex, and (4) sexual intercourse" (p. 189). Finally, parents had less influence than the media on teens' light sexual activity, about equal influence when it came to heavy sexual activity, and stronger influence when it came to their teenage child's intention to have sex (L'Engle et al.). This research suggests that the media is an influential component in teens' sexual decision making, but that peers and parents are more influential in certain aspects of teen choices about sex. Other studies suggest that in the absence of peer and parental influence on sexual decision making, adolescents tend to look to the media to decide what other teens find acceptable (Brown, Halpern, & L'Engle, 2005). This view of the media as setting norms for behavior is similar to the earlier discussion of media as constituting a "parasocial" relationship (Arnett, 1995, as cited in Giles & Maltby, 2004; Giles, 2002; Larson, 1995).

Midchapter Summary

A lot of content on media influence on adolescents has been discussed and this warrants a midchapter summary before heading into the areas of assessment, intervention, and case application. Table 8.1 provides a summary of the main points.

TABLE 8.1. Summary of Concepts and Ideas about Media in the Lives of Adolescents

General concepts related to media in the lives of adolescents

- Stokols (1999) points out that interactive media opportunities "blur" the "boundaries among one's micro-, meso-, and exosystems" (p. 343).
- Teens have unique responses to media related to variations in gender, race/ethnicity, social class, and sexual orientation as well as from the level of access a teen has to different types of media.
- When teens talk with each other about media experiences they create shared responses and meanings.
- Noninteractive media, such as television, serve as a practice arena for adolescents through which they may or may not decide how to behave in a real-life situation and try out different ways of acting with peers "without risking peer rejection" (Lloyd, 2002. p. 75).
- Interactive media have instantaneous effects, similar to words spoken out loud, once an e-mail is sent or a blog is posted it cannot be taken back. Hence, opportunities for rehearsal without risk disappear.
- Parasocial relationships with media celebrities and characters "also provide cultural materials for developing gender role identity, forming values and beliefs, and learning sexual and romantic scripts" (Arnett, 1995, as cited in Giles & Maltby, 2004, pp. 814–815).
- "Homosexual and transgendered youth rarely find themselves represented in the mainstream media. Although a few youth-targeted programs, such as *Dawson's Creek*, have recently included gay characters, what some have called 'compulsory heterosexuality' prevails" (Brown & Keller, 2000, p. 255).

Identity and emotions in cyberspace

- Agger (2004) suggests that virtual communication through cyberspace has ushered in opportunities to present or invent the self in ever-changing ways that were not possible prior to its development. He notes, "the internet opens up a new world of self-creation, storytelling, global communities, interactive instantaneity" (p. 146).
- One teen interviewed by Thomas (2007) states, "I'm not sure if anybody here [in cyberspace] totally gets to know me—I'm sort of a persona. It's a lot like me, but minus the things I don't like about myself" (p. 5).
- "real emotions and bodily reactions are intimately connected with communication, whether online or offline. Real people, experiencing real reactions are involved in cyber-communities and online interactions" (Thomas, 2007, pp. 9–10).

Body image and the media

- Researchers note the specific influence of the media on adolescent boys' body image demonstrate that advertisements portraying muscular males tend to decrease teenage boys' sense of body satisfaction (Baird & Greive, 2006; Leit et al., 2002).
- Numerous studies demonstrate a connection between media images promoting thinness as an ideal body type for women and the development of body dissatisfaction among teenage girls (e.g., Harrison, 2000).

(cont.)

TABLE 8.1. *(cont.)*

- McCabe and Ricciardelli (2005) found media influences are more potent for girls than boys over time because boys' concern with body image fades as they age while girls' does not fade.
- Body dissatisfaction has been noted as a catalyst for future eating disorders requiring mental and physical health treatment, making assessment of body image and satisfaction an important element in clinical work with teenage boys (Gentles & Harrison, 2006).

Sexuality and the media

- Eighty-three percent of teenage-focused programs contained portrayals of sex and sexuality (Kunkel et al., 2003, as cited in Epstein & Ward, 2008). Forty-four percent to 76% of music videos and DVDs contain similar content (Ward, 2003).
- Brown and Keller (2000) note that only a small percentage (9%) of television programs that provide portrayals of sex, depict situations that cover the potential risks of unprotected and early initiated sex.
- Teens report that, when it comes to their understanding of sex and sexuality, they are more influenced by friends and the media than they are by their parents (Ballard & Morris, 1998; Stodghill, 1998).
- Research suggests that about 30% of teens between the ages of 15 and 17 years indicate that they approach their parents about sexuality as a result of television exposure to sexual content (Kaiser Family Foundation, 2002, as cited in Collins et al., 2004).
- Researchers found that the adolescents who viewed television programs that contained a greater amount of sexual content indicated a stronger tendency to adopt more sexually advanced behaviors, including sexual intercourse, than the teens that saw television shows with less sexual content (Collins et al., 2004).

Considerations for Assessment

Clinical intake and assessment protocols do not typically include questions about teen media activities. Therefore, the M-E practitioner needs to develop his or her own assessment strategy. Assessing the impact of the media on adolescents' presenting concerns requires a bit of a backdoor approach because they tend to believe that they are less affected by the media than other peers their age (Scharrer & Leone, 2006). A backdoor approach includes a less formal assessment in favor of general conversation to get to know the teen's interests, including the music, television, movies, magazines, and Internet sites he or she enjoys. If asked, some teens will bring their music or magazines to a session. Also, appropriate self-disclosure on the part of the practitioner can launch conversations about recent movies and television shows the teen may have seen. Asking a teen to describe most liked or most disliked characters, musicians, and magazines may lead to clues about their potential effects. For example, as a teen describes an admired musician or television character the attuned practitioner listens for clues about the teen's "parasocial" relationship to that character (Giles, 2002). Posing questions to assess whether the adolescent's friends have similar or different tastes allows for an assessment of how the peer group may be influencing the meaning that the teen makes out of his or her media diet (L'Engle et al., 2006).

Assessing teen access to the Internet may be more complicated since electronic media such as MySpace and e-mail tend to be private and strictly age graded making it difficult for the more mature practitioner to launch conversations with appropriate self-disclosure. One option is to ask general open-ended questions about use of the Internet. It is important to keep in mind that cyberspace media experiences are as fraught with social interactions and emotions as face-to-face experiences (Thomas, 2007).

Throughout the assessment it is essential to remember that some teens use the media as a way to consider possible courses of action when interacting with peers and adults (Lloyd, 2002). Practitioners can use discussions about media to assist with teen decisions about how to behave in a real-life setting. On the other hand, teens without this kind of guidance may be at risk for making choices that lead to trouble outside of the world of television and movies.

Case Study and Clinical Application

In the previous sections we discussed how the media serve a normative function for teens. In addition, studies show that adolescents tend to think that other peers, especially those who are not friends, will be more affected by the media than themselves (Scharrer & Leone, 2006). These are concepts to consider when assessing media influences. The following case example provides an opportunity to examine how media influences the life of one adolescent girl. We encourage you to apply the content presented thus far as a means to assess her. The intervention section that follows will assist you in considering how you might work with the adolescent and her family. Questions posted at the end of the intervention section provide an opportunity for you to apply the content on media.

Marie is a 14-year-old Latina girl who lives with her father, stepmother, and two younger half-siblings, John, age 8, and Jonas, age 7. Marie's mother died from cancer when she was 3 years old and her father remarried when Marie was 5 years old. Marie and her stepmother have gotten along very well and Marie considers her as her "real mom" since she barely remembers her biological mother. However, in the past year Marie has become distant from both of her parents and family arguments occur on a regular basis as Marie asks to do things that her parents think are too grown up for her. For example, Marie wanted to take the train into the nearby city to go shopping with her friends and then to a movie. Her parents told her she can go to the local mall with her friends, but they don't think she is ready to take the 40-minute train ride into the city without an adult. Both of Marie's parents work and with the two younger boys they can't chaperone Marie and her friends on an event into the city. None of Marie's friends' parents have the time to do this either, but are willing to let their daughters go to the city on their own. As a result, Marie has been left out of many of these weekend activities with her peers.

At school these same peers are calling her a "baby" because she is not allowed to accompany them to the city. Recently, these same peers have encouraged other girls to make fun of Marie as well. Marie has not told her parents about this. Instead, after school and on weekends Marie sulks around the house spending most of her time in her room surfing the Internet, reading fashion magazines, watching her favorite DVDs, and listening to music. Since she is spending less time with her friends she now has time to surf the Internet. She's been inspired by some of the websites mentioned in her fashion magazine. There are two websites she visits every day, one with information about how to have a body like a supermodel and another that gives tips on how to get and keep a man. Each of these websites have interactive blogs and Marie has been conversing with college-age girls and brags about her older girlfriends at school as a way to make her peers jealous.

Marie's parents are *not* aware of these new sites she is visiting, but they accept her sulking and isolation in her room as part of adolescence. However, they begin to worry when Marie's usual B-plus average drops to C and they are called by the school social worker because of the way Marie is dressing and acting toward boys at school. On the day they are at school to meet with the social worker, Marie passes out after lunch during her gym class. She is in the nurse's office when her parents arrive. Her parents are shocked to see that Marie is not wearing the same shirt, sweater, and jeans that she had on when she left the house that morning. Instead, she has on a tightly fitted tank top that exposes her breasts and belly, and a short skirt. They are not sure where she acquired the outfit and this adds to the other concerns raised by the social worker.

Clinical Interventions for Media Influences on Adolescents

Building interventions that include peers and family is important because they have the power to mediate media effects on youth like Marie (Austin, 1993; Collins et al., 2003; Kaiser Family Foundation, 2002, as cited in Collins et al., 2004; L'Engle et al., 2006). Additionally, Currie's (1997) study suggests that teens can assess media messages from a logical, critical vantage point. However, she also notes that when teens are exposed to media that is beyond their developmental experiences and that media fosters ideological images such as motherhood and marriage, then the teen's critical thinking and logic flounder.

In light of the evidence just discussed, interventions that promote discussion among peers to unpack the messages of the media are indicted. Peer group critiques of the messages in advertising can be a positive way to begin since these media may be less personal to teens than music, television characters, and Internet communications. Existential-oriented interventions (Frankl, 1969; Walsh & Lantz, 2007) allow for critique, exploration of messages, and the development of choices based on new meanings. Some teens will like the idea of being smarter than the advertisements and then be willing to use this to critique the messages in other media sources beyond advertisements. Interventions based on existential or meaning-making approaches are supported by theories such as symbolic interaction (Heise & Weir, 1999; Mead, 1934; Spencer, 1999). These peer group critiques do not have to take place in formal clinical settings. In fact, school social workers and counselors are in a unique position to collaborate with teachers to create and facilitate classroom projects and discussions that foster this kind of critique. Given the propensity for today's teens to be enamored with technology, classroom discussions and projects can be enhanced with blogging. Projects and related discussions can be furthered through the use of cell phone cameras such that teens, teachers, and school social workers and counselors can take digital photos of local billboards and send them to a shared Internet site for critique and discussion. Additionally, Twittering among the teens, teacher, and school social worker or counselor can be used to alert others to the location of local billboards or to the channel for a television program or advertisement they want to critique.

Another intervention with a focus on peer-to-peer influences is the development of opinion leaders, also known as peer educators and natural helpers (Valente & Pumpuang, 2007). The use of opinion leaders to promote positive behavior arises out of public health work aimed at enhancing communitywide health behaviors, such as antismoking campaigns. Teens have been enlisted as opinion leaders in schoolwide prevention and intervention strategies (Valente & Pumpuang). Given the relative influence of peers over parents and that teens share access and knowledge of teen-oriented media, selection of the *right* teens to promote awareness of media influences in the lives of their peers may be useful. Selecting opinion leaders is challenging. First, those selected need to be teens "who influence the opinions, attitudes, beliefs, motivations, and behaviors of others" within their age group (p. 881). Opinion leaders need to be viewed as credible in the eyes of their peers. For example, Valente and Pumpuang note that problems arise when opinion leaders are not accepted by their peers either because they represent an unattainable social group or they represent an unfavorable social group. Among adolescents, this could be a problem even if opinion leaders are selected as opposed to volunteering. For example, if they are chosen by adults, such as teachers, then it's possible that their peers will view them as suspect to being teachers' pets and not *want* to have anything in common with them. If opinion leaders are selected by peer voting, then the role may be viewed as the result of a popularity contest, similar to prom dignitaries, and their peers will view them as figureheads without anything real to say.

Valente and Pumpuang (2007) provide in-depth details about 10 methods for selecting opinion leaders and the advantages and disadvantages of each method. Three of those methods, self-selection, self-identification, and staff selection, are most feasible for adolescent populations. However, each has some of the disadvantages noted above. Given the cliqueish nature of teenagers, it's possible that different opinion leaders representing different groups may need to be identified. Practitioners need to keep these points in mind as they facilitate the selection of opinion leaders.

While the intervention suggestions noted above are based in theoretical and empirical evidence, a note of caution is in order. Developing interventions aimed at group activities among peers can have negative effects if the peers are known for regular participation in high-risk behaviors. Dishion and his colleagues (Dishion, McCord, & Poulin, 1999; Dishion & Owen, 2002) provide evidence for this caution. They "suggest that social interactions among adolescents with a history of risky behavior—even in the presence of trained moderators—can have the unfavorable effect of creating a kind of 'deviancy training' producing, in some circumstances, short-term and long-term increases in risky behavior (Dishion et al., 1999; Dishion, Poulin, & Burraston, 2001, as cited in David, Cappella, & Fishbein, 2006, p. 120). In light of this, practitioners need to train peer group opinion leaders to be aware of peer comments that suggest an interest in risky behaviors. In addition to training, practitioners need to be available as an occasional cofacilitator with peer opinion leaders.

Behavioral techniques that integrate the use of popular movies and television shows as a means for behavioral rehearsal and decision making is another option for intervention. Literature that theorizes about (1) "parasocial" relationships via the media (Giles, 2002), and (2) behavior rehearsal through the media (Llyod, 2002) provide conceptual evidence for this kind of intervention. However, behavioral interventions need to enlist teens as experts in their values so that the practitioner is not viewed as teaching a particular brand of morality. Teens are apt to reject such stances. Given this, teens may best be served when practitioners serve as facilitators for peer-to-peer helping networks that focus on debunking television myths about adolescent life. One way to accomplish this is by creating parodies of television shows to demonstrate what really happens when teens make uninformed choices like the ones they see in the shows. Interventions such as this can enlist the cooperation of high school drama or art teachers to develop teen workgroups as part of their classroom teaching.

Interventions that include parents, older siblings, or aunts and uncles are also useful when it comes to media influences. Facilitating this type of intervention requires assessment of parent–adolescent and older sibling–adolescent relationships. In discussions with the parents or other family members, the practitioner listens for their openness to discussing some of the issues that arise for teens as a result of viewing different kinds of media. For example, some parents and family members are more approachable than others when it comes to their adolescent children asking them about sexuality and body image. Given the strains that occur between parents and their adolescents, the choice of trusted older siblings, aunts, or uncles may be more fruitful in this type of intervention. It may be desirable for practitioners to assist families in facilitating these discussions. However, caution is in order because all families have particular values about sexuality, images of women and men, and food-related issues. Often, teens are at odds with their parents in regard to these values. Therefore, practitioners need to be aware of the family's values and keep from being viewed as taking the side of either parents or teens in these potential values conflicts.

QUESTIONS FOR THE REFLECTIVE PRACTITIONER

1. Describe the psychological and behavior factors that might be playing a role in Marie's current issues. What information from the case study provides clues to these factors?

2. Describe the recent family and peer events in Marie's life that might be a factor in her current behavior at school and at home.

3. Marie's interaction with the media has increased as her time with her peers has become limited. How might her current behavior be influenced by the media she has been accessing?

4. What questions should the practitioner ask Marie to find out if her actions and issues are influenced by the media? Given the proclivity for teens to assume that others are more influenced by the media than they are themselves, what might be the best way to word these questions?

5. Several intervention strategies (family discussions, use of opinion leaders, and peer group projects that critique the media) and ideas for implementing them were discussed in this chapter. Based on the issues confronting Marie, which do you think will be the most useful and why?

6. Recall the types of media you interacted with as an adolescent. What messages do you recall in those media sources? Did you talk with your parents and family about them and why or why not?

7. Recall some of your most liked and disliked television characters when you were a teen. What did you like and dislike about them? Do you recall making any choices about how you wanted to act in the present or future as a result of those characters?

8. Explore the current media (music, television, magazines, and Internet sites) that are aimed at an adolescent audience. Become conversant with them so you can understand some of what your teenage clients describe to you when you conduct a media diet assessment (L'Engle et al., 2006).

Chapter Summary

This chapter focused on the influences of the media on adolescents, especially how it can affect identity, body image, and ideas about and intentions for sexuality. Research shows that media and peers tend to have a greater influence on teens' perceptions than their parents. However, it is also clear that if parents and other trusted adults are approachable, at least some adolescents will approach them with questions that result from these media influences. Additionally, cyberspace communities represent opportunities for teens to try out different identities in ways that are not allowed with non-interactive media, such as television and DVDs. Given the instantaneous communication allowed in cyberspace, teens are not able to rehearse these identities before presenting them to the public. This is riskier than when they imagine how they might act similar to or different from the characters in their favorite television shows or movies, before presenting those actions in public. The theory and research discussed in this chapter suggest that practitioners focus on the media as an area of assessment in their clinical practice with adolescents. Suggestions for assessment of media influences and possible modalities for intervention were provided.

The next chapter provides a review of protective and risk factors at each ecological level. You will meet Marta, a 14-year-old, and see how the authors would apply the M-E approach for assessment and intervention with Marta and her family.

CHAPTER 9

Assessment and Intervention at Each Ecological Level

A CASE ILLUSTRATION

Julie Anne Laser, Nicole Nicotera, Tom Luster,
and Douglas Davies

Chapter Overview

Throughout the previous chapters, you were challenged to apply the protective and risk factors for assessment and intervention at each level of the ecological model. This chapter allows you to learn how the authors apply the M-E approach to one adolescent. This is an opportunity for you to assess the skills and knowledge you've gained thus far, by comparing how you applied the content of the previous chapters to other case examples to how the authors assess and intervene in this case. Practitioners' capacity to assess and intervene at each level of the ecological model is imperative as Deutsch (2008) points out:

> Adolescents are in the process of exploring who they are, of envisioning and building a place for themselves in adult society. . . . And they are doing so within multiple, overlapping social environments . . . teens interact within and across an increasing number of contexts, from home to school to neighborhood to cyberspace. Yet too often portraits of adolescence . . . overlook the nuanced ways in which development is intimately tied to the interaction of individual youth with particular people within specific social contexts. (pp. 2–3)

146

Background Information

Marta is a 14-year-old African American girl and in the ninth grade. She is average height and weight for her age, but appears more muscular than some of the girls her age because of her longtime participation in sports. She is the only child of two working parents. Her mother is a librarian and her father is a civil engineer with a private firm in the city where the family resides. Marta has excellent scholastic skills and gets along well with her teachers and peers at school. She is respected by both the "jocks" and the "brains" at her school. She has many friends at school in all social groups. She is frequently invited to the mall to "hang out" with friends. Marta hopes to attend a prestigious university and knows that she will have to be outstanding in all academic and extracurricular aspects to be accepted. She holds high expectations for herself, as do her parents. However, when she does poorly on an exam, does not uphold her usual time when running in track meets, or loses tennis competitions she is self-critical.

Given her positive history of academic, social, and athletic skills, the school social worker is surprised when her mother calls to share the following concerns: (1) Marta is not associating with any same-age peers in the neighborhood, nor is she inviting them over to the house like she used to in the past, and (2) she prefers to watch television, listen to music, play games on the computer, and instant message or share Facebook with friends, some of whom her parents have not met. Her parents banned television, music, the computer, and cell phone use on the weekends in an effort to get Marta to have face-to-face interactions with them and with peers. Since that time she is sullen, lethargic with chores, and has been talking back to her parents.

Due to their long workdays, her parents have minimal contact with the school. They are aware of her grades, but infrequently attend school conferences or events such as Marta's track meets or tennis competitions. This is a change from when Marta was in elementary school where her mother was the school librarian. However, since she took a full-time job at the local public library, she does not have the flexibility to be involved in Marta's high school activities. Marta's father works long hours in order to meet the high demands of his firm and is almost always unavailable to attend events except on weekends. He has been made a partner in the firm and just received a large raise, which they used to help pay for their gorgeous new home.

Marta's parents are worried that she may be depressed or that her behavior could be a sign of adolescent rebellion. Marta's mother calls the social worker and explains that she did not act this way before they relocated to the new neighborhood about a year and a half ago, but that was also before she had entered puberty. Marta's mother tells the social worker that they purchased the new home to have more living space, to have a place where Marta could entertain her friends, and to be closer to their workplaces. Marta now takes the school bus to and from school each day instead of walking like she did in the past. Moving was a big decision for the family because in their old neighborhood they lived near many extended family members and longtime friends, who they considered to be part of their family as well. The mother reports that Marta tells them she prefers to stay in the house because it feels safer and not so boring. When they encourage her to invite friends and cousins over to the house she refuses and stomps off to her room. Her behavior baffles them. They thought the new home would bring them all joy.

Assessment of Protective and Risk Factors for Marta

Internal Risk and Protective Factors

Marta is blessed with internal protective factors that include good cognitive ability, good athletic ability, appropriate physical development, good social skills, good ability to make and keep friends, and high expectations for self. During the assessment phase with Marta the practitioner will want to make a determination of Marta's self-awareness of these strengths. Posing questions such as "What things do you like about yourself?" and "What school activities do you think you do best?" will allow the practitioner to assess Marta's verbal and nonverbal responses to being asked to describe her strengths. Conversely, there are a few risk factors that may undermine Marta that include being overly self-critical, needing perfectionism, and possible depression. Assessment of these internal factors may be a challenge since many teens are reticent to admit to strengths for fear of sounding conceited. They may not have the words to describe internal characteristics such as perfectionism. Therefore, the draw-a-person technique (Merrell, 2003) may be useful for assessment of Marta's internal risk factors as well as her strengths. This strategy allows the client to be at a psychological distance from self while describing both challenges and protective factors.

Family Protective and Risk Factors

Marta's parents care about and are invested in her. They have high hopes for her future. Their support, authoritative parenting, and high expectations for achievement have resulted in Marta's competent functioning in school, athletics, and with peers. However, the recent move to a new community has been difficult for Marta. Marta's sense of isolation calls attention to the loss of a rich extended family and community support system in their old neighborhood. The parents' intense involvement in their careers is a risk factor because Marta needs them more now. She is not able (or not willing) to articulate this, and her parents, while they suspect that the move has been stressful for her, do not give clear evidence that they understand its impact, nor that they need to provide her with more support. The change in environment creates a loss of stability for Marta during a developmental transition—early adolescence—when secure attachment and family stability is particularly important.

In African American families and communities, support for children comes not only from parents but also from a network of other caregivers, including grandparents, other blood relatives, fictive kin, and friends (Hatchett & Jackson, 1999). This was Marta's experience during her childhood. Now as a young adolescent she is living in a nuclear family apparently isolated from other caregivers. It may be that neither Marta nor her parents were aware how much her previous environment acted supportively *in loco parentis.* Did extended family and neighborhood cohesion mask compromised family cohesion, or, more likely, were nuclear family and extended family experienced as a gestalt, which is now fragmented because extended family is missing from Marta's daily life?

It seems clear that Marta is reacting to the loss of daily contact with extended family and her familiar childhood neighborhood. Yet Marta's mother does not seem to have put this together, and asks the school social worker for insight. Her parents are concerned about her current negativity. At the same time, since her distress "baffles" them, one wonders if they are out of touch with how she currently feels and thinks. Have the parents asked Marta how she feels about her new environment? Were her opinions about the move solicited in advance?

Marta is signaling her distress in a number of ways, and her parents want to understand her. However, teen and parents seem to be missing each other, rather than communicating directly. Marta's withdrawal from her parents raises the question of whether she is angry with them for moving but unable to express this directly. Her parents have given her a great deal, both in terms of encouragement and material advantages. It may seem ungrateful to her to directly oppose them. It will be important to ask Marta's parents how they interpret her current behavior. It will also be useful to ask how conflict is handled within the family, and to find out whether Marta has a model for speaking her mind when she is upset with her parents.

Marta expresses her feelings with withdrawal, sullenness, and talking back about small issues and this confuses her parents. They respond with coercive measures—banning her from using media—punishing behavior rather than looking at its potential sources. Marta's behavior is common in early adolescence. However, it could be a sign that she is trying to cope with a real loss, as opposed to "going through a phase" in development. There is a risk that Marta and her parents will get stuck in mutual misunderstanding of a problem that has been building for 1½ years.

That this is an African American family may be a significant issue. Positive racial socialization is a protective factor for African American youth (McAdoo, 2001). Given Marta's parents' high levels of achievement it seems likely that they have encouraged her to view her racial identity positively, but also have conveyed that as an African American she will have to work extra hard to succeed in a racist society. It is likely that Marta has internalized positive identifications with her parents on the dimension of striving to succeed. In her previous community, Marta must have received a lot of recognition as both a successful person and a successful African American. Although the case material does not describe the racial composition of her new neighborhood, general U.S. demographics suggest that primarily white professional families populate affluent suburbs with "gorgeous" houses. If this holds true for Marta's new neighborhood, what might it mean to Marta that her parents have chosen to move from a community where one's accomplishments have a positive racial valence to one where others do not validate self-esteem based in part on being a successful African American? Given Marta's apparent alienation from her current community, it is as if she has moved into a new culture, not just a new neighborhood.

The family's previous means of providing cohesion and support for Marta was through a network of extended family and familylike caregivers. Now Marta and her parents face a crisis of adaptation that they did not anticipate. The parents may be less aware of how difficult this transition has been for Marta because their individual lives continue to be organized around their work. From this perspective, it is a good sign that the school social worker was surprised to hear the mother's concerns. Apparently, Marta continues to do well in school, suggesting that school is a source of continuity for her, just as her parents' work is for them.

The practitioner should emphasize Marta's reactions to the loss of community and suggest that her parents help her to make connections in the new neighborhood. However, their encouragement will be resisted until they can initiate open conversation with Marta about what the move has meant to her. Clearly, Marta's behaviorally expressed resentment and her parents' coercive reactions are transforming Marta's internal responses to loss and dislocation into a relationship problem with her parents.

School Protective and Risk Factors

Marta's school microsystem is filled with protective factors. She is a good student, gets good grades, and gets along with all students. School is a happy place for Marta. Her only risk in this microsystem is that there is minimal interface between the school and the family microsystem. Even though Marta appears to be successful at school on many levels, it is still important for the practitioner to assess her school experiences. Since school seems to be one of the environments in which she excels, Marta may feel most comfortable talking about it. The practitioner can use this comfort level as a means to join with her in a strengths assessment. Assessment of parent involvement from Marta's perspective is important since many teens are relieved if their parents appear to be less involved in their school lives, even though their involvement remains as important as in middle childhood. Empathy for the parents' working hours will also be important in this part of the assessment so that the practitioner can join with them in order to use the relationship to encourage more involvement in school as needed.

Neighborhood Protective and Risk Factors

Neighborhood-level protective factors include collective efficacy and social cohesion, low crime rates, and higher rates of affluent residents. On the other hand, neighborhood-level risk factors include high crime rates, access to drugs and weapons, high population density, high rates of residential mobility, deteriorated properties, absence of social cohesion, and diminished attachment to the neighborhood (Jensen & Fraser, 2006). Chapter 7 stresses the importance of assessing for neighborhood social cohesion, which promotes social trust and cooperation, neighborhood collective socialization or norms for behavior, and neighborhood social disorganization, which influences social cohesion and collective socialization.

The practitioner asks Marta to describe her old neighborhood and new neighborhood so he can *listen for* the neighborhood protective and risk factors just noted. The reason he *listens for*, as opposed to asking directly, is that neighborhood protective and risk factors are full of jargon that is unfamiliar to most individuals, especially teenagers. Marta reports that she misses her old neighborhood because she lived there since she was born and had many relatives and neighbors nearby. After school she would often stop at her grandmother's home to say hello and sometimes she would see her cousins there and become involved in the spontaneous games or activities that tend to erupt when a group of similar age young people get together. There was also a small library and group of shops about three blocks from her old neighborhood. She knew the shopkeepers as well as the librarian, who often told her about new books that had arrived. She liked to run errands for her grandmother and get groceries for some of the older adults in her neighborhood to earn spending money. She also used to babysit her younger cousins who live in the neighborhood and misses doing that. She reports that she always felt safe in her old neighborhood because there were so many people she knew, so many kids to hang out with, and she liked being able to go to the library or the shops on her own. In comparison, she does not know any of the other teens in her new neighborhood. She says, "People have beautiful yards and flower gardens, but don't spend time in them." She reports that neighbors wave and smile, but they drive their cars into their garages and then she doesn't see them. She says, "There don't seem to be any other girls or boys my age in the neighborhood, everyone seems to have little kids or no kids at all." She also tells the practitioner, "There are no shops or other places that are close enough to walk to, Mom or Dad has to drive me everywhere I want to go. Once I get home from school there is really nothing to do, but watch TV, play on the computer, or listen to music. My parents tell me to invite my cousins and friends from school over to the house, but I am sure they won't want to come here, it's so boring!"

The practitioner needs to assess the cultural environment of Marta's old neighborhood and her new neighborhood. It's possible that Marta's old neighborhood had a higher percentage of African Americans in it, at least by way of her extended family that live there. While her new neighborhood may be culturally similar to her old one, if she has moved to an area where there are more white people than she was previously used to, she may be experiencing racism there. Hence the comment that cousins and friends from her old neighborhood will be bored if they visit her new home.

Media Protective and Risk Factors

You will recall from Chapter 8 that teenagers in the United States spend about 6 to 7 hours each day interacting with various media sources (Roberts et al., 2004 as cited in L'Engle et al., 2006). Therefore, the amount of time Marta spends accessing the different media her parents describe is not out of line with other teens. However, you will remember that assessing the content of the media, or the teen's "media diet," is important. Additionally, Marta's focus on the media, combined with the other internal and social challenges that her parents report is cause for assessment of her "media diet" (L'Engle et al., 2006). Using the content of Chapter 8 we know we need to assess for (1) the types of media Marta uses, (2) if she is developing virtual friendships and identities in cyberspace, (3) the content of the media she accesses (e.g., images of women and sex and sexuality), and (4) her virtual relationships to any media stars (e.g., actors, musicians).

During assessment, Marta is open and excited to talk about the new Internet sites she's discovered since she is spending so much more time alone. She tells you she found a site that is completely for girls who want to learn the ins and outs of dating boys and the kinds of fashions that are "sure to get a girl a date." She says, "Sometimes that site has guest bloggers such as the stars from a favorite television show and also a new favorite girl band." She reports that she hopes to keep running track and playing tennis but maybe will go on a diet so she can fit into the fashions she sees on the site that will attract boys. She reports that while her cousins and friends at school have experimented with kissing boys, she has not, but she hopes to now that she is learning how to attract them.

Modes of Intervention for Working with Marta

Interventions for Internal, Psychological, Social, and Emotional Concerns

In general, Marta has many positive outcomes to look forward to in her life. Because she has excellent cognitive and athletic skills, she is able to create plans to be highly successful in her future. However, "putting the bar so high" also increases her fear of failure and lack of self-tolerance of any failure or setback. If Marta is able to see only one path for being successful and any imperfections in herself undermine her continuing on that path, it causes a great deal of inner stress. The practitioner should point out that many paths can lead to her goals. This may be done simplistically by asking Marta to draw a picture of where she is now, where she would like to be in the future, and then discuss the multiple paths to get to those goals.

The practitioner should bring up the idea that "No one is good at everything, and that is OK!" Highly motivated girls are often unwilling to consider that some imperfections are normal and that no one achieves perfection in all spheres of his or her life. A positive byproduct of the women's movement is that girls believe that they can do it all, but the pressure for excellence in all areas is sometimes extreme. Girls need to learn how to prioritize what is most important for their future and then decide on the steps of getting there.

Additionally, Marta should be assessed for depression with a depression inventory, such as the Beck's Depression Inventory. Depression should be ruled out even though Marta's behavior and circumstances seem more in line with stress due to perfectionism and unhappiness over the move.

Interventions for Family Concerns

The practitioner can be optimistic that a short-term intervention would be effective because of Marta's and her parents' high levels of functioning. Given the apparent absence of a history of individual psychopathology or significant relationship difficulties the practitioner may be able to apply a problem-solving approach focused on helping Marta's parents understand her perspective. Separate sessions with Marta and the parents would be a beneficial way to begin. Then these separate sessions can be followed with some family sessions. Interventions should focus on trying, in a nonjudgmental manner, to help the parents see Marta's view of the changes in her life, and to rally them to provide empathy, understanding, and increased support. A major concern is that the parents do not seem to understand why Marta is distressed. If they can convey that they understand why moving to a new community has been difficult for her, this will help repair the relationship and reduce the family conflicts. Further, it will help Marta experience her parents as being on her side, and help her disengage from her current oppositional struggle with them.

Specific interventions with the parents include the following:

• Frame the central issue and ask the parents to consider it, with an opening statement like the following:

> "Marta seems to have been thrown off by moving away from people and a community she had always known and where she felt supported. In the long run, the move hopefully will turn out to be a good thing, but up to now she feels it's more of a loss than a gain. I got the impression she doesn't want to disappoint you. But she's showing you she's unhappy with her moods and behavior, and that is affecting her relationship with you. I don't believe she wants that, but she seems stuck in the problem. I have some ideas about what you can do to help her."

• Encourage them to explore possible differences between their goals and Marta's needs. The move to a new community may symbolize for the parents their own success and competence, and should be a source of pride. They have worked hard to provide their daughter with a materially secure life that may or may not have been part of their experiences growing up. But for Marta the move symbolizes loss of community. To help the parents think about Marta's perspective, it would be helpful to ask them to reflect on their own adjustment to the new community. Have they made friends? Do they interact regularly with neighbors? Are there ways in which they miss their old neighborhood? Their responses to these inquiries might help them better appreciate Marta's sense of isolation. In the context of this discussion, Marta's increased use of media and cell phone could be reframed not just as typical adolescent behavior, but as an attempt to remain connected with friends, and, metaphorically, to recreate a sense of community that she feels she's lost.

• Encourage the parents to imagine Marta's experience of the transition from her old neighborhood. Does she miss spending time with her cousins and longtime friends? Who and what does she miss? How does she feel as she rides the school bus from and to her new home? What does she experience on the bus? Has she held herself aloof? Has she been ignored or teased, seen as an oddity because of her race, or taunted with racist remarks? Does she identify with people she sees in the new neighborhood? When she arrives home is she alone until her parents come home from work? Does she feel at loose ends or lonely and compensate with media involvement? Is her media focus on the weekends an extension of her week-day habits? Her parents want her to connect with peers in the new neigh-borhood, but how have teens there responded to her? Has she received invitations from them?

- Perhaps Marta's parents could identify with Marta's situation if they reflected on their experiences as African Americans negotiating a pre-dominately white professional world. What have they had to learn to do that successfully? How have they coped with coworkers' and bosses' percep-tions and misperceptions of them? By analogy, what challenges is Marta facing in her new community, especially in terms of peer relationships? Marta's parents probably have a lot to teach her about how to function well as a minority person in a majority community.

Following these parent sessions aimed at helping the parents develop insight into Marta's perspective, we would shift to family sessions in which parents and adolescent would be guided to share perspectives, improve communication, and repair their relationships.

Interventions for School Concerns

The school microsystem is an area of success for Marta. There are few changes that need to be made in this venue. The only area that could use improvement is better parent–school interface. Perhaps the school could offer more flexible hours for parent–teacher conferences. Marta's parents could also ask their respective employers to flex their work, so that they could attend school conferences and sports events.

Interventions for Neighborhood Concerns

Marta is suffering from a change in residence that has taken her away from longtime friends and a supportive extended family network. This move has also decreased the amount of independence and sense of responsibil-ity she had in her old neighborhood. These changes have come during adolescence, a time when most young people crave greater independence and a sense of being viewed as a contributing member of the family and community.

The practitioner should work with Marta, her parents, and the school to explore ways in which Marta can continue to grow in skills for independence as well as ensure the continued support from extended family members in her old neighborhood. For example, since there are many young children in the current neighborhood and Marta has the skills and is interested in babysitting she is in a prime position to babysit for neighbors. This will also allow her to earn spending money like she did in her old neighborhood. The key for the practitioner is ensuring that Marta and her parents are in agreement with this idea before beginning the steps to make it happen. Additionally, the practitioner will work with Marta's parents to make sure they are acquainted with the neighbors who will need to get to know her as a trusted young woman before they'll want her to babysit. Marta will also need guidance in getting testimonials from the aunts and uncles she has babysat for and also in coming up with a reasonable fee. This intervention can assist Marta in regaining some sense of independence and responsibility in her community. The practitioner's role in this intervention is to serve as coach and advisor to the family so they can put a plan into action. Coaching and advising is important in this intervention so that the family develops a plan that is congruent with their values and aspirations for Marta.

In addition, the practitioner needs to work with Marta and her parents to ensure that she stays connected to her longtime friends and extended family. For example, there may be some days of the week when Marta can walk with her cousins and friends from school to the old neighborhood and be picked up by mom or dad after work. They might make this a Friday event so she can spend the night with her grandmother or other relatives. This second option will allow her parents not to feel rushed to get her after their work days and also give them a chance to have their own time as couple. The practitioner serves in the role of facilitator of family discussions about how to build a plan that allows Marta to stay connected to these important social and emotional resources. In this role, the practitioner may assist in resolving conflicts that occur between Marta and her parents or between the parents as a couple as they develop a plan to support Marta's needs that fits with the family's other needs.

Interventions for Media Concerns

Marta has turned to the media to fill the void left by the loss of consistent contact with relatives and friends in her old neighborhood. The first line of intervention is for the practitioner to gain a better understanding of Marta's values about being a young woman, what it means to attract and kiss boys, and the broader social context around fashion and the kinds of statements it can make about her. Additionally, the practitioner needs to learn about the messages Marta is getting from the media. Some of these messages may not be in line with her parents' values and aspirations for her. Therefore, the next line of intervention is for the practitioner to facilitate a family conversation about the media that Marta is excited about. First, the practitioner facilitates a conversation between Marta and her parents so she can share the hopes and aspirations she is gaining from the messages in the media (e.g., to run more track so she can fit into fashions that will attract boys she can kiss). The practitioner may also need to meet with the parents to talk about typical teenage development and impress upon them the importance of family conversations about values related to Marta's exploration of being attracted to boys and wanting to kiss them.

The practitioner needs to encourage the parents to stay involved in Marta's life and her choices now as opposed to waiting until she does something that is unacceptable to the family. If Marta is willing, the practitioner may want to have her introduce her parents to the sites she is visiting during a session. Depending on the parents' reactions to this, the practitioner may need to coach them in accepting that Marta is maturing and in setting limits that are in line with their values, but that keep them connected to her. Additionally, the practitioner will want to assure the parents that Marta's interests are part of regular development that they will want to be present for so they can monitor her and help her learn to make healthy choices. Finally, since Marta has close ties with her extended family, there may be an older cousin who her parents trust who may serve as mentor for Marta as she navigates this new territory in her identity development. The practitioner's role is to serve as a facilitator to help the family arrive at a plan that is consonant with their values and needs as Marta matures.

QUESTIONS FOR THE REFLECTIVE PRACTITIONER

1. Describe the internal protective and risk factors that play a role in Marta's current issues. What information from the case study provides clues to these factors? Propose an intervention for Marta at the internal level and describe how you would implement it.

2. Describe the family protective and risk factors in Marta's life that play a role in her current behavior at school and at home. What information from the case study provides clues to these factors? Propose an intervention for Marta at the family level and describe how you would implement it.

3. Marta's interactions and behavior in school suggest many protective factors. What are these factors? What steps would you take to verify these protective factors? What risk factors could be present and how would you assess for them? If an intervention at the school level becomes necessary, what would you do? How would you implement it?

4. What questions should the practitioner ask Marta to find out whether her actions and issues are influenced by neighborhood-level protective and risk factors? According to the case illustration what are the protective and risk factors in Marta's old neighborhood and in her new neighborhood?

5. What role does the Internet play in Marta's current concerns? What protective and risk factors does the Internet pose for her? How would you assess for these and what kind of intervention might be warranted at this time?

6. Work with a group of your peers to create a role play in which one of you plays the role of the practitioner and interviews Marta and her parents about the details in the case illustration. Engage the "family" in creating an ecomap to display the multiple systems that influence Marta and her family. Be sure to note which aspects of the ecomap represent protective factors and which aspects represent risk factors. Have another peer observe the role play and keep track of the spontaneous questions the "practitioner" uses in the interview. When the interview is complete discuss the process with your peers and consider how you can apply this multisystemic, ecological approach in your practice. See Table 9.1 for a summary of the areas for assessment and intervention.

Chapter Summary

This chapter provided a case example and the manner in which the authors would proceed with assessment and intervention at the varying levels of the ecological model. You are encouraged to compare how you applied the content of Chapters 1–8 to how the authors applied it to Marta in this chapter. Given that each adolescent client and his or her family will present with varying regional and cultural differences, practitioners are cautioned to remember that assessment and intervention methods must be tailored to fit the needs and specific cultural backgrounds of the teens and families they serve. The next chapter presents the role of protective and risk factors in the onset and progression of substance abuse.

TABLE 9.1. Multisystemic Ecological Levels for Assessment and Intervention

Ecological level	Description of areas for assessment and intervention
Micro-Settings:	
Do relationships provide these four types of support?	*Instrumental:* sharing, helping, and other forms of prosocial behavior.
	Esteem: statements of actions that convince people of their own worth or value.
	Informational: advice giving or guidance helpful in coping with problems.
	Companionship: a sense of belonging through shared activities (Tietjen, 1989).
Meso-Settings:	
Do relationships allow for the development of these?	*Mutual trust* between the adolescent, his or her parents, and other members of the community.
	Accurate information about the adolescent and his or her family.
	Bidirectional communication between the adolescent, his or her parents, and other members of the community (e.g., teachers, coaches, parents of peers).
	Goal consensus or agreement between the adolescent, his or her parents, and other members of the community about his or her current and future goals.
	An evolving balance of power in favor of the adolescent such that he or she takes on more initiative and self-direction as he or she demonstrates the maturity to do so (Bronfenbrenner, 1979).
Exo-Settings:	
Does the adolescent client have access, through a parent or other advocate, to sites of economic, political, and social power?	How does the adolescent client and his or her family or others in his or her life interface with the formal and informal systems of society such as employment, education, city governments, school boards, parent–teacher associations, local organizations, and informal clubs.
Macro settings:	
What kinds of macro blueprints shape the adolescent's life experiences?	Assess the social, political, and economic structures in society that can produce inequality related to social class, skin color, ethnicity, gender, ability, sexual orientation, religion, and age. How is the adolescent and his or her family impacted by these structures?
Element of time	Assess for the critical events (positive, negative, and neutral) that are unique to the adolescent and his or her family.

PART III

CLINICAL INTERVENTIONS FOR PROBLEMATIC ADOLESCENT BEHAVIOR

CHAPTER 10

Substance Abuse

Julie Anne Laser, George Stuart Leibowitz, and Nicole Nicotera

Chapter Overview

This chapter utilizes a protective and risk factor framework to understand the onset and progression of adolescent substance abuse (Hawkins et al., 1992; Jessor et al., 1995; Rutter, 1987). The chapter begins with a discussion of the definitions of adolescent substance abuse and the substances most often used by youth. The frequency and severity of substance abuse is reviewed as well as differences in substance abuse between females and males. Additionally, individual and family clinical interventions for addicts are presented. The chapter concludes with a case example and questions.

CASE EXAMPLE:
Who Are the Youth Represented in This Chapter?

The following case example represents some of the concerns related to adolescents and substance abuse. Considering the implications for this case within the context of the risk factors, theory, assessment, and intervention strategies presented in the following pages will prepare you to assess and suggest interventions for the more developed case study at the end of the chapter.

Peter is a 16-year-old European American boy who attends a suburban high school. Peter is a smart student, but often does not work very hard at his studies. He gets mainly B's in school with barely studying. He is popular with both the boys and girls at school. Peter is a great skateboarder and spends a lot of time after school at the skate park. He has visions of competing in the X Games. Recently, Peter has been smoking joints that are given to him at the park. He feels that it makes him calmer and less stressed at trying and completing big tricks. His friend Matt told him that he has become a better boarder by smoking DMT (dimethyltryptamine, a psychedelic drug) before attempting big tricks. Peter wonders if doing more drugs will improve his boarding or just mess him up. He has one friend, Ben, who has done so many drugs that he can hardly speak in coherent sentences. He remembers when Ben was a great boarder; now he is just a stoner.

Defining Substance Abuse

Adolescents who become involved in drugs are a diverse population with a variety of individual characteristics and social experiences. Researchers interested in the assessment, prevention, and treatment of substance use have tried to understand why some youth who experiment with alcohol or marijuana are at increased risk to progress to the use of more serious drugs such as opiates, heroin, OxyCotin, methamphetamine, and "club drugs" (Ecstasy and GHB [gamma-hydroxybutyrate]) and why others will not progress to "hard" drugs and will discontinue drug use after a period of experimentation (Botvin & Griffin, 2007; Petraitis, Flay, & Miller, 1995). Still other youth will become quickly addicted to marijuana or alcohol (Urschel, 2009). It has been suggested that many adolescents who experiment with drugs do not develop dependence on substances into adulthood or become drug addicts (Shedler & Block, 1990). However, approximately 10–15% of American youth will become addicted to substances (Hanson, 2008).

Historically, marijuana was not considered an addictive drug, but it has been found to be extremely addictive and the *addiction cycle*, the time between use where increased cravings and desire for the drug is manifested, may be as long as 42 days (Urschel, 2009). Therefore, addiction to marijuana may not initially be considered since the marijuana addict, unlike the heroin addict, does not need the drug daily. Due to more stringent laws regarding underage purchasing of alcohol and underage serving of alcohol to minors, alcohol is difficult for youth to obtain. However, marijuana is ubiquitous and inexpensive. Additionally, some states have reduced penalties for marijuana possession. Thus, marijuana use is on the rise in the United States with youth.

Marijuana has also been cultivated to be more potent with higher levels of tetrahydrocannabinol (THC), the psychoactive substance in marijuana. Therefore, the drug that the parents of these youth may have experimented with in their adolescence may be 10 times as potent as the drug that they used. Parents who are unaware of the changed potency of marijuana may underestimate the effect on their children.

Developmental Pathways to Substance Abuse

Adolescent substance addiction usually has its onset in late adolescence and early adulthood (Corcoran & Walsh, 2006). Adolescents who begin to experiment with drugs at an early age (prior to age 16) are at increased risk for continued drug-related issues into adulthood (Dishion & Owen, 2002; Hawkins et al., 1992; Rohde, Lewinson, Kahler, Seeley, & Brown, 2001).

From a developmental perspective, adolescence is associated with increased risk taking and experimentation. For some adolescents, experimentation with drugs and/or alcohol is part of the negotiation of transitions between adolescence and adulthood (Shedler & Block, 1990). These transitions include cognitive shifts about self, identity, sexuality, future orientation, changes in parental relationships, and increased peer group involvement (Schulenberg, Maggs, Steinman, & Zucker, 2001). In the United States, media and popular culture messages about drinking and smoking often spur experimentation with alcohol and tobacco in early to middle adolescence (Botvin & Griffin, 2007). Some adolescents may become a member of a drug subculture to find acceptance and social connection. However, a significant proportion of youth are at risk to become regular drug users, and will increase their use of a particular drug or across several drugs, and develop severe substance abuse problems (Botvin & Griffin, 2007; Kilpatrick, Acierno, Resnick, Saunders, & Best, 1997).

Gender Differences

There are different pathways to abuse for females compared with males. Generally girls/young woman progress to addiction quicker, and suffer more severe consequences from drug abuse compared with males (Harvard Mental Health Letter, 2010). Moreover, treatment programs developed without regard for gender fail to influence the trajectory of substance abuse (Califano, 2003; Molidor, Nissen, & Watkins, 2002). While conduct disorder, propensity for risk taking, ADHD, and depression are related to substance use in males, depression is significantly associated with substance use disorders among females (Whitmore et al., 1997). Girls tend to use substances to reduce stress, ameliorate depression, and improve mood. Females are also more likely to use prescription painkillers, stimulants, and tranquilizers. Males tend to use drugs to enhance social status and for sensation seeking.

Race/Ethnicity

Membership in a racial/ethnic minority group may be a risk factor for substance abuse (Felix-Ortiz, Newcomb, & Myers, 1994). Race-related oppression, trauma, discrimination, value conflicts, and decreased access to opportunities for marginalized groups can result in increased levels of drug and alcohol abuse.

Rates of Adolescent Substance Use

Despite declines in illicit drug use in the 1990s, and the recent decline in methamphetamine abuse, a number of drugs remain steady in their use among adolescents such as marijuana, as previously discussed, alcohol, and prescription drugs. Alcohol use remains prevalent among teenagers, with 72% of students reporting consumption before completing high school (Johnston, O'Malley, Bachman, & Schulenberg, 2008). Raiding the family medicine cabinet and ingesting the pills that are found within is called *pharming.* Sometimes at parties the drugs found in many medicine cabinets are put together in a bowl and then a youth takes a handful, mixing a wide variety of prescription drugs, which can have very dangerous and sometimes fatal results. Additionally, there is substantial use at high schools and college campuses of Ritalin and Adderall (both ADHD medications), which work as a powerful stimulant for those not diagnosed with ADHD.

Clinical Perspectives on Substance Abuse

Adolescent substance abuse is a particularly challenging and complex phenomenon to understand and address in clinical practice. Some clinical settings have determined that the youth first needs to get clean and sober prior to being involved in other types of therapy.

Adolescents who abuse substances often present a range of co-occurring issues: delinquency or involvement with the legal system, propensity for risk taking or sensation seeking, mental health problems such as depression, anxiety, or obsessive–compulsive disorder (OCD), truancy, school suspensions, lack of interest in school, and family problems such as the breakdown of family trust or family support (Howard & Jenson, 1999; Loeber, Farrington, Stouthamer-Loeber, & Van Kammen, 1998; Newcomb & Bentler, 1989; Riggs, 2003; Robins & McEvoy, 1990). Additionally, abused and neglected youth may be at a greater risk for substance abuse as compared to nonabused youth (Wall & Kohl, 2007). Adolescents who have experienced traumatic stress tend to score higher on substance abuse problem measures than nontraumatized youth (Hall et al., 2008).

Protective and Risk Factors Related to Substance Abuse

Developmental studies have produced a significant amount of information regarding specific risks that may increase the likelihood of developing a substance abuse problem, as well as protective factors that may mitigate the onset and course of substance problems and have important implications for recovery (Tarter, 2002).

Internal Protective and Risk Factors Related to Substance Abuse

Behaviors That Put Youth at Risk

There are particular behaviors that make youth more vulnerable to substance abuse. A youth is at greater risk for dependence if he or she binge drinks or began drug use prior to age 16 (Clark, 2004). Youth who have not found school to be a venue where they can be successful due to lack of aptitude, lack of interest in academics, or lack of involvement with school activities are more likely to be involved in substances. Additionally, youth who are sensation seekers or impulsive are at higher risk for substance use (Catalano, Kosterman, Hawkins, Newcomb, & Abbott, 1996; Dishion & Loeber, 1985; Hawkins et al., 1992; Jenson, 2004; Jessor et al., 1995). If the youth has poor coping mechanisms, he or she is more likely to use substances to self-soothe. Similarly, if the youth does not have an *internal locus of control*, the conviction that he or she can control his or her own destiny, the youth may look to external inhibitors of pain or increased pleasure through substances.

MENTAL HEALTH ISSUES

Youth who have been diagnosed with ADHD, bipolar disorder (BPD), conduct disorder (CD), depression, anxiety disorder, or OCD are more likely to use or abuse substances. Adolescents with ADHD are more likely to have co-occurring substance abuse problems. Adolescents with a CD diagnosis were 10 times more likely to have drug abuse histories than adolescents without a CD diagnosis (Kuperman et al., 2001). Youth with adolescent-onset BPD were at greater risk for substance abuse (Wilens et al., 1999). Additionally, increased levels of depressive symptoms and illicit drug abuse were found among suicide attempters compared with those who had not attempted (Windle & Windle, 1997). Interestingly, it has also been found that early-onset substance use alongside neurohormonal changes during puberty impacts brain development and exacerbates symptoms of CD and ADHD (Riggs, 2003; Rutter, Giller, & Hagell, 1998). Therefore, the substance use can make mental health issues worse.

Frequently, youth with mental health issues use substances to self-medicate prior to a mental health intervention and diagnosis. The youth knows there is something wrong and the substances numb the pain and may decrease negative or embarrassing symptoms. Occasionally after diagnosis, youth use illegal substances in lieu of their prescribed medication because they do not like the way the prescribed medication makes them feel or reduces their ability to think clearly.

Practitioners should assess the youth's history of mental health symptoms to determine the relationship between *comorbid*, co-occurring disorders, and substance abuse in order to evaluate whether symptoms of conditions such as ADHD, BPD, CD, OCD, anxiety, or depression was present during periods of abstinence. In some instances, the symptoms of drug dependency may look like mental health problems. Conversely, substance abuse problems may mask underlying mental health issues. It is considered best practice to wait until an adolescent has discontinued using substances before assessing the existence of a mental health disorder since substances can mask or intensify the appearance of a mental health disorder.

Behaviors and Characteristics That Decrease Drug Use in Youth

Youth are less likely to be involved in substances if they have good problem-solving skills, a positive orientation to school, easy temperament, good intellectual capability, and have high self-efficacy (Catalano et al., 1996; Dishion & Loeber, 1985; Hawkins et al., 1992; Jenson, 2004; Jessor et al., 1995).

Protective and Risk Factors Related to Substance Abuse in the Family Microsystem

Risk Factors

Within the family system, youth who have parents or siblings who abuse substances are more likely to abuse substances themselves (Dishion & McMahon, 1998). Youth who experience violence in the family, whether it is child maltreatment, chronic family conflict, or domestic violence, sometimes try to get away or remove themselves from the painful situation through substance use. Additionally, youth who have parents with mental health issues are more prone to use substances.

Protective Factors

The positive influence of adult caregivers has been found to be an important variable in assessing adolescent substance abuse (Dishion & McMahon, 1998). The organization and structure of the family may serve to mediate or reduce contact an adolescent has with substance-using peers. Specifically, the presence of parental guidance, support, supervision, and a clear and consistent parental message disapproving substance use can be an effective intervention for reducing substance use. Similarly, youth who spend time with their family in sports or activities are also less likely to be involved in substance use.

Protective and Risk Factors Related to Substance Abuse in the Peer Microsystem

Risk Factors

Association with peers who use substance is related to adolescent substance abuse. Similarly, spending time with youth who are involved in deviant activities increases the likelihood of substance use for that youth (Dishion & Loeber, 1985; Elliott, Huizinga, & Ageton, 1985). Youth who have a great deal of unsupervised free time to spend with other youth are also more at risk for substance abuse.

Protective Factors

Youth who spend time with peers who are future oriented are more likely not to be involved in substance abuse. Youth who are in the company of friends who possess healthy *resistance skills*, the ability to turn down drugs or alcohol when offered, are more likely not to be involved with substances themselves. Additionally, youth who spend time with friends who have a positive orientation to school are less likely to be involved in substance use.

The Problem Severity Continuum

Winters (2001) proposed that drug and alcohol involvement among youth occur on a problem severity continuum, from abstinence on one end to recovery on the opposite end; adolescents may relapse and go through the stages again. Three categories follow the abstinence category and precede the dependence threshold: *experimental use* (limited recreational use); *early abuse* (greater frequency or *polysubstance* of more than one drug); *abuse* (frequent use with adverse consequences), followed by *dependency* (signs of tolerance to the substance, cycling through the addiction cycle: pre-occupation, ritual, compulsivity, despair), and finally, *recovery* (no longer using substances). Implications for treatment for the problem severity continuum suggest interventions should reflect a continuum of care and be consistent with the severity of drug use, from least restrictive treatments for low-level users, such as harm reduction, checking sobriety through urine analysis, individual or family counseling or psychoeducational groups, to more intensive residential treatments for those youth who are polysubstance abusers or use chronically. Practitioners need to be able to distinguish between experimental use, abuse, or dependency in order to make the appropriate treatment recommendations (Burrow-Sanchez, 2006).

Substance Abuse and DSM-IV

Since many practitioners providing treatment to adolescents will be required to diagnose substance use disorders, they should be aware of the considerations and controversies regarding the use of the *Diagnostic and Statistical Manual of Mental Disorders* (DSM-IV-TR; American Psychiatric Association, 2000) with youth. Martin and Winters (1999) questioned the validity of the DSM-IV criteria for substance abuse as applied to adolescents given the fact that the criteria were developed from research on adults. They noted that symptoms such as withdrawal and drug-related medical problems are prominent only after years of sustained abuse, which may not be developmentally relevant for adolescents (Martin & Winters).

The Social Development Model

The social development model (SDM; Catalano et al., 1996) utilizes knowledge of protective and risk factors that can contribute to, or moderate, delinquency or substance abuse in youth. The SDM hypothesizes that specific socializing individuals influence a child at each stage of development, which can result in either a prosocial or an antisocial pathway. In preschool, children are more likely influenced by parents; teachers and peers during elementary school, with an increasing role of the peer group during middle school; and more complex individual and societal influences are prevalent during high school. If consistent involvement occurs during each of the stages, a child will observe and remember the behaviors of those with whom he or she is connected. In terms of protection and risk, risk factors can block opportunities for prosocial relationships at each stage, which can result in substance use and other negative outcomes, and protective factors can contribute to prosocial outcomes. According to the SDM model, positive peer group influences may potentially steer a youth away from substance use.

Externalizing Behaviors and Substance Abuse

Externalizing behaviors, antisocial behavior that involves disregard for the rights or property of others, such as stealing, graffiti "tagging," destruction of property, and rule breaking, significantly coincides with substance abuse (Feldstein & Miller, 2007; Loeber et al., 1998). In a sample of young adults, Hussong, Curran, Moffitt, Caspi, and Carrig (2004) tested the "snares" hypothesis, which suggests that substance abuse ensnares or interferes with normative decreases in antisocial behavior from adolescence into adulthood. Snares are in contrast to the effects of protective factors that serve to buffer the risk of antisocial behavior as a young person develops. Interestingly, the researchers confirmed that men who abused substances during their youth showed increased antisocial behavior above what would have been predicted given their individual patterns of behavior. That is to say, during time periods where greater substance abuse was reported, increased levels of antisocial behavior were also reported. Overall, adolescents with externalizing behaviors tend to have compromised family functioning, lower academic competencies, and increased associations with negative peers, which are also all risk factors for substance abuse.

Traumatic Stress and Adolescent Substance Abuse

Traumatic stress involves an actual or perceived threat of serious injury, or a threat to the physical integrity of self or others, and the person may respond with fear, helplessness, or horror (American Psychiatric Association, 2000). Practitioners have begun to pay particular attention to trauma exposure and PTSD symptoms, such as hypervigilance, nightmares, and flashbacks among adolescents in substance abuse treatment (Jaycox, Ebener, Damesek, & Becker, 2004). Some youth may use illicit drugs to alleviate traumatic stress symptoms. Youth diagnosed with substance abuse had greater levels of anger, had more PTSD symptomatology, and were more likely to have been sexually abused (Evans, Spirito, Celio, Dyl, & Hunt, 2007).

Child abuse may bring about PTSD and subsequent substance abuse (Cohen, Mannarino, Zhitova, & Capone, 2003). Child maltreatment affects the cognitive, social, and behavioral aspects of youth. Child abuse also negatively impacts brain functioning and plays a role in organizing neural systems in the brain that can create vulnerability (Perry, 2001a, 2001b). Some of the negative outcomes of child abuse include a range of *internalizing behaviors*, emotional problems, such as depression, and *externalizing behaviors*, behavioral disruptions, such as CD and high-risk behavior (Kisiel & Lyons, 2001; McNally, 2003). A large body of research has investigated the relationship between trauma and particular negative outcomes in adolescence: delinquency (Brosky & Lally, 2004; Finkelhor, 2008; Greenwald, 2002; Maschi, 2006; Perry, 1997; Smith, Lizotte, Thornberry, & Krohn, 1995), substance abuse (Cohen et al., 2003; Rutter, 2001; Tubman, Gil, & Wagner, 2004; Weiner et al., 2003), self-destructive behavior (Baer & Maschi, 2003), sexual behavior problems, and dissociation (Carrion & Steiner, 2000; Friedrich, Jaworski, Huxsahl, & Bengston, 1997; Leibowitz et al., in press).

Assessment and Clinical Intervention

Several areas must be considered in the assessment of and intervention for substance use in adolescents. Initial considerations include the context where drug use occurs, as well as defining *experimental use* versus *abuse/ dependence*. Several key clinical areas associated with addressing substance use have been identified for practitioners.

Creating a Therapeutic Alliance

It is important for the practitioner to developing a therapeutic relationship with adolescents in drug treatment (Hawke, Hennen, & Gallione, 2005). A working alliance between the youth and the practitioner needs to be sought. It is important for the practitioner to be authentic and realistic. A respectful, collaborative alliance with families to motivate family change is also an important ingredient (Madsen, 2009).

Assessment of Severity of Substance Abuse

It is important to assess where the youth's substance behaviors fall along the problem severity continuum, as discussed earlier in the chapter.

Assessment of Comorbid Disorders

The practitioner should assess for the presence of mental health issues such as ADHD, BPD, CD, OCD, anxiety, and depression. Additionally, the practitioner should assess for PTSD and a history of child abuse.

Clinical Interventions for Addiction

It should be remembered that addiction is a chronic disease that can be controlled but never cured. More recently, it has been found that outpatient rehabilitative (rehab) therapy is more successful than inpatient rehab therapy because the youth has to negotiate "real-life" issues while he or she is involved in therapy. Additionally, if the substance abuse has been long in duration or marked by heavy use, there may be damage to the brain that cannot be reversed by talk therapy alone (Urschel, 2009). It may be necessary for the client to be under the care of a psychiatrist to prescribe medications to help improve brain functioning or help with cravings. The practitioner should utilize a treatment approach that is strengths based, gender specific, and culturally congruent when working with recovering addicts. First, it is important to understand in which *stage of change* the client is currently situated.

The Stages of Change

Prochaska, Norcross, and DiClemente (1994) found that permanent change only happens when the individual is actually ready to change. This seems obvious, but many who enter rehab treatment are not yet ready to create change in their lives and thus fail to remain clean and sober, thereby creating another failure in their lives. By assessing what stage of change the client is in, the practitioner can determine whether the client is ready to do the work to be successful in his or her sobriety. There are six stages of change. The first stage is called *precontemplation*; friends or family may have suggested the addict get help, but the addict responds with anger or denial that there is a problem. The second stage is *contemplation*; the addict realizes that he or she has a problem, but is not quite ready to commit to making changes in his or her life. The third stage is *action*; the addict has chosen to be involved in rehab and is willing to do the work that is required of him or her to maintain sobriety. The fourth stage is *maintenance*; the recovering addict realizes that he or she has made important positive changes in his or her life and is also aware that there continues to be temptations and triggers that could put his or her sobriety at risk. The final stage is *termination*; sobriety is effortless and is simply a way of life. If the client is not in the action stage or moving from the contemplation to the action stage, real change may not yet be possible.

Fostering Prosocial Interactions for Youth

The practitioner should help the adolescent identify social support networks of youth, family members, and adults who can support him or her

in being clean and sober. It is important that youth who have abused substances do not return to the same companions that they used to drink
or do drugs with. An adage from the rehab world is that to remain clean
and sober "you need to change your playmates and playhouses." Intervention strategies that foster the development of interpersonal skills, prosocial
skills, and academic skills help youth develop attachments to positive role
models and increase their self-esteem and self-efficacy.

Activities that help the addict feel good about him- or herself and the
direction of his or her life are important. The early stages of sobriety are
not fun, and some youth may feel that their current desire to be clean
and sober is nothing but drudgery. Therefore, activities that support ath-
leticism, problem solving, and cooperation are beneficial for recovering
addicts. In many communities, organized activities for recovering addicts
such as biking, hiking, climbing, or training for a distance-running race or
a triathlon have been created to help them in their sobriety.

Exploring the Youth's Feelings of Guilt and Shame

The youth who has chosen to enter treatment often feels very guilty about
some of the activities that he or she participated in when he or she was
under the influence. Some youth have put themselves at risk or their
friends or family at risk through their involvement with substances. Some
youth may have told lies and undermined the trust of the people important
to him or her. They may have spent a great deal of energy hiding behaviors,
substances, and paraphernalia from their family or friends, and lived a
dual life, which is both physically and emotionally draining. Others have
stolen money or have stolen items from their friends or family to support
their habit and now feel very guilty about their actions. Some youth have
said hurtful things or acted in hurtful ways to friends or family and now in
their sobriety they feel embarrassed. As youth continue in their sobriety, it
is important for them to be able to confront their own feelings of guilt and
shame. When possible and appropriate, it may be freeing for the recovering addict to take responsibility for his or her past behavior, apologize to
those he or she has hurt, make amends, and move forward.

Understanding the Youth's Developmental Stage

As stated throughout this book, developmental issues are always evolving
and subject to change in youth. Consequently, intervention should consider the physical, social, cognitive, emotional, and moral issues that may
evolve during the course of the practitioner's relationship with the adolescent. Since the recovering addict is discovering who he or she is without

the substances, his or her identity may also go through a transformation. The addict may have to get to know who he or she is without the substance, including how he or she thinks, feels and interacts with others when not high or not seeking his or her preferred substance. Often, the addict had a very intimate relationship with his or her preferred substance. It may be helpful to frame the ending of this relationship as a "break up" between the addict and the substance. Since most teens have experienced the ending of a relationship, they can effectively use this metaphor.

Cognitive-Behavioral Therapy

The recovering addict must change his or her thoughts from proaddiction to prorecovery (Urschel, 2009). The practitioner should address and dispel thoughts that previously supported the client's substance abuse. These thoughts may include an inability to see consequences for his or her behavior, irrational thinking, inaccurate thoughts, jumping to conclusions, inability to think through cause to effect, inability to take another's perspective, inability to reframe a situation, paranoia, or rage directed at particular individuals or situations. Cognitive-behavioral therapy (CBT) conceptualizes substance abuse as learned behaviors reinforced by environmental contexts. It can be utilized in a group or individual format that can enhance problem solving, self-efficacy, communication, and anger management. It can help the adolescent identify *triggers* for substance use. Triggers are ideas, persons, places, music, memories, or emotional states that stimulate the desire to use substances (Urschel, 2009). Knowing what triggers drive the desire to use can help youth avoid the trigger or brainstorm in advance options of how to deal with the trigger when it occurs. Core to the notion of CBT is that the recovering addict is incapable of fully extinguishing all thoughts about the substance of choice. However, through CBT the recovering addict can change what he or she does about those thoughts. The recovering addict has the power to decide to act on those thoughts or not. A full discussion of CBT is presented in Chapter 12.

Motivational Enhancement Therapy

Motivational enhancement therapy (MET) uses *intrinsic motivation* to change behavior. Intrinsic motivation is the belief that one has the necessary attributes to complete the task and that the completion of the task is the reward itself; there are no external rewards or "carrots." The use of intrinsic motivation leads the client to initiate, persist in, and comply with behavior change efforts (Miller & Rollnick, 1991). There are five basic motivational principles:

1. *Express empathy.* This means that the practitioner needs to use *reflective listening skills.* Reflective listening skills combine respect for the client, acceptance of where he or she currently is, and supporting the process of change (Miller, 1995).

2. *Develop discrepancy.* The practitioner helps the client see the discrepancy between where he or she is and where he or she wants to be. This allows the client to begin honest discussion of the negative affects of his or her drug use and create motivation for change (Miller, 1995).

3. *Avoid argumentation.* The practitioner avoids moralizing or attacking the client about his or her drug use. The practitioner helps the client accurately see the consequences of his or her drug use. It is the client who comes to the realization that change is necessary and what he or she wants (Miller, 1995).

4. *Roll with resistance.* The practitioner helps the client understand that resistance to change is normal. The practitioner asks the client to brainstorm ideas of how to move past resistance (Miller, 1995).

5. *Support self-efficacy.* The practitioner helps the client come to know that he or she has the requisite skills to make a permanent change. The belief in him- or herself, in his or her own strength and skills, allows the client to have hope that change is possible. It also helps the client have optimism about the future (Miller, 1995).

Group Work

Though a great deal of substance abuse treatment is done in a group setting, practitioners should keep in mind that peer group interactions may occasionally increase adolescent problem behavior by providing recovering addicts an opportunity to learn and model deviant behavior from other youth who are not serious about change (Dodge, Dishion, & Lansford, 2006). However, when the group is motivated to work, groups can be extremely effective. Groups can help support positive change and buoy group members when they are feeling weak or discouraged. Psychoeducational groups can be extremely effective in helping youth understand the steps to recovery and the impediments to change.

Setting Realistic Goals and Expectations for Yourself as the Practitioner

Practitioners must acknowledge that their client may return to using substances. This can be disheartening. Some youth may not be ready to remain clean and sober. The practitioner must acknowledge the potential for relapse and not take the client's inability to stay sober as a personal affront on his or her clinical abilities (Burrow-Sanchez, 2006).

Family-Based Treatments

Most family-based models are based on family systems theory. By addressing protective and risk factors, the practitioner works to promote family engagement and increase motivation for change. The practitioner can help the family improve parenting skills, communication between family members, and better connect the family to seek supportive members in their peer, neighborhood, and school microsystems.

MULTISYSTEMIC THERAPY

Multisystemic therapy (MST) goals include improving family parenting disciplinary practices, decreasing association with negative peers, increasing involvement with prosocial youth, and developing support systems that include extended family, schools, and neighborhoods (Henggeler et al., 2002). MST practitioners generally have small caseloads and spend a considerable amount of time with the family to restructure its interactions with its various environments.

MULTIDIMENSIONAL FAMILY THERAPY

There are four domains of multidimensional family therapy (MDFT): (1) the adolescent as a member of a family and a member of a peer group, (2) the parents in their role as mother and father, (3) the family environment, and (4) the extrafamilial environments of positive and negative influence such as the school and the neighborhood (Liddle, Rodriguez, Dakof, Kanzki, & Marvel, 2005). As part of MDFT, random urine drug screens are required for the youth throughout treatment. The results of these screens make youth responsible for their behavior rather than keeping their behavior a secret from their family. MDFT employs intervention strategies in three stages within each of the four domains:

- *Stage 1: Build the foundation.* The goal of the first stage is to create engagement. Examples of work during this stage include developing a collaborative process between family members, encouraging youth to voice concerns, eliciting the family story, understanding the parents' previous attempts to develop an emotional connection to the adolescent, and investigating possible past traumatic experiences and mental health issues.

- *Stage 2: Work the themes/request change.* The work during the second stage includes working with the adolescent about ambivalence to change, addressing drug abuse directly, addressing difficulties in other environments such as school failure and delinquency, helping the adolescent imagine alternative behaviors, helping the adolescent plan to make changes, instilling hope in all family members, improving communication, working with the parents around their own drug abuse history, and emphasizing self-care strategies for all members of the family.

- *Stage 3: Progress in treatment.* In the third stage, work from stage 2 is strengthened and solidified. During the termination process, a new family story is created about the family's successes in therapy.

Case Study

Jerry is an athletic 16-year-old European American male. He was on his high school's ski team. Unfortunately, Jerry had a bad accident skiing, which left him with a broken right arm and leg. He had two surgeries that were painful and his recovery was slow. He was given Vicodin as a painkiller. Jerry at first was scared of the Vicodin because it made him feel like he was floating and made him feel nauseous, but after several doses he enjoyed the pain being taken away and the feeling of euphoria it gave him. He continued to use the Vicodin, even when he no longer experienced pain, but told his doctor he continued to have pain so that his prescription was renewed. As he healed, Jerry realized he would miss the following competitive ski season and that made him feel sad, he would miss both friends who skied with him, and he would miss the sport he loved. Jerry's identity had been centered on his being a competitive skier. Jerry was not sure who he was if he was not a skier.

Jerry felt lonely and sad and began to use marijuana to soothe those feelings. As Jerry smoked more marijuana, he felt more relaxed about his lack of skiing and began to make friends with others who used marijuana and other drugs. Jerry began to skip school with his new friends to get high or get stoned at lunch. Jerry had moved from being in the jock group at school to the stoner group. Jerry was gaining a reputation for being a wild partier and he dabbled in selling weed as well. Jerry had always done relatively well at school with minimum effort, but he was now in danger of failing a class.

When Jerry missed an entire day of classes without an excuse, the school social worker called Jerry's dad, Edward, at work. Edward had dropped off Jerry at school that morning and was dumbstruck. Edward called his wife, Margaret, who had just returned home from work. Margaret went through

Jerry's bedroom and found a small pipe and some weed in a plastic bag at the bottom of his sock drawer. Margaret called her family physician, who referred the family to a local substance abuse treatment center. That night at dinner, Margaret showed Jerry what she found in his room. At first, Jerry denied that the pipe and the marijuana were his. When he realized that his secret was out, he began telling his parents about his marijuana use and how it had gotten out of control. Jerry agreed to attend the intake appointment at the substance abuse treatment center.

Jerry is currently in outpatient rehab treatment. He attends a weekly psychoeducational group, as well as individual and family counseling with his mother and father.

QUESTIONS FOR THE REFLECTIVE PRACTITIONER

1. What risk factors does Jerry have?
2. What protective factors does Jerry have?
3. If you were Jerry's practitioner, how would you begin working with him?
4. How could you help Jerry maintain sobriety?
5. How would you work with Jerry's family to support his sobriety?
6. How would you create a more supportive social network to improve Jerry's functioning?
7. Do you think Jerry will maintain sobriety?

Chapter Summary

The chapter discussed the protective and risk factors related to adolescent substance abuse. The various pathways to adolescence substance abuse were also investigated. Additionally, the rates of substance abuse and the current drugs of choice by youth were explored. Interventions for addicts were discussed, which included both individual interventions and family interventions. In the next chapter, sexual orientation is discussed.

CHAPTER 11

Sexual Orientation
and Gender Identity Development

Chapter Overview

We discuss sexual orientation identity, transgender identity development, and clinical implications for working with gay, lesbian, and transgender (GLT) adolescents. Protective and risk factors in the lives of gay, lesbian, and trans-identified teens and case examples for clinical assessment and intervention are also presented.

CASE EXAMPLE:
Who Are the Youth Represented in this Chapter?

The following three case examples represent some of the concerns of GLT adolescents. Considering the implications for each case within the context of the risk factors, theory, assessment, and intervention strategies presented in the following pages will prepare you to assess and suggest interventions for the more developed case study at the end of the chapter.

Jana, a 15-year-old European American, is a controversial figure in her high school. She is artistic, overweight, and male identified. She declares, "I don't fit in with any girl group!" She spends most of her time with a few boys who do not fit in either. They dress in Goth fashion, dye their hair, and have tattoos and piercings (Fish & Harvey, 2005, p. 76).

Joey, age 16, Asian American, figured out he was gay by surfing the Web for information about why he felt so different. He is close to a few girls in his Spanish class and told one of them about his sexual identity long before he told anyone else. He has a gay uncle, but the family has no contact with him. (Fish & Harvey, p. 75).

Kathy, age 14, African American, is experiencing feelings of depression and distress as a result of unwanted feelings of same-sex attraction. She comes from a supportive evangelical Christian family and her parents have told her that in spite of biblical teaching against same-sex behavior their love for her is unconditional and they will not reject her. Although Kathy states that she believes her parents, she is unable to extend that level of acceptance to herself. She is plagued by guilt, shame, and condemnation fuelled by her fear that God sees her as "dirty." Her fear that God does not love her is distressing and compounds her feelings of depression because she is so strongly identified with Christianity (Yarhouse & Tan, 2005, p. 532).

* * *

We often think that sexual orientation applies only to gays, lesbians, and bisexuals. The idea that heterosexuals also have a sexual orientation is often dismissed because it is considered to be *normal* or "relegated to unconsciousness in a heterosexist society as a result of 'normative' assumptions about heterosexuality" (Fassinger, 2000, as cited in Worthington, Savoy, Dillon, & Vernaglia, 2002, p. 496). However, scholars are calling attention to heterosexuality as a developed sexual orientation and identity (Eliason, 1995; Mohr, 2002; Sullivan, 1998; Worthington et al., 2002).

Sexual orientation is a person's sexual attraction to a particular gender. For example, adolescent girls who are sexually attracted to teenage boys are heterosexual and adolescent boys who are sexually attracted to teenage boys are homosexual. However, the term *homosexuality* is considered old-fashioned. Members of the gay community typically prefer to be called gay, lesbian, bisexual, or queer. The term *queer* is most often used among adolescents who identify as gay, lesbian, or bisexual or transgendered because it is more inclusive of the wider community of GLBT people. Their use of this term is indicative of how different generations "reclaim" words that in former usage were viewed as pejorative labels. The term is used in this chapter as a more efficient way to refer to members of the population, male, female, and transgender. Practitioners are encouraged to listen for how the queer youth they serve self-identify and to use the same term each client uses to refer to him- or herself.

"Transgender is a term used to describe individuals who exhibit gender-nonconforming identities and behaviors, or in other words, those who transcend typical gender paradigms" (Ryan & Fetterman, 1997, as cited in Grossman & D'Augelli, 2006, p. 112). While sexual orientation and gender identity are presented together in this chapter, a person's gender identification is not linked to a person's sexual orientation. For example, a person can be gender identified as male and be sexually attracted to either males or females. In fact, Savin-Williams and Diamond (1999) point out the importance of not "assuming that sexual orientation and gender atypicality [girls acting as tomboys and boys acting effeminate] are the *same phenomenon* or that they should be taken as generalizable indicators of each other" (p. 245). Some girls are labeled tomboys and in their adult lives viewed as *athletic,* but have heterosexual orientations and some boys are effeminate in their childhoods and retain these characteristics into adulthood and have heterosexual orientations.

The prevalence of gay-, lesbian-, and queer-identified individuals is difficult to count because conditions of homophobia and heterosexism cause some queer people to be closeted. The 2000 U.S. Census attempted to count gay and lesbian couples and found that the percentage in the United States ranges from .97 to 1.13% of all couples (*www.gaydemographics. org/USA/2000_Census_Total.htm*). These percentages are widely critiqued as inaccurate because some couples fear repercussions if they admit to being gay on a U.S. Government form. Others question the U.S. Census definition of what constitutes a gay, lesbian, or queer couple (*www.gaydemo-graphics.org/USA/2000_Census_Total.htm*). In contrast to sexual orientation, gender identity is defined as a person's expression of the characteristics viewed as socially acceptable for males or females within a particular culture. Culturally, we assume that one's gender expression will match one's biological sex, that is, whether a person has female or male genitalia. However, there is not always a direct match between a person's gender identity and his or her biological sex characteristics. Sometimes a person is born into a male biological body, but as he ages he realizes that how he feels and thinks within his body doesn't fit with what people expect of him as a boy. Similarly, sometimes a biological girl comes to realize that how she thinks and feels within her body does not resonate with the behavioral expectations for girls. The prevalence of trans-identified people is difficult to measure because "in most Western cultures . . . social structures assume a binary classification of gender [rendering this population nearly invisible]" (Grossman & D'Augelli, 2006, p. 112). The revised fourth edition of the *Diagnostic and Statistical Manual of Mental Disorders* (DSM-IV-TR; American Psychiatric Association, 2000) states that "there are no recent epidemiological studies to provide data on the prevalence of Gender Identity Disorder" (p. 579). The gender identity disorder (GID) diagnosis is controversial within different communities. However, trans-identified people must seek a GID diagnosis if they want surgery to alter their biological sex characteristics. However, not all transgender people seek surgery. Regardless, once a person makes the transition from the gender to which he or she was assigned at birth, based on biological sex characteristics, to the gender he or she feels most aligned with, then that person is always referred to as the gender to which he or she has transitioned, even if you are referring to him or her in the past prior to the transition. For example, a person who was born biologically a boy but transitions to live as a woman in all aspects of her life, is referred to as girl, even when talking about her childhood.

There is a difference between feeling that one's biological body does not match society's expectations for gender expressions and the transitory experience of a young girl who is viewed as a "tomboy" or the young boy who likes to play with dolls. These transitory experiences are referred to as gender-atypical behavior (Savin-Williams & Diamond, 1999). Gender-atypical behavior is more acceptable for girls than for boys. Savin-Williams and Diamond speculate that "in a society that values masculine over feminine traits, gender-atypical boys are problematized far more consistently than and fervently than gender-atypical girls" (p. 246). In contrast to gender-atypical behavior, transgender people experience confusion and discomfort when they realize that how they think and feel in their body does not line up with society's expectations for their biological sex. Jennifer Boylan's (2004) memoir of beginning life as biologically male and her later transition to womanhood echoes Green's (2004) description of the "transgender childhood as one in which the child unconsciously (at first, and perhaps consciously later) expresses gender characteristics or behaviors that are typically associated with those of the opposite sex to the point of making other people uncomfortable or otherwise acutely aware of the dissonance" (p. 13). A quote from Boylan's memoir makes this idea obvious. She recollects the following conversation with her mother when she was 3 years old. She was watching her mother iron her father's shirts when her mother said: "Someday you'll wear shirts like this" (Boylan, 2004, p. 19). Boylan narrates her thoughts about this with the following words:

> I just listened to her strange words as if they were a language other than *English*, I didn't understand what she was getting at. *She* never wore shirts like that. Why would I ever be wearing shirts like my *father's*? Since then, the awareness that I was in the wrong body, living the wrong life, was never out of my conscious mind—*never*, although my understanding of what it meant to be a boy, or girl, changed over time. . . . At every moment as I lived my life I countered this awareness with an exasperated companion thought, namely, don't be an *idiot*. You're *not* a girl. Get over it. (2004, pp. 19–20)

Ecological theory (Bronfenbrenner, 1979) calls attention to the social and cultural dynamics that affect gay, lesbian, and transgender teens. We raised similar dynamics in Chapter 2 when we discussed how racism affects adolescents of color because the person they can be within the family and within their cultural-ethnic group may be more genuine than the person they are perceived to be by a dominant social structure imbued with racism. They may ponder, "Do I have the same identity in the minority community as I do in the majority society?" As noted in Chapter 2, Du Bois (1903, 1996) wrote about African American experiences of their families' and communities' high expectations within a context of the racist images of an oppressive white society (hooks, 1981).

> It is a peculiar sensation, this double-consciousness, this sense of always looking at oneself through the eyes of others, of measuring one's soul by the tape of a world that looks on in amused contempt and pity. One ever feels his twoness—an American, a Negro [*sic*]; two souls, two thoughts, two unreconciled strivings; two warring ideals in one dark body, whose dogged strength alone keeps it from being torn asunder. (Du Bois, 1903, 1996, p. 5)

Research demonstrates that racism negatively influences the behavioral and mental health of adolescents of color (Surko, Ciro, Blackwood, Nembhard, & Peake, 2005). Similarly, heterosexism, homophobia, and transphobia create unique challenges for queer youth "in addition to the typical challenges for adolescence (e.g., identity formation, career planning, independence from parents)" (Rose, Boyce Rogers, & Small, 2006, p. 132). One difference between queer adolescents and teens of color is that teens of color have families that validate their identity, while GLT youth's families hold the same heterosexist, homophobic, and transphobic views as the rest of society. In effect, their families and the majority of their peers do not offer a respite from the stigma prevalent in society. In fact, within the gay and lesbian community, transgender people are often misunderstood and shunned.

GLT youth are stigmatized within the macrosystem. These stigmas are perpetuated at the other ecological levels through discriminatory policies (exosystems) and meso and micro expectations for compulsory heterosexuality and binary gender identity. Thus, queer teens are exposed to numerous risk factors at every level of the ecological model. In fact, research demonstrates that queer youth experience mental and behavioral health problems "largely because of victimization experiences and lack of support rather than sexual orientation on its own" (Williams, Connolly, Pepler, & Craig, 2005, p. 479).

Risk Factors for GLT Adolescents

Macrosystem and exosytem environments built on cultural blueprints for heterosexism, homophobia, and transphobia create risks for queer youth. Supportive, accepting, and caring individuals and policies can mediate these risks. Practitioners can serve as important supports for GLT teens and their families. Additionally, "a validating family system can be crucial for youth who, on a daily basis, encounter shame and ridicule from the broader society because of their sexual orientation or transgender identity" (Morrow, 2006, p. 187). Queer youth are protected if they have prosocial skills, a likeable disposition, an affirming and sustaining faith, and a family and school environment that are able to offer support and validation (Morrow). However, supports are minimal because peers, family members, teachers, school administrators, and policy makers are steeped in macro blueprints that perpetuate stereotypes, prejudice, and discrimination.

Intrapersonal Risk Factors

Teens who are questioning their sexual orientation or gender identity are at heightened risk for emotional distress, isolation, depression, substance abuse, suicide, pregnancy, sexually transmited diseases (STDs), and internalized homophobia and transphobia (Morrow, 2006). This risk is not surprising because there are few protections from the negative images and misinformation about GLTs. Queer youth tend to apply these messages as meaningful definitions of themselves or to internalize homophobia and transphobia unless they have the support to counter them (Morrow). Some youth take on an "exaggerated heterosexual image" (p. 181) as a way to hide their sexual orientation. As a result, "some gay male teens father children, and some lesbian teens become pregnant in seeking social validation by 'passing' for heterosexual" (p. 187).

Transgender teens face health risks if they acquire hormones from nonmedical providers (e.g., street dealers) to support the development of a male or female appearance. Without the support and knowledge of trained healthcare providers, these youth are liable to (1) use hormones improperly and cause "serious health problems that may have impact on their pubertal growth," and (2) inject the hormones with shared or unclean needles and become infected with HIV (Grossman & D'Augelli, 2006, p. 114).

Family Risk Factors

Research indicates that 33% of the queer teens surveyed admit to being verbally abused in their homes and 10% have been physically assaulted by family members (Pilkington & D'Augelli, 1995). Transgender youth who exhibit obvious nonconforming gender expression are more likely to report that their parents verbally and physically abused them in adolescence and middle childhood (Grossman, D'Augelli, Howell, & Hubbard, 2005). Clearly, not all families verbally and physically abuse their GLT teens. How-

ever, parents tend to have minimal accurate knowledge—yet lots of culturally transmitted misinformation and stereotypes—about sexual minority
groups" (Morrow, 2006, p. 186). Some families enter a crisis period upon
learning of their child's sexual orientation or transgender identity. Family
rejection adds to societal rejection and increases risk. Many teens are alone
with the struggle of facing a society and family that pressures them to deny
and/or hide their sexual orientation and gender identity development.

Research indicates that teens' comfort with expressing their gay or lesbian sexual orientation is related to parental characteristics. For example,
lesbian adolescents who perceived religion as important to their parents
were less apt to express their sexual orientation identity (Waldner-Haugrud
& Magruder, 1996). However, this factor did not play a role in gay male
teens' expression of their sexual orientation. Instead, for the gay teenage
boy, parents' political stance as liberal or conservative played a role in their
level of expression. The teenage boys who perceived their parents as politi-
cally conservative were less apt to be open about their gay sexual orientation (Waldner-Haugrud & Magruder).

Peer and School Risk Factors

During adolescence, peers and school are inseparable because they spend
a great deal of time together in school. Queer youth are at risk for being
ridiculed and bullied. Transgender youth may have faced taunts prior to
adolescence because children as young as 5 years have well-defined understandings of what it means to be a boy or girl. At this early age "children
express stereotypic ideas of what each sex should do, wear, feel, and react
approvingly or disapprovingly toward each other, according to their choice
of sex-appropriate toys and play patterns" (Perrin & the Committee on
Psychosocial Aspects of Child and Family Health, 2002, p. 45).

The peer and school environment can be fraught with tension
because youth will ridicule and bully anyone they suspect is gay, lesbian,
or transgender. Internet technology allows this tension to extend beyond
the school day. Adolescents are in near constant contact with each other
through e-mail, instant messaging, Twittering, and networking websites
such as Facebook and MySpace. The faceless nature of electronic communication can intensify ridicule and bullying.

Morrow (2006) notes that "pejorative words like fag, dyke, queer, lez-
zie, and homo are common [in schools], and those terms often go unchal-
lenged by teachers and administrators in ways that similar pejorative terms
against other groups of students would never be tolerated" (p. 181). In fact,
the National School Climate Survey (2003) notes that "the average student
of diverse sexuality hears eight homophobic insults per day with one third
from faculty and staff" (as cited in Sweet and DesRoches, 2007, p. 173).

The 2007 National Climate Survey reported that "Almost a third (32.7%) of [GLT] students missed a day of school because of feeling unsafe, compared to only 4.5% of a national sample of secondary students" (Gay, Lesbian, Straight Educators Network, 2009, p. 3). Even if they have the courage to share their pain with a parent, teacher, or other trusted adult, queer teens are left without recourse when schools don't have policies that protect them and don't have educational policies aimed at reducing the kind of ignorance that perpetuates cruel treatment.

Many queer adolescents may be afraid to come out to parents, teachers, or other helping professionals causing them to not report ridicule and bullying. As a result teens are at risk for truancy, academic failure, and dropping out of school all together in addition to the concerns already mentioned (Morrow, 2006). Other factors affect a teen's willingness to share this pain. For example, lesbian teens who placed a higher value on school and school-related functions are less likely to be open with peers about their sexual orientation. In contrast, gay male teens who placed a higher value on their heterosexual friends were not as open with their peers about being gay (Waldner-Haugrud & Magruder, 1996).

Sexual Orientation Identity Development

Heterosexual adolescents and adults are often unaware of how they develop their sexual orientation because society assumes that heterosexuality is the norm. The heterosexual teen just knows he's attracted to one girl or another and does not label himself; he's *just normal*. The heterosexually oriented girl just knows she wants that certain boy to pay attention to her; she has no sense that there is a name for that attraction; she *just fits in*. In contrast, the queer teen is aware that he or she is different from his or her peers and from all the displays of relationships he or she sees in the media. These teens may not have a word or label to describe their same gender attractions and may not even be fully aware of what that means for them, but they know they are *not just normal* and *do not just fit in*. This sense of difference may vary depending on the teen's exposure to individuals and media sources that support or reject their same-sex attractions. As Savin-Williams and Diamond (1999) state:

> Children do not wonder "why am I gay" but "why am I different?" These feelings often eventuate in feelings of marginality, alienation, and isolation from family, peers, and the larger society. The feelings may become especially salient . . . [as puberty progresses and] . . . what were once feelings and thoughts such as *she's my best friend forever* turn to feelings and thoughts such as *why do I feel like I want to kiss her?* (p. 244)

Macro-, exo-, meso-, and microsystem expectations for heterosexuality influence the sexual orientation identity development of all teens. In fact, Worthington and his colleagues (2002) state that "homonegativity is so pervasive at both macro and micro levels of the social ecology that it undoubtedly has impact on the sexual identity development of both males and females" (p. 508). You will recall from Chapter 2 that we discussed Erikson's developmental stage of identity development versus role confusion and Marcia's (1966, 1991, 1993) stages of identity formation (identity moratorium, identity foreclosure, identity diffusion, identity achievement). Neither Erikson nor Marcia appeared to have considered how their theories would apply to sexual orientation identity development. However, their ideas provide a foundation for understanding it and Worthington and his colleagues extend Marcia's (1966) work to explain the five statuses of heterosexual identity development: unexplored commitment, active exploration, diffusion, deepening commitment, and synthesis. A summary of each status is provided in Table 11.1.

Sexual orientation development for queer youth stems from the identity statuses noted in Table 11.1 with the outcome of active exploration resulting in a gay/lesbian sexual orientation as opposed to a heterosexual orientation. Cass (1979) suggests the developmental phases these youths might experience as they work through Worthington et al.'s (2002) stage of active exploration. Cass's phases are noted alongside of Worthington et al.'s pertinent identity statuses in Table 11.2.

Heterosexism and homophobia at all levels of the social ecology from macro blueprints and exosystem policies to micro relationships influence a teen's active exploration of his or her sexual orientation. This influence combined with the teen's internal need for cognitive and emotional congruency can lead to the social and emotional risks noted earlier in this chapter (Waldner-Haugrud & Magruder, 1996). Teens in this predicament may tend toward depression and low self-esteem (Maylon, 1982). Lack of support can compound the teen's internal confusion as well as social isolation (Dietz & Dettlaff, 1997). In fact, a recent study demonstrates that teens who are confused about sexual orientation identity (i.e., those who were unsure and had not declared themselves as gay, lesbian, bisexual, or heterosexual) are more likely to (1) be delinquent, (2) use illicit substances, (3) report running away overnight, (4) report more depression, and (5) report more suicidal thoughts (Rose et al., 2006). The questioning adolescent who has access to trusted adults, and a belief that those adults care about him or her as well as the capacity to do well in school, will be protected from some of these risks (Rose et al., 2006; Rotheram-Borus, Rosario, Van Rossem, Reid, & Gillis, 1995).

TABLE 11.1. Identity Statuses of Heterosexual Identity Development

Identity status	Summary of status characteristics
Unexplored commitment	Characterized by a naïve commitment to heterosexual identity in which "most heterosexually identified individuals . . . are likely to experience little conscious thought about their adoption of compulsory heterosexuality" (Worthington et al., 2002, p. 515). "People at this level of identity development are likely to assume that non-heterosexuals do not exist in their microsocial contexts (e.g., familial and immediate social circumstances) and believe they do not know anyone who is [GLB gay, lesbian, bisexual]" (p. 516). Hence, they often have a limited understanding of [GLB] people, based on the stereotypes present in society.
Active exploration	This status is marked by "purposeful exploration, evaluation, or experimentation of one's sexual needs, values, orientation and/ or preferences for activities, partner characteristics" (Worthington et al., 2002, p. 516). During this exploration individuals question the normative expectations for heterosexuality. "Although some individuals in this status may consciously experiment with [imagined] or real sexual activities with same-sex partners, most seem to [still maintain that they are heterosexual]" (p. 517); however, some individuals in this identity status might question their fit with a heterosexual identity and wonder if they might be gay, lesbian, or bisexual.
Diffusion	Individuals often enter this status as a result of a crisis and those in this status are likely to be confused about a number of their identities, not just sexual orientation. This status is marked by individuals being "intentional in their nearly random willingness to try or be almost anything [related to their sexual orientation], however this intentionality is with respect to rejection of social conformity for its own sake rather than toward a specific set of experiences or outcomes" (Worthington et al., 2002, p. 518).
Deepening commitment	This status resembles Marcia's (1987) achieved identity in that the youth makes a commitment to heterosexual orientation through, for example, the experience of dating opposite-sex peers. However, given the "strong social forces that create sets of narrowly defined expectations for sexual identity [e.g., heterosexuality]" (Worthington et al., 2002, p. 519), many enter this commitment status without experiencing active exploration. Some people will maintain this status, others may move back to diffusion or active exploration, while others may move forward to synthesis.
Synthesis	This status is characterized by the integration of one's heterosexual orientation with the other identities (e.g., gender, race/ethnicity, religious). Worthington and colleagues (2002) suggest that this status might not be achieved without active exploration through which the youth is able to question the social mandate for heterosexuality, in effect reflecting on the question "Am I heterosexual?" or "What makes me heterosexual?"

Note. Based on Worthington, Savoy, Dillon, and Vernaglia (2002).

TABLE 11.2. Identity Statuses Integrated with Model of Gay/Lesbian Identity Development

Worthington et al.'s (2002) identity status	Cass's (1979) identity phase	Summary of Cass's identity phases
Active exploration	Identity confusion	*"Could I be gay?"* Marked by denial and confusion due to compulsory heterosexuality.
	Identity comparison	*"Maybe this does apply to me."* Marked by social isolation and a sense that it's just this one person, otherwise I like the opposite sex.
	Identity tolerance	*"I'm not the only one."* Marked by beginning acceptance of probability of being gay, experience of internalized heterosexism and stereotypes combined with awareness of gay community/culture.
Deepening commitment	Identity acceptance	*"I will be OK [if I am gay]."* Marked by acceptance of self as gay, attempts at coming out to selected peers and adults.
	Identity pride	*"I've got to let people know who I am!"* Marked by immersion into gay/lesbian identity and culture with a sense that only other gay people are relevant friends and supports.
Synthesis	Identity synthesis	Integrates gay/lesbian sexual orientation as one aspect of self with other identities (gender, race/ethnicity, religious). Values all peer and adult supports, both gay and heterosexual.

Note. Based on Worthington, Savoy, Dillon, and Vernaglia (2002) and Cass (1979) as adapted by Young (1995).

Transgender Identity Development

There is minimal research and theory on the process of transgender identity development (Mallon, 1999). However, one study reports age-graded experiences of coming to recognize transgender identity (Grossman et al., 2005). Trans-identified youth reported an awareness of "feeling different from others" as early as 7 years old. Girls who transitioned to boys reported that at around the age of 6 years they heard others refer to them as different, but boys who transitioned to girls were around 9 years old when they experienced this (Grossman et al.). Ridicule experiences related to being called either a "tomboy" or a "sissy" as a result of their gender nonconforming behavior began at an average age of 6 years for girls and an average age of 8 years for boys.

By an average of 9 to 10 years old the youth in this study reported that their parents asked them to "stop acting like a tomboy or sissy" (Grossman et al., 2005, p. 4). However, their parents did not ask if they were either gay, lesbian, or transgender until they reached an average age of 12 to 13 years old. The youth also reported that at around this same age their parents suggested that they needed counseling for their gender nonconforming actions (14 years for females who transitioned to male [FTM] and 11 years for males who transitioned to female [MTF]). The youth began to label themselves as transgender between 13 years old (MTF) and 15 years old (FTM) and told someone else for the first time that they identified as transgender at around 17 years old (FTM) and 14 years old (MFT) (Grossman et al.).

While more research is required, the Grossman et al. study (2005) highlights the early inklings of difference described in Jennifer Boylan's (2004) memoir of growing up and into transgender identity as male to female. It also confirms that transgender youth experience ridicule and pressure as they struggle with societal expectations on their gender expression.

The GLBT Adolescent's Family

Teens are often fearful of how their parents will react to them when and if they announce that they are gay, lesbian, bisexual, or transgendered. Their fear is well founded because parents react to this news within a social and cultural context of pervasive heterosexism, homophobia, and transphobia. Parents may have never imagined that stereotypes and prejudices about queer people would apply to their child (Saltzburg, 2004). Saltzburg and other researchers (Boxer, Cook, & Herdt, 1991) demonstrate both parental and teen experiences of the coming out process. Teens typically are nervous about letting their parents know about their sexual orientation and some will hide it from them as long as they can. For example, a young man in Boxer et al.'s study noted, "When I am older I will be able to be more like myself. Like I will not have to make up stories about where I am going and who I am with . . . " (p. 63). Sometimes both the teen and his or her parents accept this denial. For example, one 15-year-old girl stated, "I overheard my mom tell my dad that she thought I was a lesbian because of what she read in my diary," but noted that neither of them had brought this up pointing out, "No, it's never mentioned. It would be too scary to tell your mom . . . " (p. 70).

Youth who have been raised to value honesty, especially within their families, are stressed by hiding their identity (Boxer et al., 1991). Some teens come out to their parents because the secrecy is too stressful. For example, one young woman in Boxer and colleagues' study said, "I was so frustrated from hiding that I just told her, so it wasn't that hard. But, at that point I didn't care anymore. She thinks I am totally wrong and that I am making a big mistake" (p. 70). Other teens experience acceptance after coming out to their parents such as the young man who noted, "I think she [his mother] may have realized that when I came out I needed her most . . . she has met my boyfriend and likes him. I don't know what she thinks about gays. . . . You see, my mother doesn't treat me as an issue. She regards me as her son who is gay and not as her gay son" (p. 74). Whereas some teens experience rejection and others acceptance, still others have parents who appear to be in denial. For example, this 16-year-old boy notes, "She doesn't accept it as being the truth. She sees me as her asexual child. She said, 'you're too young to think one way or the other.' I left it alone. I didn't feel like dealing with it. We never talk about it now" (p. 80).

Teens' stress about coming out to parents is related to their perception of how their parents will react. Teens aspire for loving acceptance and assistance during what may be a difficult time. However, many may be met with rejection and even emotional and physical violence (Morrow, 2006). In fact, D'Augelli, Hershberger, and Pilkington (1998) found that of those who came out to their families, 50% experienced rejection from mothers and siblings and 75% experienced rejection from their fathers.

Parents also experience the disclosure as a stressful adjustment. Some parents question their parenting and others feel guilty if their initial response was negative (Boxer et al., 1991). Whatever the reaction, studies demonstrate that parents move into a self-reflective mode upon hearing their child is gay or lesbian. Saltzburg (2004) uses her research to conceptualize varying responses of parents. The parents in her study indicate an early awareness that their child was different and wondered if he was gay or she was a lesbian. One of the mothers in the study made the following statement, "When he was in sixth grade, I went up to his room one day and you know those *Teen Beat* magazines and they have pictures of the boys? The whole wall was filled with popular actors—cute boys. I mean, I'm thinking, 'He should have pictures of girls on the wall!' I knew really then. I didn't want to really know . . . " (Saltzburg, p. 112). Regardless of this early "awareness of difference" (Saltzburg, p. 112), parents were not prepared when their child came out to them. As one parent stated, "I think that the first year of really knowing—you know having it out in the open—

is really, really hard. It's like the death of a child that you thought was going to grow up in the way you always thought about. All your dreams for this kid—you know, marriage, the whole bit—none of that is going to happen and it all turns so suddenly" (Saltzburg, p. 113). Other researchers note similar parental experiences. For example, a parent in Boxer et al.'s study (1991) reported the following: "Like most parents I was concerned for his happiness. Was he going to have a satisfying life? It was the social aspects. We knew about the criticisms, discrimination and harassment of gay men. We didn't want that for our child" (p. 81).

Parents must also come to terms with the stereotypes they have learned from the pervasive heterosexism and homophobia (Boxer et al., 1991; Saltzburg, 2004). A parent in Saltzburg's study said, "I can't stop the thoughts I have about homosexuality. This is what I've learned and what I believe. And now these apply to my child. It's awful to have these thoughts about one of your children. . . . I felt shut down from her and felt so empty" (p. 113). Parents also realize the limits to their liberal values noting how these values were "challenged for the first time" when their child came out (Boxer et al., p. 85).

Saltzburg (2004) labels these parental experiences as "fears of estrangement" (p. 114). Parents in her study expressed a sense of loss that their child was part of a "subculture that they could never be part of" (p. 114). Parents felt so different from their gay or lesbian teen that they wondered what role they could play in mentoring and teaching him or her how to navigate life's perils (Saltzburg). Parents in this position can find support from other parents who have experienced the same thing. They can also get to know adult members of the gay community as means for support as well as to unlearn negative stereotypes (Boxer et al., 1991; Saltzburg, 2004). Saltzburg suggests that "The primary structure for helping them overcome their emotional anguish is knowing someone gay and meeting other parents of gay and lesbian adolescents" (p. 114). The parents in Saltzburg's study reported that connections with gay men and lesbians "helped to diminish their fears of the unknown and begin to restore a sense of connection to their children" (p. 114).

Assessment

Assessment should focus on risk factors such as depression, substance abuse, school difficulties, and the degree to which internalized homophobia and/or transphobia has influenced the teen's self-concept. Assessment of where a teen is in regard to his or her sexual orientation or gender identity development is also important. The theories and research on developmental progression of sexual orientation and gender identity serve as a reference guide for this part of the assessment. However, practitioners should proceed with caution as the theories and research should not be universally applied to all adolescents.

Assessment should include peer and family relationships as well as macro- and exosystem influences. The skills necessary for this assessment are similar to the skills applied in all clinical assessments with adolescents. However, practitioners who work with queer youth must be fully aware of their own attitudes toward this population as teens are sensitive to verbal and nonverbal judgments, even when unintended. Since practitioners are embedded in the macro blueprints of homophobia, heterosexism, and transphobia and will need to unlearn the same negative messages their clients internalize in order to effectively assess and intervene in a supportive and empowering manner.

Intervention

Numerous professional associations state that it is unethical and harmful to attempt to "change a person's sexual orientation from lesbian, gay, or bisexual to heterosexual" (Morrow, 2006, p. 185) (e.g., American Association of Marriage and Family Therapy, n.d.; American Psychiatric Association, 1998; American Psychological Association, 2004; American School Counselors Association, 2004; National Association of Social Workers, 2000). Some interventions that make this attempt are called conversion or reparative therapies. We do not espouse the use of these interventions and agree with the professional organizations that view them as harmful and unethical.

The most basic intervention requires accurate information about sexual orientation and transgender identity. Morrow (2006) echoes this and suggests that "GLBT-affirming clergy may be helpful resources for families [and others such as teachers, peers, school administrators] whose religious values may conflict with understanding sexual orientation and gender identity" (p. 186). Additionally, the research demonstrates that queer adolescents may be experiencing depression and suicidal thoughts. These teens long for a trusted, nonjudgmental adult who can listen and talk about these issues (Ciro et al., 2005).

Individual Intervention

Lemoire and Chen (2005) recommend the person-centered approach for clinical work with queer adolescents. It allows the teen to be in charge of self-exploration as he or she seeks to understand his or her sexual orientation and/or gender identity development. In a social and cultural environment characterized by homophobia and transphobia, it is imperative that adolescents experience unconditional positive regard and a nonjudgmental attitude as they navigate the questions surrounding their sexual orientation and/or gender identity. As such, the practitioner encourages the teen to be self-directed as he or she explores what his or her sexual orientation and/or gender identity mean for his or her self-concept while providing a supportive environment without regard for the outcome of the exploration. This support, without expectation for outcome, is paramount to the teen negotiating a world of pressures from peers, family, teachers, coaches, school, and clergy (Lemoire & Chen). In some instances, the practitioner may be the single adult in a teen's life who listens without judgment or personal agenda.

The person-centered approach may be especially useful for working with teens who struggle with a faith foundation that is contrary to their identity. For example, Yarhouse and Tan (2005) note that these youth may be seeking to resolve fears that (1) God no longer loves them, (2) they no longer feel positive about God, or (3) they can't be allowed to have faith in God and a queer identity. The person-centered approach allows the practitioner to support the teen's exploration of: his or her religious orientation and the strengths it may offer; any negative feelings he or she has about God or fears that God has negative feelings about him or her and how the teen came to understand these as pertinent in his or her life (Yarhouse & Tan). Yarhouse and Tan recommend that practitioners refrain from disputing teen's and family's religious tenets and values. The person-centered approach that is client directed and nonjudgmental offers the guidelines necessary to respond to this recommendation.

Additional elements should be added to person-centered work with queer adolescents (Lemoire and Chen, 2005). One of these is assessing the risks for a teen who decides to disclose his or her sexual orientation and/or transgender identity. For example, practitioners need to ask the teen to describe the relationship with the person to whom he or she wants to disclose his or her identity. Questions should include asking the teen how much contact that person has with the gay or transgender community and what kinds of things that person says when the topic of gay marriage or other issues arise in the news or other media. Some clients may find it helpful to role play the interaction with the practitioner before disclosing in real life. The empty chair and role reversal techniques (Sheafor & Horejsi, 2003) are recommended for this type of role play. The empty chair technique encourages the teen to talk to the person he or she intends to come out to as if he or she was in the empty chair across from him or her. The role-reversal strategy allows the teen to consider not only how he or she might feel during the disclosure, but also how the person he or she intends to come out to might experience the conversation (Sheafor & Horejsi).

Lemoire and Chen (2005) also suggest adding a peer-support group to the individually oriented person-centered approach so that teens gain a sense of support from peers facing similar challenges. This may require helping the teen to locate a peer-support group or if none exist, the practitioner may need to develop one. In rural areas, where there may be few "out" teens and/or no resources for the youth, the practitioner can assist the teen in finding safe and reputable online supports.

Family Intervention

Saltzburg (2004) points out that while most parents, over time, accept their gay and lesbian children, "the precarious nature of adolescence calls for vital timing of interventions in response to crisis" and other reactions to learning that their teenager is gay, lesbian, or transgender (p. 110). Intervention at the family level needs to assist family members in gaining appropriate information since they will have misinformation and negative stereotypes (Morrow, 2006). Additionally, parents may be comforted by joining a support group of parents with queer teens (Saltzburg, 2004).

The literature does not suggest any particular form of family intervention beyond the 2 interventions just noted. However, Heatherington and Lavner (2008) note that family characteristics, such as disengagement and cohesion, and parent–child relationship quality influence family responses. Therefore, we encourage practitioners to assist the family in finding a balance of cohesion and distance. For example, Heatherington and Lavner suggest that families marked by a sense of cohesion or togetherness are likely to be more supportive of their teenagers. However, some teens who have cohesive relationships with their families may fear the loss of that closeness if members react negatively to their coming out. In light of this the practitioner can first assess the quality of the adolescent's relationship with his or her parents and ask about any fears related to losing a close relationship. Armed with this knowledge the practitioner can facilitate a heartfelt conversation between the youth and his or her parents pointing out the strengths of the closeness as a means to assist the parents in coping with the teen's disclosure.

School Intervention

School-level interventions should focus on policy and education (Goldstein, Collins, & Halder, 2007; Taylor, 2007). McCaskell and Russell suggest that efforts to "suppress individual actions through rules and discipline . . . [is] like pressing down on the top of an ice cube in a bowl of water (2000, p. 248). These strategies do not change the overall school culture of homophobia and transphobia; they just send it underground (McCaskell & Russell). If the school community culture espouses negative and stereotypic views of queer youth, then protective policies will have minimal influence on the psychological and physical safety of the youth (Goldstein et al., 2007).

Education to assist students, parents, teachers, and administrators in unlearning a culture of oppression is one step in the process. In some communities these efforts may be welcome while in others they may be met with outrage (Taylor, 2007). Therefore, practitioners need to carefully assess the general attitudes in a community. Educational efforts can be backed by policies, especially "legal framework[s that] give authorities support when they encounter resistance or fear [on the part of other community members]" (p. 166). Taylor also suggests that "testimonies of [GLBT] students and the spectacle of them under attack by homophobic bullies" go a long way in moving communities from outrage to support (p. 166). Some communities have organizations, such as Parents and Friends of Gays and Lesbians (PFLAG), that have speaker's bureaus that include older teens and young adults who tell their stories in a panel format. Educational programs and policies must be developed within a school community in order to meet the needs most relevant to individual schools. Suggestions for developing safe school environments can be found at the Gay, Lesbian, and Straight Education Network *www.glsen.org/cgi-bin/iowa/all/home/index.html.*

Case Study

The following case studies will assist you in developing clinical assessments and interventions for two adolescents, Alberto and Nathan. Application of the information on protective and risk factors, and theories and research on sexual orientation and transgender identity development, as well as the more specific suggestions for assessment and intervention, will allow you to assess and suggest interventions for Alberto and Nathan.

Case 1

Alberto, a 13-year-old Latino, has been experiencing problems with peers who have been teasing him because of the things he wants to do and the ways he has been acting. The teacher reports that when the students did a talent show, Alberto lip-synced to the song, "I Enjoy Being a Girl." He also has poor relationships with other boys and prefers to spend his free time with the girls in his class. While the majority of both his male and female peers make fun of him, the girls he spends time with are accepting of him. He comes to school dressed in feminine-type pants, shirts, and colorful scarves and recently told one of the girls he spends a lot of time with that he knows God made a mistake when he was born because he is sure he is really meant to be a girl (adapted from McIntyre & Von Ornsteiner, 2001).

Case 2

Melinda is the parent of a bi-racial 16-year-old boy, Nathan, who came out to her about 6 months ago. She suspected he might be gay and was relieved when he told her and they could talk about it. Melinda had an uncle who was gay, but he never told anyone. He was killed in what appeared to be a hate crime when Melinda was 20, but the crime was never solved or proved to actually be a hate crime.

Melinda is worried about her son because he is moody and angry, always pointing out heterosexually oriented ads on TV and walking out of the room in a huff. He refuses to attend history class because all they ever talk about is "het history." He got beat up at school because he wore a gay pride shirt. Melinda says, "I am fine with him being gay, I just don't see why he has to show it off to everyone and let it get in the way of his schoolwork and school friendships. I wish I could get him to calm down about all of this."

QUESTIONS FOR THE REFLECTIVE PRACTITIONER

1. Describe all the psychological and behavior factors that might be playing a role in the current issues affecting Alberto and Nathan. What information from the case studies provides the evidence for these factors?

2. Describe the recent family and/or peer events in the lives of Alberto and Nathan that might be a factor in school and home behaviors.

3. How might Alberto's and Nathan's current behaviors be influenced by the macro- and exosystem factors related to homophobia and transphobia?

4. What should the practitioner listen for as Alberto and Nathan tell their stories to assess for identity development and the effects of internalized transphobia and homophobia?

5. Intervention strategies with suggestions for practitioners at the individual, family, and school levels were discussed in this chapter. Based on the issues confronting Alberto and Nathan, which do you think will be the most useful and why?

6. When did you first have a sense of your sexual orientation or your gender identity? Did you talk with your parents/family about this and why or why not?

7. What stereotypes about GLBT people are prevalent in your community? What are some of the supports for GLBT people in your community?

Chapter Summary

This chapter introduced the development of sexual orientation identity, transgender identity, and protective and risk factors in the lives of queer adolescents. Areas for assessment and intervention were also discussed. Case studies provided the opportunity to apply the content of the chapter for clinical assessment and intervention. In the next chapter we address mental health issues such as depression and suicide.

CHAPTER 12

Mental Health Issues

DEPRESSIVE SYMPTOMS, PERSONALITY DISORDERS, SUICIDAL BEHAVIOR, AND SELF-INJURIOUS BEHAVIOR

Chapter Overview

This chapter utilizes an ecological perspective to understand depression, suicide, personality disorders, and self-injurious behavior (SIB), such as cutting. We discuss risk factors that increase the likelihood of mental health disorders, and protective factors that help to reduce mental health problem outcomes. Specific components for assessment of suicidality are also presented. Treatment interventions that are useful for youth with mental health issues are discussed, such as cognitive-behavioral therapy (CBT) and dialectical behavior therapy (DBT). Additionally, information on medication is also presented.

CASE EXAMPLE:
Who Are the Youth Represented in This Chapter?

The following case example represents some of the concerns related to adolescents and mental health issues. Considering the implications for this case within the context of the risk factors, theory, assessment, and intervention strategies presented in the following pages will prepare you to assess and suggest interventions for the more developed case study at the end of the chapter.

James is 17 years old, African American, and attends a public magnet high school specializing in math, science, and technology. His academic abilities for advanced sciences and math contribute to his desire to be a physician, like his mother who is a surgeon and his father who has a private medical practice in family medicine. James had an older sister, Jenny, who was also a promising science student, but she committed suicide when she was 19 after failing one of her premed courses in college. James confesses to a friend that ever since he began to apply to colleges, he's been dreaming about Jenny. He tells his friend that in the dreams Jenny is talking to him, warning him not to study medicine. In these disturbing dreams, Jenny tells him the details of what it felt like when she committed suicide and tells him, "Don't do what I did, drop out of school and see the world before it's too late for you too!" James does not want to stress out his parents about his dreams and therefore has not shared the dreams with them. However, he has been thinking about the dreams a lot and they are getting in the way of completing his college essays.

Using the Ecological Perspective
to Assess Mental Health Issues

Risk factors for mental health issues exist at the internal level, as well as in the environments where adolescents spend much of their time, including the family, peer group, school, and neighborhood (Fergusson & Horwood, 2003; Luster & Small, 1997; Werner & Smith, 1998). Because of the inherent emotionality of the adolescent stage of development, youth can experience real or felt challenges in any of these environments.

Practitioners should assess what is happening in each of the spheres of the youth's life and become aware of any changes and how the teen feels about the changes. Is he or she frustrated, disappointed, uneasy, embarrassed, harassed, misunderstood, lonely, anxious, or feeling ostracized in a particular sphere of his or her life? How long has the youth been feeling this way and what is the depth of the feeling? Are these feelings also accompanied by sleep changes (either sleeping more than what he or she normally sleeps or having difficulty sleeping), eating changes (either loss of appetite or using food to soothe him- or herself), energy level decreases (lack of enthusiasm for typical activities and/or trouble getting going), or decreases in normal social behaviors (lack of desire to connect with friends or family members or involvement in social activities in which the youth would normally be an active participant)? If there are changes in behaviors along with negative feelings, it may point to depressive symptoms.

It is not uncommon for teenagers to move quickly from the depths of despair to giddiness and excitement. However, eccentric, dramatic, emotional, erratic, anxious, or fearful behaviors are the basic components of a personality disorder (American Psychiatric Association, 2000). The practitioner needs to evaluate whether these emotional swings are reactions to external events, particular triggers, or whether the youth seems to have become more emotionally charged without a clear precipitating event. The practitioner should also assess whether the behaviors have become more pervasive over time, which may indicate the presence of a personality disorder.

Defining Adolescent Depression, Personality Disorders, Suicidal Behavior, and SIB

Depression

Depressive symptoms include feelings of sadness, loneliness, suicidal ideation, and self-dislike. These problems may not be apparent to anyone but the individual who experiences them, in contrast to externalizing behaviors. A major depressive episode is diagnosed by having five of the following symptoms within a 2-week period: depressed mood or agitated mood, diminished interest in activities, significant weight loss or loss of appetite, fatigue or loss of energy, feelings of worthlessness or inappropriate guilt, diminished ability to think or to concentrate, feelings of restlessness, recurrent thoughts of death with no concrete plan, or insomnia or sleeping all of the time (American Psychiatric Association, 2000).

Personality Disorders

Personality disorders is a general term for mental health problems that refer to the way an individual thinks, perceives situations, reacts to situations, and relates to others. There are several types of personality disorders: paranoid personality disorder, schizoid and schzotypal personality disorder, antisocial personality disorder, borderline personality disorder, histrionic personality disorder, narcissistic personality disorder, avoidant personality disorder, dependent personality disorder, and obsessive–compulsive personality disorder (American Psychiatric Association, 2000). Frequently, these patterns of thinking and behaving make it difficult for the individual to relate well to others, and also make others have difficulty relating to the individual. Behaviors may include rapidly fluctuating mood from elation to irritability several times a day; being aggressive or explosive to peers, teachers, or relatives; becoming singularly focused on particular activities or needs; withdrawing; not taking pleasure in activities most youth do and calling them boring; engaging in high-risk behaviors (dangerous driving, promiscuity, drug use); difficulty maintaining friendships; altercations at school or run-ins with the law; difficulty getting to sleep and trouble waking; or diagnosed with attention disorder or depression but does not respond to treatment (Fassler & Papolo, 2009). Individuals with personality disorders often realize that they have trouble connecting to others, but they are unable to see how their thoughts and behaviors contribute to that distancing.

Suicidal Behavior

Suicidal behavior has three components: *suicidal ideation*, which can vary from weak to strong; *suicidal intent*, which varies from low to high; and *suicide plan*, which varies from vague to specific. Suicidal ideation is the amount of time that the youth thinks about suicide and believes that it is a real solution for his or her problems. Suicidal intent is the strength of the desire to carry out the suicide and its level of lethality. For instance, if a youth takes five aspirins, his or her intent was probably low to actually carry out the suicide. Suicide plan is the level of specificity of the plan: How does the youth plan on carrying out the suicide? When? Where? How? Has he or she written a note? Has he or she left his or her possessions to others? Has he or she made "peace" with those around him or her and said good-bye? The more specific the plan the more likely that the youth will carry out the suicide.

Self-Injurious Behavior

There are nine categories of SIB: cutting, biting, abrading, severing, inserting, burning, ingesting or inhaling, hitting, and constricting. These categories vary by frequency and severity. SIB is different than suicide because it is not intended to cause suicide, therefore the motivation is different (Epps, 1997). SIB has also been called nonsuicidal self-injury (NSSI; Armey & Crowther, 2008; Nock & Mendes, 2008).

There have been a wide variety of proposed rationales for SIB that include clinical depression (Epps, 1997; Weierich & Nock, 2008), attention-seeking behavior, copycat behavior through seeing others doing SIB, a coping mechanism for dealing with an excessively controlling environment (Epps), wanting to have an effect on others, a manner by which to express difficult emotions, an arousal in response to stressful events, decreased ability to tolerate distress or persist in a task, deficits in problem-solving skills, low self-efficacy (Nock & Mendes), escaping unpleasant affective states (Armey & Crowther, 2008; Weierich & Nock), escaping negative self-appraisals, shame, ruminating (Armey & Crowther), childhood sexual abuse, histrionic personality disorder or borderline personality disorder (Weierich & Nock), PTSD (Weierich & Nock; Yates, Tracy, & Luthar, 2008), excessive parental criticism especially for males, youth alienation to parents, general distrust of others, pressure to contain emotions, and pressure to perform at a superior level (Yates et al., 2008). In the great majority of these rationales, the youth engages in hurtful behaviors to relieve emotional pressure or pain.

Prevalence of Adolescent Depression, Personality Disorders, Suicidal Behavior, and SIB

Depression

Recent research has found that symptoms of depression are most prevalent in late adolescence (Wight, Sepúlveda, & Aneshensel, 2004). Twenty percent of youth acknowledge symptoms of depression. However, only 30% of those recognizing symptoms of depression have sought treatment (SAMHSA, 2008).

Differences in depressive symptoms have been linked to gender (Kistner, David, & White, 2003; Schradley, Turner, & Gotlib, 2002). Late-adolescent females are the most at risk for developing depression (Duggal, Carlson, Sroufe, & Egeland, 2001; Rutter & Sroufe, 2000)

Personality Disorders

A recent Columbia University study (2008) stated that nearly one in five American youth have a personality disorder. However, less than 25% of those suffering from a personality disorder seek treatment (SAMHSA, 2008).

There is some discussion about the prevalence of personality disorders in males versus females. Historically, personality disorders were thought to be more common in females. More recently, research shows that some personality disorders are more common for females such as borderline personality disorder and histrionic personality disorder, and narcissistic, antisocial, and obsessive–compulsive personality disorders are more common in males (Golomb, Fava, Abraham, & Rosenbaum, 1995).

Suicidal Behavior

For the past 13 years there has been a decrease in suicidal behavior in youth until 2008 when it increased (Hung & Rabin, 2009). The current rate of youth suicide is 8% in the United States. Suicide is the second cause of death after accidents in the 18–24 age group.

The greatest increase in suicidal behavior has been in females ages 10–14 years (Hung & Rabin, 2009). Overall, there are more females who attempt suicide but more males who complete suicides. Therefore, suicide is frequently more deadly for males than females since males often choose suicide methods that are more lethal such as using guns or hanging.

Self-Injurious Behavior

Over the last several years there has been an increase in the incidence and severity of SIB (Armey & Crowther, 2008). Adolescents and young adults are at highest risk for having completed a SIB. The rate of SIB in adolescence is reported at 12–21% of the adolescent population (Weierich & Nock, 2008). Thirty-eight percent of college students report having completed an SIB and 75% of these college students report more than one episode (Yates et al., 2008).

Nearly one-third of privileged youth acknowledged having completed an SIB and greater than three-fourths of these did so repeatedly (Yates et al., 2008). Therefore, SIB may be most prevalent in higher-socioeconomic-status (SES) youth. Particularly, rates were elevated among upper-middle-class suburban youth for SIB (Yates et al., 2008). It is hypothesized that the pressures imposed on the higher-SES youth are more than they can support and that their status makes it difficult for them to acknowledge weakness or seek help. Gender differences in SIB rates were more modest and were not statistically significant (Yates et al., 2008).

Protective and Risk Factors
Related to Mental Health Issues

Some protective factors may reduce the likelihood of mental health issues from occurring and some risk factors may exacerbate mental health problems.

Protective Factors

Easy Temperament

At the individual level, easy temperament has been linked to better functioning among youth (Chess & Thomas, 1996; Compas, Connor-Smith, & Jaser, 2004). The lack of easy temperament was also predictive of depressive symptoms for both genders (Laser et al., 2007b). The lack of easy temperament has also been linked to greater difficulty in negotiating and adapting to change and eliciting positive responses from peers and adults (Chess & Thomas), which may in turn increase mental health problems.

Positive Relationship with Parents

Within the family microsystem, a positive relationship between the youth and his or her parents has been predictive of better adjustment (Masten & Coatsworth, 1998; Roth & Brooks-Gunn, 2000).

Supportive Friends

Extrafamilial factors such as positive experiences in the peer group play a pivotal role in youth's healthy functioning. Supportive friends are viewed as a strong protective factor. Friends act to buffer the youth from the full impact of negative events and help him or her cope with adversity (Galambos, Leadbeater, & Barker, 2004; Greenberger, Chen, Tally, & Dong, 2000; Werner & Smith, 2001).

Strong Partner Relationship

The creation of a strong partner dyad is very important for resilient outcomes in youth. Studies show that involvement in a secure, committed relationship is an important protective factor especially if the individual has experienced difficulties in his or her family system (Higgins, 1994; Quinton, Rutter, & Liddle, 1984; Werner & Smith, 2001).

Risk Factors

Severe Illness

A history of severe illness is predictive of more problematic outcomes (Werner & Smith, 2001). A long-standing physical illness or a series of illnesses may be a significant stressor in and of itself, but it may also interfere with other activities that are important to youth such as time with peers, involvement in sports, and missed classes. This may contribute to anxiety about school, social withdrawal, and difficulties in making and maintaining friendships.

Confusion over Sexual Orientation

Confusion over sexual orientation has been found to have a deleterious effect on adolescent adjustment (Lam et al., 2004; Remafedi, Farrow, & Deischer, 1991; Savin-Williams, 1994). Confusion over sexual orientation may undermine the development of a genuine identity (Erikson, 1968; Marcia, 1993). An adolescent who is struggling to find an identity, one that includes a sexual identity, may have increased depressive symptoms.

Lack of Parental Involvement

Lack of parental involvement in the youth's life has been found to be a significant risk factor for a variety of outcomes (Fergusson, Horwood, & Lynskey, 1994; Repetti, Taylor, & Seeman, 2002). Youth had more mental health problems if they perceived their parents to be uninvolved or uninterested in their lives (Laser et al., 2007b).

History of Parental Mental Health Issues

A history of parental mental health difficulties is associated with vulnerability in their offspring. The link between parental mental health issues and mental health symptoms in youth may be due to shared genetic vulnerability, problematic family relationships stemming from parental mental health issues, or a combination of genetic vulnerability and family dynamics (Dugall et al., 2001; Garber & Little, 1999; Luthar, Cushing, Merikangas, & Rounsaville, 1998).

History of Frequent Corporal Punishment

Greater vulnerability in youth is often found when there is a dysfunctional family environment. In particular, if the youth had been frequently disciplined by corporal punishment, his or her functioning may be compromised (Emery & Laumann-Billings, 1998; Fantuzzo & Mohr, 1999). The relationship between corporal punishment and mental health symptoms has been noted (Garbarino, 1995). A history of corporal punishment was a stronger predictor of mental health problems among males more than females (Laser et al., 2007b).

Parental Favoritism of Sibling

An additional family risk factor for mental health symptoms is parental favoritism of a sibling (Dunn & Plomin, 1990; Rutter, 1987). Youth seem to be acutely aware of the treatment they receive from parents relative to their siblings throughout childhood (Dunn & Plomin). Respondents who felt that parents favored their siblings reported more mental health symptoms (Laser et al., 2007b).

History of Being Bullied

Being bullied by peers as a child has been found to be a risk factor for mental health symptoms during adolescence (Cleary, 2000; Duncan, 1999; Laser, 2006). Not surprisingly, being harassed by one's peers increases symptoms for both sexes (Olweus, 2001a, 2001b). Peer acceptance is of paramount importance for youth. Thus being victimized by peers contributes to feelings of loneliness, sadness, lack of self-worth, and self-doubt.

Some of the protective and risk factors are associated with the individual's sense of acceptance, importance, and worth. Fundamental to adolescent development is a sense of self-identity and group identity with a strong family base from which to launch (Zaff & Hair, 2003). Many of these risks undermine the ability to create an authentic identity, especially when family dynamics have not nurtured the individual's development and the peers have bullied him or her.

Particular Signs Associated with Suicidal Behavior

Since suicide assessment is really a matter of life or death, there are some particular signs the practitioner needs to be aware of and assess with youth. However, there are times when a suicide has occurred and there have been no signs. If the youth exhibits any of these signs, further inquiry with the youth needs to take place. If there are multiple signs or a particular sign points strongly to the youth who is considering suicide, a *suicide intervention* needs to take place. A suicide intervention requires that the youth be fully assessed by trained personnel in an appropriate mental health setting (inpatient hospital or outpatient mental health facility). The suicide intervention plan should include who will take the youth to the assessment and who will talk to the parents. Practitioners who work in schools or community centers may have specific intervention protocols.

Changes in Behavior and Verbal Comments That May Suggest a Youth Is Considering Suicide

• *Positive fantasies about dying.* The youth refers to dying as a relief or a better option than his or her current situation.

• *Positive fantasies about pain inflicted on others.* The youth is relishing the idea that his or her death would devastate another.

• *Perfectionism–high-achieving behavior–fear of failure.* Perfectionism coupled with a need to be high achieving in all spheres of his or her life and an overarching fear of failure creates the inability to tolerate any personal failure. The youth is particularly vulnerable for suicidal ideation if he or she has just experienced a major failure especially at school or work. The youth has not had the opportunity to learn the skills to "bounce back" from a setback and may feel that he or she is no longer worthy of living if he or she is not perfect. It should be added that this is a very good reason to allow children and youth to have some failures along the way so that they learn how to cope with failure.

- *Low self-esteem.* The youth is unhappy with him- or herself and does not feel he or she is worthwhile or deserves to live.

- *Hopelessness.* The youth does not have hope or optimism that the future will be any better than the present.

- *Early childhood trauma/loss.* The youth experienced a major loss of a loved one early in his or her life. He or she misses that person and wishes he or she was with this person now during difficult adolescent times.

- *History of suicide of a family member/close friend.* The youth is particularly at risk if he or she has experienced the loss of a family member or a close friend by suicide. Having a member of the family or a friend commit suicide puts the suicide option "on the table" as a method of coping with difficulties.

- *Lack of acceptance of sexual orientation.* Those who are closest to the youth who do not accept his or her sexual orientation can cause a great deal of pain for the youth. Some youth think that it is better to no longer live than to be at odds with their relatives about their sexual orientation and do not see that this will change in the future. If a youth has recently "come out" and his or her family or friends were very cruel or unaccepting of his or her sexual orientation, it is imperative that the youth has the opportunity to be involved in a support group or has the opportunity to talk with a hotline GLBT worker.

- *Communication problems.* The youth has increasing problems communicating with his or her family and friends. He or she is no longer able to share his or her thoughts or feelings with others.

- *Rapid changes in behavior.* The youth's behavior is very erratic and different from what is normally expected. Substance use should also be ruled out.

- *Breakdown of a family relationship.* The family, which had been a source of stability for the youth, is imploding perhaps because a member in the family system is no longer available due to death, separation, divorce, incarceration, severe illness, substance abuse, or debilitating mental health issues. Without the family support the youth feels lost and hopeless.

- *Social withdrawal and isolation.* The youth is isolating him- or herself from activities and people with whom he or she normally likes. Social support is available to him or her, but the youth is incapable of accessing it. Friends may be concerned about the youth or put off by his or her behavior.

- *Eating/sleeping problems.* The youth is either under- or overeating and either hardly sleeping or sleeping a great deal. Any behavior that is not consistent with prior behavior should be inquired about and substance abuse should also be ruled out.

• *Decrease in self-care.* The youth is no longer concerned about his or her physical appearance and is not bathing, putting on clean clothes, or fixing his or her hair. Once again, substance abuse should be ruled out.

• *Emotional behavior out of the norm.* The youth is emotionally charged for unknown reasons. The youth cries easily, is intolerant of other's behavior, or is engaging in physical fighting or verbal arguments for no apparent reason.

• *Getting personal items in order.* The youth is giving away important personal possessions and returning borrowed possessions. He or she may want the people who are important to him or her to remember the youth after he or she is gone through the possessions he or she has given them.

• *Visiting loved one to say good-bye.* The youth may make a special effort to see loved ones to tell them how much he or she loves them, to hug them one last time, or to say good-bye. The youth may be very emotional about this exchange and the loved one may not understand the finality of it. It may be only in retrospect that it is understood, which can be devastating for the survivors.

• *Increased frequency of drug or alcohol use.* If the youth has been using substances, his or her use increases, or is using multiple substances or a larger quantity of substances. The increased substance use can distort thinking, increase feelings of guilt or shame, or make him or her withdraw from sober people who could support him or her.

• *Creating an organized plan.* The youth is collecting pills, buying or obtaining a gun, or purchasing rope, duct tape, and so forth. The youth is planning a place for the suicide and has a date in mind.

• *Recent loss of family member or friend or the anniversary of death is approaching.* The youth may want to meet the deceased "on the other side" and is having a difficult time continuing to live with the deceased gone. Death anniversaries can be very difficult for survivors because the youth remembers the events of that horrible day and wants to dull the pain.

• *Health problems.* Recent diagnose of a debilitating or terminal illness or worsening of a chronic or terminal illness may make suicide an option. The youth prefers to think of leaving the world in his or her prime rather than after his or her body has been wracked by the illness.

• *Severe argument with family, friend, or significant other.* A severe argument with a family member, friend, or significant other creates the fear that the argument cannot be overlooked and will end the relationship. The youth believes that he or she cannot live without the relationship and the relationship has been irreparably destroyed.

• *Feelings of extremely disappointing a family, friend, or significant other.* The youth believes that something he or she said or did will never be forgiven by a family member, friend, or significant other and cannot live with that disapproval and lack of relationship.

• *Previous suicide attempt.* If the youth has attempted suicide in the past, he or she is at much higher risk for attempting suicide in the future.

• *Psychiatric history.* If the youth has a psychiatric disorder and is not in care, his or her behavior may be very erratic and he or she may not be thinking clearly. If he or she was rational suicide would not be an option, but in an altered state it may seem an option.

• *Medications creating severe depression.* Some medications for depression, anxiety, or acne can increase depression in youth. Youth who are receiving medication should be educated about the side effects of the prescription. Additionally, the youth's family should also be educated about the side effects of the youth's medication by the doctor and should be told to alert the doctor if they see any changes in the youth's behavior. The youth should also be made aware that stopping medications "cold turkey" may also cause severe depression.

• *Impulsivity.* If the youth is very impulsive, he or she needs to slow down to think about his behaviors and feelings so that he or she does not act rashly and without thinking.

Clinical Interventions with Adolescents with Mental Health Issues

Cognitive-Behavioral Therapy

The practitioner can use CBT to help the youth gain insight into how he or she gathers and supports his or her beliefs about an incident or a situation. By doing so, the youth can perceive the incident differently and then react differently both emotionally and behaviorally in the future. Through CBT, the youth can learn how to change the conclusions he or she draws about an event and thereby change his or her beliefs (Beck, 1995). The youth begins to understand that his or her prior conclusions often had errors in his or her own logic (Dobson, 2002). Thus the painful feelings associated with those erroneous conclusions are no longer necessary. The youth learns how to think differently about an issue and therefore changes his or her behavior and feelings about an issue. The real or perceived interaction no longer holds the power it once did; it no longer elicits the emotions or behaviors it once did.

CBT-Specific Helping Methods

THOUGHT RECORDS

To help the youth gain insight some specific techniques can be used. First, to begin to assess the triggers that are associated with the behavior and the subsequent thoughts and emotions, it is often helpful to ask the youth to complete a thought record that includes information such as date, situation, behaviors, emotions, thoughts, and responses (Dobson, 2002). The process of keeping a thought record can be very insightful for the youth to reflect on when the situation occurred and how he or she reacted to the situations in the past and how he or she could change his or her reactions to the event in the future. Questions that should be asked by the practitioner include When a trigger in the past happened how did he or she react? How could he or she act differently? How could he or she perceive the incident differently? If the youth perceived the incident differently, then how would this change his or her reaction to the incident? What were his or her feelings about the situation? How can the youth use those past feelings to interpret what is happening for him or her now? How does changing the youth's thinking about the event change his or her behavior and feelings?

As an example, Mary (16 years old), a very shy and introverted young woman, often perceived that a girl in her class, Betsy, was trying to intimidate her when Mary was called on by the teacher. When looking at her thought record, it became clear to Mary that she only had these feelings when she was being called on in class and not in other social situations. She was able to become aware that the anxious and humiliating feelings were being generated as a response to her being requested to participate in class and not by a perceived threat to her by Betsy. When she understood the situation differently, Mary was able to change her behavior and her feelings about the classroom experience. As Mary began to understand that she had the inner strength to answer the teacher's question, especially since she knew the answers, the self-doubt was vanquished and she was able to more fully participate in class without worrying about her classmate's perceptions of her.

AFFECTIVE EDUCATION

Affective education is teaching how to learn to recognize, label, and develop a vocabulary to talk about emotions. Frequently, in the United States, we do not provide our male youth with ample vocabulary to express his emotions effectively and therefore he becomes cut off from his emotions and often does not understand how his emotions are affecting his behavior. Through affective education, the youth can learn to understand that there are many emotions other than anger, which he may feel is the only emotion he is "allowed" to express. He can learn to understand the multitude of emotions in himself and in others. Affective education can be taught by observing people, by viewing pictures or movies, or reading scenarios. Ask the youth to name the emotion and why he believes it is that emotion. As this continues, it can be a game that he enjoys playing. Additionally, ask him When does he feel the emotion being discussed? What does he do when he feels the emotion? How does his body feel when he feels the emotion? Then ask him When does he see the discussed emotion in other important people in his life? How do they behave when they experience the emotion? With this knowledge, the youth can better assess his own emotions and assess the emotions of others.

BODY AWARENESS

It is also helpful to work with the youth to understand what his or her body is telling him or her when he or she is stressed. Therefore, techniques such as tensing up one's body and relaxing one's body is helpful to gain an understanding of how the youth can assess when he or she is feeling stressed. The youth can also learn to self-soothe through relaxing his or her muscles especially in his or her back, arms, jaw, and forehead. Similarly, breathing techniques can be used. First help the youth become aware when he or she is breathing heavily and then monitor and control his or her breathing.

SELF-MONITORING

Over time, the youth can begin to self-monitor when stressful situations are occurring and to think through how to deal with the situation. The youth can assess his or her feelings, what his or her body is doing, why he or she is feeling that way, and then think about how he or she will react rather than just reacting. One technique I have found effective when a youth is feeling stressed or anxious by a particular situation is to help him or her remember to say to him- or herself "Doubt the doubt" thereby instead of the youth undermining or second guessing his or her own ability to persevere, he or she can push those doubts out of his or her mind and continue forward.

PROBLEM-SOLVING TECHNIQUES

Another CBT technique that is useful is to help the youth use problem-solving strategies. The youth can be taught problem-solving techniques initially through modeling or role play and then by internalizing the strategies.

First, the youth needs to define what the problem is. If they are in family therapy, the parent also needs to define what the problem is. This may take some time since frequently the trigger and the underlying problem are different issues. As an example, Sandy lives alone with her father, Mike, and is experiencing a breakdown of communication. The trigger could be that when Sandy talks to her father, her father does not act like he is listening to her. The underlying feeling for Sandy is that she feels that her father does not care about her or her life. Then, when Mike wants to spend time with Sandy, Sandy is dismissive of her dad's request and claims she already has plans. The underlying feeling for Mike is that Sandy no longer wants to spend time with her dad. Through practice, they can learn how to do this, but may need some help in understanding what the core problem is.

Second, the youth needs to generate as many solutions to the problem as possible. If they are in family therapy, the parents should also generate solutions. As the practitioner, you should write down these solutions on paper, so they can be kept. In the case of Sandy and Mike, they might suggest that they have a specific time every day where information is shared, information is shared with the TV off, they eat dinner together, they have a father–daughter night monthly, Mike acknowledges that he heard what Sandy said after she speaks, Mike asks questions about Sandy's life, and so on.

Then a solution that is agreeable to everyone needs to be chosen from the list that was created. It may be difficult to choose one solution, but a commitment to a solution is necessary to solve the problem. In the case of SIB youth, research has found that they can often generate many solutions, but have great difficulty committing to a solution (Nock & Mendes, 2008). The commitment to a solution is extremely critical for SIB youth.

Finally, the youth and/or the family commits to use the solution for the next week. Then when the youth and/or the family returns the following week, they assess the solution's effectiveness at solving the problem, agree to continue with that solution, or mutually agree to another solution off the original list or generate new solutions that they can agree upon. As the youth and/or family improves his or her or their ability to problem solve, the activity will seem more second nature and less a difficult and forced process.

RELAXATION TECHNIQUES

Through increased self-awareness of both one's mind and body through CBT, it is helpful for the youth to discover ways of reducing stress and anxiety. Centering activities (like yoga, meditation, or quiet reflection), prayer, massage, or a warm bath can be strategies that the youth can use to reduce stress in his or her life. Additionally, visioning activities, also called a "1-minute vacation," are helpful when the youth is feeling stressed to take a moment to envision him- or herself in a serene location (beach, forest, looking at a mountain, near a waterfall, etc.; anywhere he or she feels comfort and at ease). Help the youth to think about what it looks like, feels like, smells like, and sounds like in that location; how does he or she feel in that location? and can he or she bring those positive feeling to his or her present situation? When practiced these techniques can be very effective in helping to reduce stress.

It should be noted that there are some disclaimers about the use of CBT. If the youth's cognitive or emotional development is severely stunted, CBT may not be effective since the youth must possess the cognitive skill of thinking about thinking. Therefore, the youth needs to have reached formal operations (as discussed in Chapter 2) to be able to effectively use CBT. Second, the youth's social and cultural context needs to be considered (Dobson, 2002) to assess whether his or her patterns of thinking are due to culturally prescribed viewpoints. Additionally, some clinicians believe that youth with severe personality disorders are unable to achieve the needed level of personal insight necessary to make CBT successful.

Dialectical Behavior Therapy

DBT is a particular form of CBT. It has been found to be particularly effective in persons with personality disorders (Linehan, 1993) and who have made suicide attempts or self-injury (James, Taylor, Winmill, & Alfoadari, 2007; Katz, Cox, Gunasekara, & Miller, 2004; Woodberry & Poepenoe, 2008). DBT emphasizes four areas: *mindfulness, interpersonal effectiveness, emotional regulation*, and *distress tolerance* (Linehan, 1993; Woodberry & Poepenoe, 2008). Through a series of sessions on each of the components, the client is able to change both his or her thinking and behavior. Through mindfulness training the client is taught how to live in the moment and to experience his or her emotions with all of his or her senses. Interpersonal effectiveness teaches clients how to become better problem solvers in interpersonal communications and issues. It helps them learn to think about what they can change in relationships, what they cannot change in relationships, and how to differentiate between the two and not to lose themselves or their integrity in relationships. Emotional regulation is basically affective education training as previously discussed in the CBT section. Distress tolerance is a continuation of mindfulness skills in which the client is taught to see him- or herself as a survivor of a negative event and to use skills such as self-soothing, thinking of pros and cons of the prior event, and to accept oneself for who he or she is. Other such skills acquired through distress tolerance are to learn how to say what he or she means and mean what he or she says, and how to improve the current moment of his or her life. Both of these later skills are often worked on through role playing and self-imagining what the client might do in particular scenarios in his or her life. DBT works to change the client's current thinking so that he or she can function better in the present.

Interventions for SIB

There have been several interventions that have been found to be beneficial for youth involved in SIB. A recent study by Nock and Mendes (2008) concluded that clients benefited from therapy that helped them select adaptive solutions, rather than to generate solutions. They found that SIB youth were often able to generate a myriad of solutions, but were often unable to pick a solution that was most appropriate, as discussed previously. Therefore, techniques such as CBT could be of great use to SIB youth but with the added emphasis of choosing a solution and then using that solution.

Additionally, interventions that incorporate the family system into the treatment of SIB youth have been found to be effective (Yates et al., 2008). However, if the stress the youth is feeling is mainly being generated by the parent, it may be advisable for the youth to receive counseling individually before beginning family therapy. Parent education of positive parenting techniques has also found to be effective for parents of SIB youth (Yates et al.).

Medication

Some mental health issues are not ameliorated by talk therapy alone. It is always preferable to begin with talk therapy, like CBT, but in some instances it is not effective on its own. Practitioners do not have the option for prescribing medication, but they may work beside or have access for consultation to medical or psychiatric doctors who do prescribe. It is important to help the prescribing physician know the presenting symptoms and any underlying circumstances that may be contributing to the symptoms for the youth. For instance, if a youth recently experienced a loss, the behaviors that he or she may be exhibiting are not typical behaviors for him or her. It is also very important for the youth to understand the possible side effects or complications of any medication. Youth who experiment with substances must be aware of the interaction effect of the medication and his or her substance of choice.

Case Study

Isabela is a Latina 16-year-old sophomore at an urban high school. Last year, Isabela's grandmother died. Isabela and her grandmother enjoyed watching movies together and baking. She had been a major support for Isabela since her mother often works long hours at two jobs and is frequently emotionally unavailable to her. Isabela's mother is still angry about the divorce and blames her ex-husband for making her life so hard and unhappy. Isabela's father had divorced her mother several years ago and has since remarried and has two small children with his new wife. Isabela has not seen her father, stepmother, or half-brothers for over 2 years.

Isabela does not have many friends at school. She has no one to confide in at school. She is very shy and often students are unaware of her. None of her teachers have reached out to her. She often feels invisible at school. Isabela is not involved in extracurricular activities because she has no one to pick her up after school. Isabela also does not like sports because she feels uncoordinated and overweight.

Isabela has experimented with cutting on her fingers mainly to see that she is bleeding and still alive. She feels a sense of relief when she sees the blood. She often feels like if she did not experience some pain, she would not know she was alive. No one at school has noticed she has been cutting.

Isabela feels that no one really has taken the time to get to know her other than her grandmother and she is gone. She spends a great deal of time watching television and most recently has begun writing and drawing in a journal. Isabela spends long hours alone at her house. When her mother comes home she is often tired or in a bad mood and not interested in talking. Isabela does not feel that her mother knows her. She spends some time online and chats with a variety of people she has met online. Most recently there has been a guy, Mark, who seems nice. Isabela is thinking about meeting him.

QUESTIONS FOR THE REFLECTIVE PRACTITIONER

1. What mental health risk factors does Isabela have?
2. What mental health protective factors does Isabela have?
3. As a school social worker, you notice the marks on Isabela's hands when she changed classes in the hall. What should you do?
4. Is Isabela depressed? Why or why not?
5. How do you connect Isabela with other youth?
6. How do you improve Isabela's relationship with her mother?
7. Is Isabela in danger of hurting herself? Why or why not?

Chapter Summary

This chapter presented various mental health concerns among adolescents from depression and suicide to personality disorders and SIB. The prevalence of these issues among teens was discussed, as well as the protective and risk factors related to them. The particular signs associated with suicide were presented. These signs can serve as areas for assessment when a practitioner believes a teenage client is at risk for committing suicide. In addition, however, each reader is highly encouraged to talk with their clinical supervisors and professors to learn more about the specifics of assessing and reporting concerns about suicide. CBT and DBT, as well as medication, were presented as intervention modalities for adolescent mental health concerns. Treatment of mental health issues is challenging and practitioners in training are encouraged to discuss their ideas for intervention with a clinical supervisor who can guide their work. Chapter 13 discusses sexual activity in youth.

Sexual Behaviors, Sexually Transmitted Diseases Including HIV/AIDS, and Pregnancy

Julie Anne Laser, Shannon Sainer, and Nicole Nicotera

Chapter Overview

This chapter covers the issues that encompass teen sexual activity. Particularly rates of teen sexual activity, sexual behaviors of teens, STDs, HIV/AIDS, and teen pregnancy are discussed.

CASE EXAMPLE:
Who Are the Youth Represented in This Chapter?

The following case example represents some of the concerns related to adolescents and sexual activity. Considering the implications for this case within the context of the risk factors, theory, assessment, and intervention strategies presented in the following pages will prepare you to assess and suggest interventions for the more developed case study at the end of the chapter.

Lorenzo is a sophomore Latino male. Lorenzo has a girlfriend, Samantha, who is a freshman at his high school. They have been going out for the last 5 months. Last weekend, Lorenzo was at a party with friends where he "hooked up" with a senior girl, Linda, who was drunk. She gave him a "blow job" in the bathroom at the party. Lorenzo feels really guilty that he was with Linda, but she was willing to give him a blow job, whereas Samantha refuses. This week at school Lorenzo heard that Linda had also been with four other guys at the party, and has quite a history of "servicing" the football team. Lorenzo wonders if he could have caught an STD from Linda and whether he could pass that on to Samantha. Lorenzo and Samantha are planning on having intercourse for the first time this weekend. Samantha is a virgin.

Using an Ecological Perspective to Better Understand Adolescent Sexual Behavior

When discussing sexual activity of youth, we cannot underestimate the influence of the environment on shaping behavior. Teens may model their sexual behavior by the behaviors of their peers or from the popular media. Research shows that family and school environments are most important for activities that define adolescent future orientation, but peers become increasingly more influential in activities that define their present activities and behavior (Lau et al., 1990). Small and Covalt (2006) have found that youth who believe that their peers are all sexually active are more likely to be sexually active themselves. Therefore, the old adage "Birds of a feather fly together" could not be more apropos to adolescent sexual activity.

Practitioners who work with adolescents should ask, "What percentage of the kids you hang out with are sexually active?" This gives you an idea of the youth's sexual activity, but you may need further clarification regarding particular sexual behaviors. Often asking whether they are sexually active will generate different answers than asking if they are having intercourse or having oral or anal sex, as will be discussed more fully later in the chapter.

The question about peers' sexual behavior opens up the dialogue to discuss a topic that frequently youth do not discuss with adults, namely, sex: in particular their feelings about sex, their insecurities about it, pregnancy scares, bad experiences that they may have had, and any need for information about birth control or STDs. It has been our experience that the information that youth receive about sex is often incorrect or has been only partly understood. With many schools no longer teaching sexual education in the classroom, this information has been left to parents who often feel uncomfortable, are unsure, or are unable to have the important discussions about sexual activity and STDs with their youth. One-quarter of teens ages 15–17 report that they have never had a conversation with parents regarding sex, birth control, or STDs (Kaiser Family Foundation, 2006). Therefore, much of their information about sexual activity is received from other teens. Though somewhat humorous if the consequences were not so tragic, we have been told by pregnant teens that they understood that they could not get pregnant if they had intercourse standing up, had intercourse when they were menstruating, if the male pulled out prior to ejaculation, or if she douched with coca-cola after intercourse. Obviously, none of these are legitimate birth control methods, but they sounded plausible to the young women. If youth do not have sufficient information sources about birth control or STDs, they may look to the practitioner for information.

Practitioners should be familiar with their agency's policy related to discussing sexual activity, birth control, and pregnancy options with youth. Some organizations forbid practitioners to have these discussions with youth. When the agency allows open discussion of sexual topics, it is advisable to have a list of names of local organizations that can give youth more information, receive birth control, or test for STDs.

Sexual Activity Rates

The National Youth Risk Behavior Surveillance (YRBS: 2007) survey (CDC, 2007a) found that nearly 33% of ninth graders have had sex and 7% of students participating in the YRBS report having had sex before the age of 13. A recent poll from MSNBC and *Time* magazine found that 41% of youth 15 and 16 years of age acknowledged they are sexually active (MSNBC, 2005). Additionally, by 18 years of age the number of sexually active youth rises to over 70% in the United States (Santrock, 1998). Therefore, during the adolescent years most American youth are becoming sexually active. Moreover, the rates of sexual activity as studied by race/ethnicity and rural/urban populations have found that though the rates of sexual activity are lower in rural settings, minority status, especially in rural communities, puts individuals more at risk for early sexual activity (Hensel & Anderson, 2006).

Gender Differences

Some differences have been found in the rates of sexual activity between male and female teens. Santrock (1998) reports that boys acknowledge that they are sexually active at higher rates than girls in every year of mid- to later adolescence: 15-year-olds (boys 33%, girls 27%), 16-year-olds (boys 50%, girls 34%), 17-year-olds (boys 66%, girls 50%), 18-year-olds (boys 72%, girls 69%), and 19-year-olds (boys 86%, girls 75%). These findings may not be completely representative because it has been suggested that males frequently exaggerate their sexual activities and females often diminish the frequency of their sexual interactions. Some have suggested that rates are at greater parity, but that traditional cultural morays around acknowledging sexual activity account for the difference. Therefore, "nice girls" are not stating that they are sexually active and males who are "studs" but perhaps not sexually active are stating that they are sexually active.

Interestingly, higher SES in teen males was associated with both more sexual partners and more frequent sexual activity, but decreased the probability of childbearing. However, males who worked more hours after school were also more likely to be sexually active, but were also at higher risk for being adolescent fathers (Santelli, Lowry, Brener, & Robin, 2000). Therefore, males with more disposable income or males who worked more hours were both more likely to be sexually active, but were very different in their level of birth control use.

Youth who participated in sports were generally less involved in sexual risk taking. However, males, especially African American males, who considered a central component to their identity as being a "jock," were much more likely to be involved in higher levels of sexual risk taking (Miller, Farrell, Barnes, Melnick, & Sabo, 2005). Therefore, in the schools coaches should be educated about comprehensive sexual education so they can educate their student athletes.

For females, their rate of sexual activity increased significantly when they were involved with boys who were 3 or more years older than they were (Gowen, Feldman, Diaz, & Yisrael, 2004).

Effectiveness of Programs Aimed at Reducing Sexual Activity Rates

Due to United States' high rate of teen sexual activity and the highest rate of teen pregnancy in the industrialized world (Child Trends, 2002) there has been a desire to reduce these numbers. Adults (73%) and teens (56%) in the United States also continue to believe that youth need more information about abstinence and contraception, rather than merely an "either or" mentality (National Campaign to Prevent Teen and Unplanned Pregnancy, 2008). Most of the sex-education programs have centered around the "just say no" philosophy for reducing sexual activity. Few have actually been successful in changing judgment or personal considerations (McCave, 2007; Yampolskaya, Brown, & Vargo, 2004). Programs that have been successful have found that repeated and sustained discussion with teens can change risk behaviors, but it needs to be an ongoing program and not simply a short-term academic unit (Coyle et al., 2006).

One area that does seem to actually impact rates of sexual activity is to give parents clear and concise information to consistently share with their teenagers (Eisenberg, Sieving, Bearinger, Swain, & Resnick, 2006; Meschke, Bartholomae, & Zentall, 2000). Particularly, girls who had received strong consistent messages from their mothers about delaying sexual activity were much more likely to do so; however, this did not hold true for mothers speaking to their sons or to fathers speaking to their sons or daughters. Finally, there is increasing evidence that programs for parents of adolescents can lead to greater parent–teen communication about sexual behavior and to actual changes in adolescent sexual behavior, especially if the adolescents are also involved in such programs (Kirby, 2007).

It has been found that youth who have higher levels of religiosity are more likely to delay sexual activity than those with low levels (Hardy & Raffaelli, 2003), which supports the idea that religiosity can help delay sexual activity, but will not in itself keep youth from becoming sexually active. Additionally, youth who are more engaged in school and have high aspirations for the future are more likely to delay sexual activity.

Interestingly, neighborhood collective efficacy (neighbors who watch out for each other's children and let parents know if they have seen their child act inappropriately) has been found to be an effective influence for delaying sexual activity for both males and females (Browning, Leventhal, & Brooks-Gunn, 2005).

Another area that has been studied regarding teen sexual activity is time use by adolescents. American teens have the world's highest levels of free time (Larson, 2001). However, how they use that time often puts them into situations where there are greater levels of risk behavior. When controlling for gender, age, race, and SES it was found that the greatest predictors of problem behavior were family time and peer time. With increased family time, sexual activity was reduced, however, increased time with peers led to increased sexual activity (Barnes, Hoffman, Welte, Farrell, & Dintcheff, 2007). Sexual activity rates were highest if the friends that they were spending more time with were also involved in high-risk behaviors (La Greca, Prinstein, & Fetter, 2001).

Abstinence-Only Programs

A recent (2007) government study found that students who had participated in abstinence-only programs were just as likely to be sexually active as those who had not received the training. Abstinence-only programs are ones that teach only abstinence, and do not teach the effectiveness of condoms and contraception. It was found that abstinence-only education did not reduce the likelihood of engaging in vaginal intercourse. Additionally, adolescents who received comprehensive sex education were significantly less likely to report teen pregnancy than those who received no formal sex education, whereas there was no significant effect of abstinence-only education on pregnancy rates (Kohler, Manhart, & Lafferty, 2008). This is particularly concerning since the U.S. government spends $176 million annually on such programs.

Programs Proven to Be Effective in Reducing Sexual Risk-Taking Behavior

Thanks, in part, to decades of research in effective HIV-prevention programming and more recently in teen pregnancy-prevention research, there is now a body of evidence on which interventions do work in reducing sexual risk-taking behavior. There are now several programs that have been proven to change sexual risk-taking behaviors and reducing teen pregnancy or HIV. These programs are considered to be "evidence-based" or "science-based" programs because they were evaluated using rigorous evaluation methodology, replicated, published in peer-reviewed academic journals, and shown to reduce sexual risk-taking behavior for a sustained period of time. Some evidence-based programs have been shown to delay sexual activity or increase safe-sex behaviors for up to 3 years after the program implementation. Studies of these programs suggest that when the original programs are implemented with fidelity in similar settings with similar populations of young people, their positive effects on reducing sexual risk-taking behavior are also replicated (Kirby, 2007). Evidence-based programs for reducing sexual risk-taking behavior deliver clear messages to youth on delaying (or abstaining) from sexual activity, in addition to information on contraception and condom use if youth are sexually active. Mediating factors, such as knowledge, attitudes, perceptions of peer norms, self-efficacy, and intentions, have also been studied to see which factors have changed for the youth due to involvement in the programs and in turn how those factors affect behavior. There is good evidence that interactive video-based and computer-based interventions can be effective in reducing sexual risk-taking behavior. Additionally, some controversial policies such as providing emergency contraception to girls and young women in advance of having sex have promising evidence of reducing sexual risk-taking behavior (Kirby).

Birth Control Usage

Fifty-three percent of female teens and 45% of male teens acknowledge that they had a discussion with their partner regarding contraception before first intercourse. The greater the youth's knowledge about condom usage and their greater general communication with their parents were strong predictors that contraception would be discussed prior to first intercourse (Ryan, Franzetta, Manlove, & Holcombe, 2007). Increased information about condoms and other forms of birth control increases the likelihood that teens will discuss and use birth control prior to being sexual active. Additionally, it underscores the parents need to be educated about birth control. Condom use by 9th to 12th graders is at about 63%, which is the highest since it has been studied (Kaiser Family Foundation, 2005). However, more recently there has been a decline in condom use (CDC, 2007a) and a recent study found that condom use is overreported by youth (Rose et al., 2009). Nevertheless, the great majority of youth consider condoms the best way to prevent pregnancy (94%) and HIV and STDs (98%) (Kai-

ser Family Foundation, 2005). Therefore, youth are hearing and understanding the message about condoms.

However, 17% of females and 9% of males between the ages of 15 and
19 admit that they used no form of birth control the last time they had
sexual intercourse (Kaiser Family Foundation, 2005), underscoring the
need for the message to be repeated often.

Sexual Behaviors of Teens

Dating versus "Friends with Benefits" or "Hooking Up"

The trend toward "hooking up" (sexual liaisons without emotional commitments) and "friends with benefits" (friends, not romantic attachments,
with whom the youth is engaging in sexual activity) has trickled down from
college campuses into high schools and middle schools. This is seen as a
way of gaining sexual experience without the emotional attachments, time
requirements, exclusivity, or financial obligations of dating. Cell phones
and the Internet have made hooking up that much easier, whether in Chicago or Golden, Colorado (Boies, Knudson, & Young, 2004). However, it
has been found that hooking up is particularly prevalent in the suburbs,
in that more suburban 12th graders than urban students have admitted
to sexual relationships outside of a romantic relationship (43% compared
with 39%, respectively) (Denizet-Lewis, 2004). A recent study found that
of the 55% of 11th graders who acknowledged having intercourse, 60% of
those stated that their partner was a friend and not a romantic partner.
That number would perhaps be higher if the study asked about oral sex
because many teenagers have simply replaced intercourse with oral sex
(Denizet-Lewis).

It has been suggested that hooking up undermines the ability of teenagers as young adults to create and sustain intimate relationships (Stepp &
Shaver, 2008). This is particularly concerning since Erikson (1959, 1968)
understands that the primary responsibility of early adulthood psychosocial development is to establish intimacy with another. However, Bogle
(2008) has found that many of the individuals who were involved in hooking up developed more traditional forms of dating after college. Since
hooking up is a newer phenomenon, the long-term effects are unclear
because many youth who have been involved in hooking up have not yet
reached adulthood.

Still, many teens date. When teenagers do date, they often do so in
ways that would be unrecognizable to their parents, or even their older
siblings. A "formal date" might be a trip to the mall with a date and some
friends. Teenagers regularly flirt online first or through texting and then
decide whether to do so in real life (Denizet-Lewis, 2004).

Oral Sex

Oral sex has become the norm of many sexual interactions between teens. Seventy-seven percent of the teens surveyed agree that oral sex is sex, however, over half stated that even after oral sex they believe they are still virgins (MSNBC, 2005). One study found that nearly 55% of adolescents (ages 15–19) have engaged in oral sex (Lindberg, Jones, & Santelli, 2007). Oral sex was more likely to occur among teens who had initiated vaginal sex, compared to those who had not. According to this study, 82% of youth reported engaging in oral sex within 6 months of first initiating vaginal sex (Lindberg et al., 2007).

Oral sex seems to be more frequently occurring by girls performing oral sex on boys rather than boys performing oral sex on girls or performing on each other (Robinson, 2009). Additionally, there seem to be differences in oral sex by race and ethnicity, with higher rates of white males performing (81.4%) or receiving oral sex (81.4%) than Latinos performing (70.7%) or receiving oral sex (73.2%) or African American males performing (50.5%) or receiving oral sex (66.3%) (Rathus, Nevid, & Fichner-Rathus, 2000).

Anal Sex

It is estimated that 10–16% of youth have had heterosexual anal sex (Lindberg et al., 2007). Some girls prefer to have anal sex so that they remain a vaginal virgin. Teens should be aware that they are at increased risk from contracting an STD from anal sex due to the higher incidence of bleeding.

Biting

With the recent popularity of vampire movies, biting during sexual activity has become an activity of some teens. Teens should understand that biting can cause bruising and infections. Some teens using biting as a way of "marking" their sexual partner.

Sex-ting

Another new development of the technological age is that adolescents are sending nude or seminude pictures of themselves electronically or posting them online. This sex-ting (sex texting) has been found to occur in about 22% of teen girls and 18% of teen boys. The recipients of these sex-tings are 33% teen boys and 25% teen girls (National Campaign to

Prevent Teen and Unplanned Pregnancy, 2008). Many have suggested that this communication is used to help create hook-ups for the future. However, it also puts these youth in danger for sexual victimization and the possibility that someone other than the intended recipient will view these photos.

Practitioners working with a youth who is sex-ting should help him or her to understand that anything he or she may send or post will likely not remain private, which could cause embarrassment or even humiliation. Additionally, youth need to understand that they may be putting themselves in danger of being victimized. It should be added that there have been a few cases in the United States where the sender of a sex-ting message was prosecuted for pornography and when convicted was included in the National Sex Offender Registry. Though this seems extremely punitive for a poor choice, it underscores the need to think about the ramifications of their behavior before acting.

Platonic Opposite Sex Relationships

The vast majority of young adults seem to see such friendships as a natural thing: A 2001 Match.com poll of 1,514 members found that 83% believe men and women can be just friends (Paul, 2003). Until recently, such friendships, when they existed, usually faded away after one of the pair got married, at which point cozying up to pals of the opposite sex no longer seemed appropriate. Today, people not only form more cross-sex friendships, but they also include their best mates in their weddings and maintain the friendships long after the wedding day (Paul, 2003).

A Word about Clinical Interventions

The best way a practitioner can work with youth regarding the discussion of sexual activity is to offer both information and to be a nonjudgmental sounding board for youth's emotional responses to sexual activity. Information gives the youth the ability to make informed choices of whether to be sexually active or not, and to be prepared and safe if he or she chooses to be sexually active.

Helping the youth become aware of the emotional issues connected to sexual activity is also very important. Sexual activity involves their bodies, their minds, and their emotions. It is important that youth understand that sex is not merely a physical event. The practitioner should help youth become aware of the level of maturity that is needed to untangle the emotional feelings from the physical desire of sexual activity.

Dating Violence

Nearly one in five sexually active teenage girls in the United States say they have been physically abused by a date in the past year (Harvard School of Public Health, 2003). Some girls see this behavior as a reaction to being jealous and a display of their partner's love for them. However, there is nothing romantic about this violent behavior. Some teenage girls believe that their partner's anger and angst can be assuaged by love and understanding; however, this is rarely effective and can often cause these girls to be treated like a "punching bag." The best advice these girls can receive is to distance herself from her violent partner.

Additionally, it has been suggested that 10.3% of American teen females and 4.8% of American teen males have been forced to have sexual intercourse on a date (Howard, Wang, & Yan, 2007). It is important to let both girls and boys know that they should never feel pressured to have sex or to feel that they need to have sexual intercourse or perform a sexual act on their partner to remain in their current relationship.

Sexually Transmitted Diseases

Adolescents are at greater risk for STDs than adults because they have a perceived invulnerability due to their good health and anticipated long life. Youth frequently underestimate their chance of getting an STD or HIV. However, teens are getting STDs at extremely high rates. A recent national study found that 26% of American females ages 14–19 have at least one STD (Centers for Disease Control and Prevention [CDC], 2007b). The most common STDs in youth are human papillomavirus (HPV), trichomoniasis, and chlamydia. Nearly two-thirds of all chlamydia cases go undiagnosed with the majority of chlamydia cases being asymptomatic. Additionally, the majority of gonorrhea cases are asymptomatic, and most cases are undiagnosed. It is estimated that twice as many new STD infections occur each year than are reported (CDC, 2007b). One in two sexually active youth will contract an STD by the age of 25 (American Social Health Association [ASHA], 2005).

STDs and Females

Females bear the greatest burden of STDs, suffering more frequent and more serious complications than males. It has also been estimated that 30–40% of preterm births and infant deaths are related to maternal STDs (CDC, 2000). Additionally, if females have not received proper medical treatment for an STD, it can render them infertile in the future.

STDs and Racial–Ethnic Minorities

STDs occur more frequently in minority youth than Caucasian youth. However, there may be some bias in the data since more minority youth frequent public health centers where STDs are reported more completely than with private healthcare providers. It has also been suggested that minority youth may lack access to screening and prevention programs (CDC, 2000).

Risk Factors for STDs

Adolescent risk behaviors vary by race and gender for sexually transmitted diseases but do not necessarily correlate to STD prevalence. Using drugs, heavy drinking, smoking, and multiple partners were noted risk factors for STDs; however, African American female youth were less likely to be involved in these activities, but were more likely to be diagnosed with an STD (Halpern et al., 2004). Therefore, awareness of the risk factors is important to curb STD rates but may miss important populations. It is generally understood that reducing the number of sexual partners and reducing concurrent sexual partners is important in reducing STD risk (Kirby, 2007).

There is a lot of misinformation by youth about how one protects oneself from STDs. Forty percent of youth believed that a pill or a shot protects them from STDs and HIV. Others believed that they could not become infected with an STD if they were having oral sex. Finally, the majority of youth believed that as part of their annual physicals they were being tested for major STDs and if they had not been told by their medical provider that they had an STD, they were free of disease (ASHA, 2005). This misinformation is alarming and can contribute to the spread of STDs.

Prevention of STDs

It is important to help teens know what behaviors put them at risk for STDs: using drugs, heavy drinking, smoking, multiple partners, concurrent sex partners, and not using condoms. All of these risk behaviors make youth less inhibited sexually and less likely to think about having safe sex. Therefore, these behaviors put youth at greater risk for participating in unprotected sexual activity.

However, just because they may not be participating in any high-risk behavior and think they are safe from disease, their partner may be or may have been involved in high-risk behavior or may have been involved sexually with someone who had an STD. Practitioners should help youth understand that if he or she is sexually active, anyone who his or her partner was ever sexually active with is a possible source of disease transmission. Therefore, if the youth is not consistently using a condom, he or she is putting him- or herself at risk for STDs.

If the youth has been sexually active, especially with multiple partners, the practitioner should suggest that the youth, as part of his or her annual physical, ask to be tested for STDs. Additionally, the practitioner should suggest that female adolescents be vaccinated for HPV.

HIV/AIDS

An estimated half of all the new HIV infections occur in people under the age of 25. Minority youth are particularly hard hit by HIV/AIDS. African American youth represent 65% of the HIV/AIDS cases and Latinos represent 20% of the cases between 13 and 19 years of age. Additionally, girls made up 51% of the HIV/AIDS cases between 13 and 19 years of age. Most youth who are HIV positive were infected sexually (Kaiser Family Foundation, 2006). Racial and ethnic differences were also found in the level of HIV prevalence of adolescent males who were having sex with males (Celentano et al., 2005). Therefore, it is extremely important that prevention and testing programs be sensitive to cultural differences.

Risk Factors for HIV

There are several risk factors that have been associated with HIV transmission. They include early age of sexual initiation, coming from a disadvantaged population, substance abuse, having an STD, lack of knowledge about HIV, poverty, and dropping out of school (CDC, 2008). Many of these risk factors are in fact societal issues and issues that characterize many of society's problems.

Effective Prevention Strategies for HIV

Recent research has found that an effective strategy for HIV prevention is to teach adolescents strategies for the prevention of HIV in groups of friends (Morrison et al., 2007). Another effective strategy is to have health education programs directed to youth who live in high-prevalence STD/HIV neighborhoods, which resulted in reduced rates of infection in both males and females (Sieverding et al., 2005). Better educating parents about HIV/AIDS helps them communicate information correctly to their youth (Nappi, McBride, & Donenberg, 2007).

Other groups that need prevention programs particularly tailored to their own personal circumstance include minority youth, sexual minority youth, runaway youth, and homeless youth. Schools should be important partners in disseminating comprehensive information about sexual health and educating youth about prevention of HIV. Along with education, more routine HIV testing can prevent HIV transmission and prevent reinfection of HIV.

Teen Pregnancy

Rates of Teen Pregnancy

During the 1990s, there was a decline in the birth rate among adolescent females in the United States. However, more recently there has been an increase in teen pregnancy rates with teen births increasing in 26 states (CDC, 2009). For 14 years, the United States experienced a dramatic decline in teen birth rates, with a 34% decline in the teen birth rate for 15- to 19-year-olds between 1991 and 2005. However, between 2005 and 2007, the teen birth rate for this age group increased by nearly 5%. Data from 2007 marked the second consecutive year that the teen birth rate increased nationally (Hamilton, Martin, & Ventura, 2009).

It is unclear why this increase in teen birth rate is occurring. There have been some theories proposed, but more research is needed to confirm or refute these theories. Stories have been presented in the popular media that girls have purposely colluded with their friends to become pregnant. Earlier research was presented that high levels of sexually explicit television programming influenced pregnancy rates but was later refuted (Chandra et al., 2008). Nevertheless, the birth rate to adolescents in the United States continues to be much higher than it is in most other developed countries (Child Trends, 2001). Countries with very low birth rates (e.g., Japan, Italy, Spain) have fewer than 10 births per 1,000 teenage females. Teens in the United States are less likely to use contraception consistently than teens in most other developed countries, and has been found to be the primary reason why other developed countries have lower birth rates among teens than the United States (Jones, Darroch, & Henshaw, 2002). Additionally, the abortion rate of U.S. teens has decreased significantly since the 1990s (Kaiser Family Foundation, 2005). Hence, more pregnant teens have chosen to give birth rather than terminate the pregnancy.

Using an Ecological Perspective to Better Understand Teen Pregnancy

Adolescent mothers are diverse. They come from all racial, ethnic, and income groups. There are adolescent mothers who are honor students and others who are in special education classes. Some adolescent mothers are well adjusted, and others are troubled or depressed. The birth rates to teens differ by race with the highest number of adolescent mothers being Latina adolescents (92 per 1000), followed by African American (82 per 1,000) and non-Hispanic whites (30 per 1,000) (Child Trends, 2002).

Risk Factors Associated with Teen Parenting

Many studies show that adolescents who become parents have some characteristics that are different from their nonpregnant or parenting teens. Adolescents who are struggling in school, score low on standardized tests, or who have dropped out of school are at risk for early childbearing (Hotz, McElroy, & Sanders, 1997; Jaffee, Caspi, Moffitt, Belsky, & Silva, 2001; Moore, Miller, Glei, & Morrison, 1995; Rauch-Elnekave, 1994). Those who become adolescent parents are more likely than their peers to have a history of sexual abuse, and to abuse alcohol or other drugs (Boyer & Fine, 1992; Butler & Burton, 1990; Luster & Small, 1997; Moore et al., 1995; Musick, 1993). Acting-out behavior in childhood is predictive of teenage pregnancy (Kessler et al., 1997; Kovacs, Krol, & Voti, 1994; Miller-Johnson et al., 1999; Zoccolillo, Meyers, & Assiter, 1997; Zoccolillo & Rogers, 1991). Additionally, 42% of teen mothers experience a second pregnancy within 24 months (Raneri & Weimann, 2007).

Family risk factors also contribute to increasing the chance of becoming a teen parent. Adolescent mothers are more likely to have problematic relationships with their parents than their nonparenting peers (Luster, 1998). A sibling who had a child as a teenager increases the risk of early pregnancy for her younger siblings (East & Jacobson, 2001).

Environmental risk factors also increase the odds of becoming a teen parent. A disproportionate number of teenage mothers live in single-parent households, in families living below the poverty line, with parents who obtained low levels of education, and with mothers who had their first child as a teenager (Hotz et al., 1997; Kahn & Anderson, 1992; Luker, 1991). Therefore, the issues that affect many teen moms are intergenerational.

Additionally, neighborhood risk factors contribute to teen parenting. Adolescents who become mothers are more likely to come from impoverished neighborhoods and to attend schools where rates of adolescent pregnancies are high (Brewster, 1994; Musick, 1993). The future the youth envision for themselves may be strongly influenced by what they observe in their neighborhoods and communities.

Risk factors in the peer network also play a part in higher rates of teen parenting. Adolescents may be influenced by the behavior of their peers and partners. Early parenthood may seem more appealing if friends gain attention, independence, and adult status from having a baby. Male partners may also pressure adolescents into having a child early as they see it accentuates their virility.

Adolescent Parenting

How well adolescents deal with the challenges of parenting likely depends on protective factors that they possess both internally and in their environment.

Frequently, the mother's family steps in to give support and to help with child care. However, it should be cautioned that social support that does not strengthen the mother–child relationship could actually undermine that lifelong relationship. Some studies showing that motvhers who received higher levels of support were not the primary individual involved in the raising of their own child (Barratt, Roach, Morgan, & Colbert, 1996).

The father of the child or the mother's current partner can be a very positive influence if he is involved. He may provide financial support for the family, emotional support for the mother, and care for the child. However, frequently the father of the child plays only a peripheral role in the new family. This may be due to his lack of maturity, if he is also a teen.

Parenting teens may use some of the same practices that were used in their family of origin to parent their child, and in other cases, they may make a conscious choice to do things differently from the way they were parented. Certainly, adolescent mothers who were the recipient of poor parenting in their family of origin will not inevitably follow the same path. However, it may be difficult to provide optimal care for children if abusive or neglectful parenting is all that the young mothers have experienced, because they truly do not know what they should do. Therefore, practitioners should connect young mothers to parenting classes and online resources that discuss parenting, appropriate developmental milestones, and methods of dealing with the everyday stressors of parenting. Additionally, it is important to help mothers brainstorm about ways they can help alleviate stress in their lives.

Case Study

Beverly is a 17-year-old European American female. She was born in Wisconsin to a mother who lost her parental rights when Beverly was 6 years old. Beverly's mother had been physically, sexually, and emotionally abused as a child. Beverly experienced the same abuse in her mother's care at her mother and mother's boyfriend's hands. Beverly was in seven foster care placements over 6 years. Eventually she was adopted when she was 12 years old.

A single mother, Helen, who is a high school math teacher, adopted Beverly. Helen loves Beverly deeply, but often has trouble connecting to her. Beverly often does not share her life events with her adoptive mother. Helen wants to be included in Beverly's life, but often feels like an outsider. Helen still hopes that Beverly will come to trust her and to love her. Currently, Helen believes that Beverly sees her current adoptive home as a safe place to stay until she becomes an adult, but does not consider Helen her family. This saddens Helen, who yearns for a relationship with Beverly. Recently, Helen has been concerned about Beverly's coming home late. She now requires Beverly to wake her when she returns home. Sometimes when Beverly comes into Helen's bedroom to say goodnight she smells like beer and cigarettes.

Beverly craves healthy positive attention. She is quite cute: She has long blonde hair, blue eyes, and has a healthy athletic body. She likes participating in sports at which she excels. She has difficulty maintaining eye contact and feels anxious if people stare at her. Beverly takes great care of her personal hygiene. She spends a great deal of time on her hair and will not leave home until it is perfect.

Beverly is very good at sticking up for herself and sometimes misunderstands her peers' joking and takes offense. She has a reputation at school for being a bit of a "hot head." She has only a few girl friends even though she plays on several sports teams. She has many male admirers with whom she sometimes hooks up, but does not see any of them as a "boyfriend."

Beverly actively pursues sexual relationships with boys. She has had sex in her car with boys that she has met at the mall. She has also sent topless pictures of herself to potential hook ups. She frequently has unprotected intercourse and gives blow jobs to boys after school or in the movies. She laughs at her behavior and thinks it is funny. When the girls at school call her a "ho" she believes they are just jealous of her and would get more action if they were not so "frigid" and hung up about their sexuality.

Beverly is extremely moody when boys reject her. She often tries to cover this up by creating negative rumors about the boy who has rejected her and moves quickly to the next hook-up. She does not like to think about the ramifications of her behavior on her physical or mental health and avoids the topic.

QUESTIONS FOR THE REFLECTIVE PRACTITIONER

1. What are the risk factors for Beverly?
2. What are the protective factors for Beverly?

3. How can you as a practitioner support Beverly in using safe-sex practices?
4. How can Helen be more involved in Beverly's life?
5. Why do you think Beverly is acting so recklessly?
6. How can you as a practitioner impact risk-taking behaviors of youth?
7. How can practitioners support pregnant and parenting teens?

Chapter Summary

This chapter presented information regarding frequency of teen sexual activity, sexual behaviors of teens, STDs, HIV/AIDS, and teen pregnancy. In the following chapter, delinquency is discussed.

CHAPTER 14

Delinquency

Julie Anne Laser, George Stuart Leibowitz,
and Nicole Nicotera

Chapter Overview

This chapter uses an ecological perspective to understand adolescent delinquency. Pathways to delinquency and antisocial behavior are explored, as well as differences between male and female delinquents. By the end of the chapter, you will be able to understand the many factors that contribute to adolescent delinquency and be able to apply that information to assess and intervene in the case study at the end of the chapter.

A teen does not simply wake up one morning and look in the mirror and say, "I think I will be a juvenile delinquent today." There are many risk factors that contribute to delinquent behavior. Adolescents who engage in delinquent behavior are a diverse group. Their behavior differs by severity and causes.

Risk factors for delinquency are found at the individual level, as well as in the key contexts where adolescents spend much of their time including the family, peer group, school, and neighborhood (Fergusson & Horwood, 2003; Luster & Small, 1997; Ungar, 2004; Werner & Smith, 1998). Additionally, the media influences some youths' involvement with delinquent behavior.

CASE EXAMPLE:
Who Are the Youth Represented in This Chapter?

The following case example represents some of the concerns related to adolescents and delinquency. Considering the implications for this case within the context of the risk factors, theory, assessment, and intervention strategies presented in the following pages will prepare you to assess and suggest interventions for the more developed study example at the end of the chapter.

Eric, a bi-racial 16-year-old, attends a charter high school focused on helping youth who have learning differences and have not been successful in their neighborhood school. About a month ago, Eric entered outpatient rehab counseling for marijuana. He has been clean and sober since he entered counseling. He seems to like his program and is motivated to change. However, he still hangs out with his friends in the neighborhood who he has been in trouble with in the past. In addition to an addiction to marijuana, Eric has a history of tagging, truancy, theft, racing cars, and running away from home. Eric lives with his father and younger brother.

Defining Delinquent Behavior, Conduct Disorder, and Antisocial Behavior

There are several definitions that are important to understand regarding delinquency: delinquent behavior, conduct disorder, and antisocial behavior. These three definitions are related to each other but are distinct.

Delinquent behavior can be defined by but is not limited to shoplifting, theft from family members, peers, teachers, or strangers, vandalizing or "tagging" (graffiti art) on public or private property, intimidation of peers or adults, involvement with gangs, and fighting (with or without weapons) with peers, teachers, parents, or strangers. These behaviors could cause involvement with the police or the criminal system. There is both a continuum of behavior and severity of behavior.

Conduct disorder is the psychiatric diagnosis found in DSM-IV-TR that involves delinquent behavior (American Psychiatric Association, 2000). It includes aggression to people or animals, destruction of property, lying, stealing, and rule breaking (American Academy of Child and Adolescent Psychiatry, 2004).

Antisocial behavior is the disregard of social customs and standards of behavior. The disregard for social customs and standards of behavior creates the opportunity for delinquent behavior. Therefore, delinquent behavior and antisocial behavior are interconnected.

Individual Protective and Risk Factors for Delinquency

At the individual level, several protective factors have been found to be important for decreasing delinquency.

Internalized Moral Development

Many researchers have suggested that internalized moral development is an important protective factor (Jessor et al., 1995; Kumpfer, 1999; Laser et al., 2007a). Internalized moral development means that youth, whether anyone is watching or not, chooses ethical behavior. Lickona (1991) noted that moral development is triadic, with the components of moral knowing, moral feeling, and moral action all being pertinent to the formation of good character. Therefore, delinquency occurs because of deficiencies in one or more of these three areas: lack of knowledge, low levels of empathy or guilt, or behaviors that show disdain for social mores. The lack of internalized moral development increases the likelihood of antisocial behavior. As a practitioner, you can help youth understand what constitutes moral behavior, increase empathy by helping the youth understand the other's viewpoint, and give them opportunities where they can act morally, like volunteering.

Easy Temperament

Easy temperament has also been found to reduce involvement with delinquent behavior and difficult temperament increases delinquent behavior (Dodge & Petit, 2003; Frick, 1998; Loeber et al., 1998). This makes sense in that youth who can "go with the flow" are less likely to get angry or frustrated and act out due to changes and difficulties that they face, as compared to youth who have difficulty with change and new situations.

History of Sexual or Physical Abuse

A history of sexual or physical abuse has also been related to delinquent behavior (Laser et al,, 2007a; Parker & Herrera, 1996). Though less severe than physical abuse, youth who had received frequent corporal punishment (e.g., spanking) were also more likely to be involved in delinquent behavior (Laser et al.).

Due to the youth's past victimization, he or she may have learned some maladaptive behaviors that put him or her at greater risk for delinquent behavior. These behaviors include a heightened sensitivity to any threat (real or imagined), difficulty with *cognitive appraisals* (gathering correct information about the situation he or she is facing), *impaired judgment* (difficulty making good decisions), prone to use substances, and *compromised self-protective abilities* (putting him- or herself in risky situations or with unsafe people). However, it is important to note that not all victims of abuse are involved in delinquent behavior, nor do all youth who have been involved in delinquent behavior have an abuse history (Finkelhor, Turner, & Ormrod, 2007).

Alcohol, Tobacco and Early Sexual Activity

Other individual behaviors put youth at risk for delinquency such as alcohol consumption (Hagan & Foster, 2003), tobacco use (Simmons-Morton & Haynie, 2008), and early sexual activity (Brooks-Gunn & Paikoff, 1997). Each of these behaviors may point to problems with decision making, risk taking, and peer pressure.

Family Protective and Risk Factors for Delinquency

Family functioning has been cited as an important predictor of delinquency (Loeber & Dishion, 1983; Loeber et al., 1998). Within the family microsystem, a positive relationship between the youth and his or her parents has been predictive of better adjustment (Laser et al., 2007a; Masten & Coatsworth, 1998; Roth & Brooks-Gunn, 2000).

Mother–Son Relationship

A healthy relationship between mother and son has been found to be particularly important to reduce delinquency and increase a greater sense of well-being in youth. The mother–son relationship gives boys a sense of support, eases distress, and helps to increase career aspirations (Field, Lang, & Yando, 1995; Laser et al., 2007a; O'Koon, 1997; Taylor, Lerner, & von Eye, 2001). Therefore, as a practitioner you should consider the importance of improving the mother–son relationship through family therapy as helping to prevent delinquency.

Lack of Father Figure

The lack of a father figure present in the life of youth is a risk factor (Fergusson et al., 1994; Fergusson & Horwood, 2003; Henry, Caspi, Moffitt, & Silva, 1996; Sameroff, 2000). Additionally, children who were raised in homes where there were constant changes in the configuration of the parental unit were at greater risk for later criminality (Henry et al., 1996). As a practitioner, you should try to connect youth with a mentor who is committed to be involved throughout the youth's teen years.

Neglectful or Permissive Parenting

Parents who are not aware of their youth's activities increase delinquent behavior (Laser et al., 2007a). Neglectful or overly permissive parenting has been found to put youth at risk for delinquency (Farrington, 1995; Fergusson et al., 1994; Garmezy, 1993). Parents who do not know where their youth are, who they are with, or what they are doing create an environment for their youth where greater risk taking can occur. Even though it may not be popular with youth, supporting parents to monitor their youth's activities is an important activity for practitioners working with youth and their families. The need for parental monitoring extends throughout adolescence.

Witnessing Domestic Violence

Witnessing domestic violence as a child or as an adolescent puts youth at risk for delinquency (Eckenrode, Powers, & Garbarino, 1997; Laser et al., 2007a). Male adolescents, in particular, who had witnessed domestic violence had greater delinquent behaviors than their peers who had not witnessed domestic violence (McGee, Wolfe, & Wilson, 1997). It has been hypothesized that adolescent males who had witnessed domestic violence used delinquent behaviors as a means of coping with their circumstances (Aymer, 2005).

Peer Protective and Risk Factors for Delinquency

Negative peer relationships have the opportunity of occurring in many venues. There is a contagion effect that happens for children and youth who associate with more delinquent peers who then become more delinquent themselves (Dodge et al., 2006). The youth's delinquency increases with ongoing delinquent peer association. The contagion effect has been found to be more pervasive with younger less serious delinquent youth. This makes sense developmentally in that younger adolescents who do not have a strong sense of personal identity may be more influenced by others with strong personalities around them. Conversely, youth who have friends who avoid trouble are more likely to stay away from trouble themselves.

School Protective and Risk Factors for Delinquency

Sense of Belonging

A sense of belonging at school plays a pivotal role in youth's functioning. A sense of belonging reduces feelings of disengagement and alienation (Bogenschneider, 1998; Garcia-Coll et al., 1996; Maughan, 1992; Roth & Brooks-Gunn, 2000; Wang et al., 1994). Students who feel that they are connected to their teachers, classmates, instructional programs, and school functions are better equipped to handle adverse circumstances (McMillan & Reed, 1994; Wang et al.). Therefore, youth are much less likely to be involved in street gangs or become isolated and antisocial if they are connected to others at school.

Negative or Punitive School Control

In school settings where negative and punitive systems continually respond to student behavior there is an increase in the effect of delinquency contagion. Students in these situations band together in defiance of what they find to be unfair policies or feel that punishment inflicted is unnecessarily harsh.

Frequently Changing Schools

Frequently changing schools is a risk factor for delinquency (Cicchetti et al., 2000; Laser et al., 2007a). Youth who changed schools several times a year were also more likely to be maltreated by their parents and more likely to be isolated from peers (Cicchetti et al.). This sense of isolation and lack of belonging is deleterious for positive youth development.

Neighborhood Risk Factors for Delinquency

Living in a neighborhood that is not safe has been found to be a risk factor for delinquency (Laser et al., 2007a). Hawkins and colleagues (1992) found that population density, high mobility, physical deterioration of the neighborhood, and high levels of crime put the adolescents and young adults who live in those neighborhoods at risk for delinquency and substance abuse.

Media Risk Factors for Delinquency

Exposure to violent movies, songs, television, and video games has been associated with delinquent behavior. Increased viewing of violence is related to delinquent behavior (Jenson & Howard, 1998; Laser et al., 2007a). Watching violence or listening to music that promotes violence may lull youth into thinking that violence is an acceptable way of solving problems or dealing with unpleasant emotions. It also may desensitize youth from the real painful outcomes of violence. As an example, when I worked with a youth who was romanticized the "gangsta" lifestyle, he stated that "a gunshot just felt like a bee sting." His inability to see gun violence for what it is kept him from realizing how dangerous and deadly it could be.

The Development of Delinquency

Delinquency and antisocial behavior can be seen as a developmental process that begins in early childhood and continues in adolescence and adulthood. Patterson, DeBaryshe, and Ramsey (1989) outlined a developmental model of delinquent behavior that emphasizes a sequence of experiences from early childhood to late childhood and adolescence that can result in problem behavior.

Initially, inconsistent parenting, parenting that vacillates between overindulgent and permissive to rigid and inflexible although consequences are not often enforced, is the first stage in the progression toward conduct disorder. The youth's first understanding about trust and healthy relationships happen in the home. Inconsistent parenting practices teach the child not to trust his or her parents or the world around him or her.

The second phase of the model highlights how problem behavior among children can be exacerbated by academic failure, which creates feelings of inferiority at school (Hernandez, 1999) and peer rejection by mainstream peers. These two failures in middle childhood can result in a greater relationship to a deviant peer group since the mainstream group has ostracized him or her. The final outcome of this model is delinquency.

Based on the development model one can see the importance of intervening early with the child before the delinquent behavior has a chance to take a foothold. For example, parenting classes that emphasize consistency, following through, and logical consequences for misbehavior are important for young children and their parents. In middle childhood there may be problems of parent–child interactions that can be remedied through family therapy. In middle childhood the parent and child are generally still committed to work together. Often by later adolescence, parents have surrendered their ability to effectively interact with the delinquent youth, and may be less inclined to be involved in the process.

The Biopsychosocial Model

Dodge and Petit (2003) developed a biopsychosocial model of the development of delinquent behavior. There are three initial components: biological, cultural values, and child development. Biological influences are genes and natural predispositions such as cognitive ability and temperament. Cultural values are the values and morays of the culture where the youth resides. Child development is the youth's progress across the domains of development: emotional, social, cognitive, moral, and physical. Parents, peers, social organizations, schools, and religious organizations then influence the initial components. With positive influences, youth reduce the risk of developing delinquent behavior even if they have the genetic predisposition or the socio-cultural influences that make delinquency more probable. However, negative influences on the initial components make delinquency more likely. Therefore, each individual is endowed with certain characteristics but then is influenced by a myriad of social factors.

The Multiple Pathways Model

The multiple Pathways model suggests that there are three pathways to delinquency: *overt, covert,* and *authority conflict* (Loeber et al., 1998; Loeber & Hay, 1997). Each of these pathways describes a different developmental pathway to delinquency. The multiple pathways model shows a progression from less serious to more serious behavior.

The first pathway is an overt pathway, which begins when a child engages in minor aggression (bullying and annoying others) progressing to physical fighting (especially gang-related fighting) and culminating in more serious violence (rape or assault). The second covert pathway begins with minor covert behavior (frequent lying, shoplifting, stealing from friends or family) and then progresses to property damage (vandalism, tagging, fire setting) culminating in moderate to serious delinquency (fraud, burglary). The third authority conflict pathway, which begins with a pattern of stubborn and defiant behavior before age 12, progresses to defiance and disobedience and culminates in authority avoidance (runaway, truancy, incorrigible behavior).

Delinquent youth who follow the overt pathway tend to decrease delinquent behaviors over time as they progress to adulthood and few move to more severe antisocial behavior. Conversely, the covert pathway delinquent youth increase in severity with age. This may be because the overt problem youth have more opportunities to change their behavior because attention is drawn to them, whereas the covert delinquent youth spend much of their time "flying below the radar." The delinquent youth who follow the authority conflict pathway are a mixed group; some will outgrow their delinquent behavior in their late teens and others will continue to exhibit antisocial behavior.

Gender Differences in Pathways to Delinquency

Sex differences in delinquent behavior have been an underexplored area (Moffitt, Caspi, Rutter, & Silva, 2001). Research has shown that delinquency has different dynamics in females versus males (Kravitz, Cavanaugh, & Rigsbee, 2002). It is known that males account for a greater number of antisocial offenses than females. Violent crimes and property offenses are disproportionately committed by males, with the highest occurrences of crimes being committed during adolescence. It is noteworthy, however, that 29% of juveniles arrested were female (Snyder & Sickmund, 2006). Within arrests of violent female offenders, 28% were juveniles (Robinson, 2009). Therefore, nearly a third of all juveniles arrested are females and a third of all females arrested are juveniles.

Many female delinquents differ from male delinquents in their exposure to childhood sexual abuse (Acoca & Dedel, 1998). Females had higher levels of sexual abuse and were abused at younger ages than their male counterparts (Matthews, Matthews, & Speltz, 1989). Additionally, female delinquents were different than their male peers in their level of mental health issues. It was found that 84% of females had mental health needs in comparison to 27% of males who had mental health needs who were involved in the criminal justice system (Timmons-Michell et al., 1997). These findings can be interpreted as a cry for help by delinquent females. Practitioners working with female delinquents should assess for both abuse histories and mental health issues. It may be that the primary issue is not delinquency, but rather the other underlying issues that affect female juvenile delinquents.

The negative influence of family criminality is more deleterious for female youth than male youth. In studies of violent girls, criminal behaviors among their family members had a greater influence in the development of delinquent behavior in females than in males (Cloninger Christiansen, Reich, & Gottesman, 1978; Funk, 1999).

Delinquent males were more influenced by peers who were involved in delinquent activities than females (Cloninger et al., 1978; Funk, 1999). Therefore, the contagion effect of delinquency for females is related to the youth's family and in males it is related to their peers.

Adolescent Onset versus Childhood Onset of Delinquency

There are two distinct patterns of delinquent behavior: life-course persistent, which begins in childhood, and adolescent onset (Moffitt, 1993; Moffitt et al., 2002). The childhood-onset group exhibits problems early in life with organization, planning, trouble understanding cause and effect, difficulty changing strategies or thinking in a novel way, and poor judgment. The childhood-onset group also has highly problematic parent–child interactions. In contrast, the adolescent-onset group develops delinquent behaviors during the adolescent years. Until their teen years, the adolescent-onset group does not have any behaviors that are of concern.

The majority of delinquent behaviors are limited to the adolescent period (Moffitt, 1993). The delinquent acts of male youth usually occur when they are with peers and involve less severe delinquent acts. Most of the adolescent-onset delinquent behaviors decrease by their late teens.

However, the childhood-onset group of delinquent youth exhibits more violent delinquent acts over time. The childhood-onset group's behavior began before adolescence and extends into adulthood. The childhood-onset group is a much smaller group of offenders than the adolescent-onset group; however, many have lifelong involvement with the legal system. For the great majority of juvenile delinquents their behavior is merely an unfortunate response to a stage of development and not a lifelong pattern of behavior.

For the practitioner who is sitting with the 16-year-old client, it may be helpful to gain a timeline of when the delinquent behavior began to better understand if his or her behavior developed during the adolescent years or before adolescence.

Clinical Interventions with Delinquent Youth

Building a Positive Therapeutic Alliance

Delinquent youth are more responsive and compliant when they share a stronger therapeutic alliance with their practitioner. Similarly, a practitioner who acts as coach by both encouraging positive behavior and making the youth aware of negative behavior can be helpful for delinquent youth.

Behavioral Therapy

Some delinquent and conduct-disordered youth need to have firm parameters for what constitutes appropriate and inappropriate behavior. Clear behavioral goals should be established that progressively shape behavior in the areas of concern. Consequences for inappropriate behavior need to be applied consistently and fairly, and a system of monitoring should be in place to ensure the accomplishment of goals. This approach, called *contingency management* (Masters & Burish, 1987), can assist the youth in making behavioral changes by rewarding prosocial behavior and reducing antisocial acts. Some youth with more severe antisocial behavior requires that the practitioner work as a coach, who both encourages positive behaviors and discourages negative behavior. This is in contrast to psychotherapy, which emphasizes the importance of the therapeutic relationship where the youth comes to understand his or her behavior over time.

Contingency management is more direct than psychotherapy and guides the youth to distinguish prosocial from antisocial behavior. The youth should begin therapy with a discussion of the rules and the consequences for not following the rules. If the youth chooses to act inappropriately, he or she will receive a negative consequence for his or her behavior. If he or she acts appropriately, he or she will be rewarded. The youth learns that good things happen when good choices are made, and bad things happen when bad choices are made; it is all about his or her choices. He or she also learns that he or she will be held accountable every time. The youth cannot complain that he or she was not aware of the consequences of his or her negative behavior or that he or she "really did not mean it."

Sometimes delinquent youth play the "unknowing victim." In this situation the practitioner can emphasize what behaviors cause negative consequences to extinguish this role. Additionally, opportunities for positive behavior need to be made so that the youth can get positive regard and acknowledgment for appropriate behavior. It is important for the youth to know that adults are aware when he or she is acting appropriately and making gains.

Over time, the repertoire of negative behaviors will decrease and prosocial behaviors will increase. Incentives for prosocial behaviors need to be found that are both appropriate and something that the youth is interested in working toward. A practitioner needs to find the "carrot" that the particular youth will be motivated to continue in positive behavior, especially when he or she is in the company of youth who may not exhibit appropriate behavior.

Motivational Interviewing

Motivational interviewing (Miller & Rollnick, 1991) has been found to be successful with delinquent youth in clinical practice. A full discussion of motivational interviewing is found in Chapter 10.

Multisystemic Therapy

MST is an intensive treatment model that addresses multiple risk factors and contexts that contribute to delinquent behaviors (Swenson, Henggler, Taylor, & Addison, 2005). These contexts include family, peers, community, school, and neighborhood. The techniques of MST are derived from family therapy (Haley, 1976; Minuchin, 1974). The goal of MST is to address parenting practices, improve family relationships, decrease adolescent involvement with delinquent peers, improve academic performance, and provide an extended network of caregivers that may include family and friends. The therapist becomes involved in all the contexts of the youth's life and tries to get the different contexts to better support the youth and more effectively communicate with each other. As you might imagine this is very labor intensive and demands that the practitioner is available, or at least on call, 24 hours a day. An MST therapist generally has a very small caseload of four to six client families. The average length of treatment is 4 months (Mihlalic, Fagan, Irwin, Ballard, & Elliot, 2002; Saldana, Swenson, & Letourneau, 2006).

Cognitive-Behavioral Therapy

CBT has been found to be effective with delinquent youth. Helping the youth understand his or her thoughts and emotions, and how they affect his or her behavior is an important insight for delinquent youth. See Chapter 12 for details.

Connecting Delinquent Youth with Nondelinquent Youth Mentors

Just as the contagion effect works to infect negative behaviors for some youth, positive role models work as an inoculation for delinquent youth. Therefore, it is helpful to pair youth with students who are both strong in their values and able to share those values with others.

Changing the Practitioner's Mindset: Risk Prevention versus Reoffense

The practitioner needs to think about how he or she can emphasize the need for prevention of deviant behaviors, rather than not reoffending. It is important to emphasize that the youth is not simply trying to stay out of trouble, but permanently changing his or her patterns of behavior to prevent future negative consequences. This may seem like just jargon, but the practitioner needs to believe in the ability of the youth to change his or her behavior and not simply become better at hiding behavior to stay out of trouble.

Mental Health Staff versus Correctional Staff

The practitioner should see him- or herself as an agent of help and positive change rather than an individual who controls and polices youth. The practitioner should see him- or herself as someone who is giving the youth tools to make positive changes in his or her life, rather than bending the will of the youth to make him or her behave.

Case Study

Charlie is a 15-year-old who is currently in a residential home. He is in the ninth grade. He is a tall, lanky, European American male and his long hair covers one of his brown eyes. Both his mother and stepfather frequently abused alcohol and meth. They severely physically and emotionally neglected Charlie and his sister, Marie, during early childhood. Charlie and Marie were exposed to extreme domestic violence between his mother and stepfather. Several times, the neighbors called the police due to the violent noise. Once his stepfather was arrested for assault, but his mother took him back. His mother and stepfather physically and emotionally abused Charlie and Marie.

When Charlie was 7 and Marie was 5, they were taken into foster care. Since that time, Charlie has been in eight foster homes. On one occasion, when he was 13, reunification was tried. Charlie was returned to his mother's home because she had left his stepfather. However, shortly after he returned home, he began arguing with his mother and the arguments escalated into violence. Charlie's behavior was beyond his mother's ability to control it, and Charlie was then placed in a residential home. Charlie has not seen Marie for a number of years. His mother has not visited the residential home for a number of months. The last time Charlie saw his mother she was distraught and under the influence of meth. Charlie's mom had been involved with a man who committed suicide in front of her. Charlie does not believe his mother ever loved him. He has no known extended family, nor does he know the whereabouts of his biological father. When he becomes 18 he hopes to find Marie again.

Charlie has done well in school even though he has been in many schools over the years. He has a full-scale IQ of 115. He does particularly well in math. Charlie has a great deal of difficulty making friends. Most of the time he is by himself. He does not have a plan for his future.

Charlie has engaged in animal cruelty, stealing, physical aggression, verbal abuse, destruction of property, and fire setting. He never cries and smiles infrequently. He lacks empathy and genuine care for others. Charlie has struggled with enuresis (bedwetting) throughout his life and it continues to be a problem. He sometimes has terrifying dreams and often wakes up to find he has wet the bed. He hides this from the other boys at the home. He has a tendency to minimize his negative behaviors and projects blame on others. His foster care worker has told him that he will not be allowed to return to his mother's home as a juvenile. The permanency plan for Charlie is to be in long-term foster care until he ages out. He is stoic about this plan for his living arrangements.

QUESTIONS FOR THE REFLECTIVE PRACTITIONER

1. What risk factors does Charlie have?
2. What protective factors does Charlie have?
3. How would you intervene with Charlie?
4. Do clients like Charlie make you nervous?
5. Do you have concerns for your own safety around a client like Charlie?
6. How would you establish a relationship with Charlie?
7. What clinical techniques would you use with Charlie?

Chapter Summary

Delinquency arises from issues in multiple contexts: family, peers, school, neighborhood, and the media. Developmental pathways that lead to delinquency were presented. The risk factors that contribute to delinquent behavior and protective factors that may serve to alleviate such behavior were also discussed. Clinical strategies for working with delinquent youth were presented. The following chapter, 15, is the final chapter of the book, which reviews the resilience and ecological approaches to working with adolescents.

CHAPTER 15

The Joys of Working with Adolescents

Chapter Overview

Practitioners by definition must assess and resolve *problem* situations, therefore, they sometimes may miss the wonderful qualities adolescents possess. We conclude this book by emphasizing the positives and by reminding you that it is the strengths and resilience of adolescents that ultimately helps them succeed. This is what makes working with them such a pleasure! They are growing and developing and are on the brink of adulthood. It is a very exciting time of life. All too often parents and teachers focus on the negatives: "Why did you get that C?" "I notice that you are sleeping late almost every morning!" or "Why can't you get a job to save up to buy a car?" The youth hearing these questions repeatedly may begin to have serious doubts about him- or herself. These doubts can become self fulfilling and cause him or her to give up without trying. He or she may also feel that nobody understands. However, when adults use a tone of curiosity and interest in helping to pose the same questions, the parent and teacher may learn that possible medical issues, worries about a friend's use of alcohol, or anxiety about college applications may be underlying the problematic behavior. The mind-set of the adults who interact with teens can make a tremendous difference in the nature and quality of the interaction. This chapter intends to put a positive spin on working with adolescents in the belief that a strengths-based approach has the greatest likelihood of success, and it certainly engenders positive feelings in both the practitioner and the client.

In this final chapter we present the Nguyen family as a culminating example of the M-E approach. We also present examples that represent the positive attributes of adolescents as active contributors to society. These constitute some of the joys of working with adolescents and the strengths they bring to the wider society.

Review of Theoretical Approaches

The ecological theory forms the foundation for the M-E approach to working with adolescents. This approach allows practitioners to work with teenagers and all the contexts that influence their development: self, family, peers, school, neighborhood, media, and cultural and societal structures, such as racism. The terms *microsystem, mesosystem, exosystem,* and *macrosystem* sum up these concepts. Each system influences adolescent development across all of the domains addressed in Chapter 2: physical, cognitive, moral, emotional, identity, and social. For example, we note in Chapter 1 that the M-E approach compels practitioners to assess and intervene beyond a teen's internal reasons for the acting out. This expanded assessment might account for experiences of racism, bullying, or homophobia as contributing factors to acting out. A strengths-based approach joins with the youth in acknowledging that although others may be putting him or her in a position of "victim," he or she does not need to accept their incorrect biased judgment. Having established the basis for a helping relationship, the practitioner will then be in a better position to engage the youth in figuring out how to fight these unfair personal attacks. This acknowledgment of and intervention into the broader influences on the day-to-day actions of the adolescent client constitutes an ecological approach to practice. The experiences of Shahir as a refugee growing up in the United States provided an excellent example of the M-E approach to understanding how context shapes behavior and the multiple points for assessment and intervention.

Resilience theory is also integral to understanding the protective and risk factors that impact the life journey of each adolescent. Early renditions of resilience theory focused on assessing an individual's risk factors. As the theory developed, scholars determined that this sole focus on risk factors made it impossible to account for youth who succeeded even in the face of great risks. This led researchers to also assess for protective factors or individual and environmental strengths that promote youth development and sometimes ameliorate negative events. No longer was youth development a liturgy of how to avoid risks that increased the chance of vulnerable outcomes, but rather the exploration of positive influences that supported healthy development or resilience. Clients were no longer "doomed" to have negative events undermine their growth and development; events could trigger growth, have no influence on growth, or as previously thought make growth more difficult. Shahir is an excellent example of how protective and risk factors work together to influence outcomes and explain how he could develop in positive ways even after the losses he experienced because of having to escape a war-torn country.

The combination of ecological theory and resilience theory allows the practitioner to understand a teenager's struggles from multiple perspectives that address psychological and internal factors and also accounts for the contextual influences on those internal experiences. In fact, in Chapter 3 we point out the connection between the two theories noting that protective and risk factors combine a mixture of individual attributes and the social and cultural context of those relationships, supports, and opportunities. An assessment of the social and political context of Shahir's new life in the United States, combined with the risks related to his personal and family losses serves as the foundation for suggesting interventions that also take account of the protective elements of a strong family system, the boy's cognitive and athletic abilities, and positive peer relationships. The M-E approach addresses each of the ecological levels and thereby offers a more complete assessment and indications for treatment planning.

Case Example: The Nguyen Family

The Nguyen family represents the combination of strength and hardship described in resilience theory. The family and its current concerns also represent the various levels of ecological theory, thereby providing a good example for assessment of the family concerns from the M-E approach.

The Nguyen family resides in Los Angeles, California, where they began their lives after escaping Vietnam in 1972. The Nguyen household includes Mr. and Mrs. Nguyen, who were born in Vietnam, and three of their children, Jenny (age 17), Gary (age 15), and Greg (age 9), who were born in the United States, and Mrs. Nguyen's parents. Their oldest son Jimmy (age 19) lives in the dorm at University of California, Berkeley where he is a freshman in college. Jimmy was also born in the United States. Mrs. Nguyen is an only child. Mr. Nguyen's parents died during the Vietnam War in 1971. His older brother was a soldier in the war and died in 1968. His younger sister still lives in Vietnam, but they lost contact when the family fled to the United States. Prior to the war, Mr. Nguyen's father was a wealthy businessman in Vietnam, but the family lost everything when the Communists came into power. With the death of his parents and the loss of the family business and fortune, Mr. Nguyen came to the United States with minimal assets. He and Mrs. Nguyen met in a refugee camp and fell in love. They share the same values and Buddhist beliefs, which they hoped to pass on to their children. They were married when they reached North America. Since that time, Mr. Nguyen makes a good living from the media store he owns and has been successful in moving the family into the middle class.

The family resides in an ethnically diverse, middle-class neighborhood and Jenny, Gary, and Greg attend the local public schools. The family is proud of their oldest son, Jimmy, who they have just sent off to attend university in northern California. They have great hope that the other three children will follow in Jimmy's footsteps. The family values education and they have tried to impart that to their children.

There have been stressors within the family as Mrs. Nguyen's parents have needed increased care in their older years and Jenny and Gary are testing family limits more than Jimmy ever did. More specifically, Jenny (17) is not interested in Vietnamese culture and is dating a young man who is European American, and Gary (15) has become distant from his parents, not sharing his ideas with them the way he used to in the past. He always has his head buried in his computer or is texting his friends from his cell phone. Everyone in the family misses Jimmy's presence in the home, but no one in the family is talking about this fact. In addition, Mrs. Nguyen's father is in the early stages of dementia.

Mr. and Mrs. Nguyen became especially alarmed when the following sequence of events occurred. On Saturday night Grandma picked up Jenny's coat and a bag with condoms fell out of the pocket. She showed them to Jenny's parents. When Jenny got home her parents yelled at her and told her she had shamed the family. Jenny insisted that she has no use for condoms and that the school had handed them out to all the students. Her parents are outraged that the school handed out condoms because they want to be in charge of these matters. Mrs. Nguyen states that she is going to call the school principal to complain about this and let the other Vietnamese families in the school know about it so they can also complain. Upon hearing this, Jenny confessed that she found them under Gary's bed when she was doing her chores, but Gary denies this. Mr. and Mrs. Nguyen do not know that Gary and Jenny have been arguing ever since the school passed out condoms because Jenny does not believe in sex before marriage, but Gary told her that all of his friends are sexually active and he is planning to make use of the condoms as soon as he finds a girlfriend. He tells her that he is tired of all of his friends teasing him for being so innocent and prudish. Jenny secretly hopes her parents will find out about this, but keeps her brother's secret because he kept her secret about dating her boyfriend until she was ready to introduce him to her parents. Jenny wishes Jimmy were in town because he would know what to do; she doesn't call or e-mail him because she does not want to interfere with his studies. Mr. and Mrs. Nguyen feel that they have lost hold of their children. They feel this even more now that Grandma found the condoms and Jenny introduced them to her white boyfriend. They are not sure which child, Jenny or Gary, is telling the truth about the condoms (adapted from Chadha, 2008).

Review of Context

Internal Characteristics

Chapter 4 presented the key internal characteristics that serve as protective factors in the lives of youth include (1) intelligence—not just the kind that fosters learning in school, but also the multiple intelligences (Gardner, 1993) that support skills for decision making, resourcefulness, and social-emotional expression; (2) the capacity to face adversity by building meaning from religious and spiritual beliefs; (3) commitment to goals; and (4) a sense of hope. Lerner, Brentano, Dowling, and Anderson (2002) sum up these internal characteristics as the "five C's" of positive youth development (competence, confidence, character, connection, caring). Note that these characteristics all have positive connotations.

Both Jenny and Gary have protective factors in that they appear to care about each other and the other family members. The fact that they talk with each other about important life events such as dating and sexuality is indicative of their capacity for social and emotional expression. Jenny is committed to her values around sex before marriage and also loyal to her brothers. Gary is also loyal to his sister, but is at risk because he feels compelled to cave into peer pressure about sexual decision making.

Further assessment of their spiritual beliefs and whether they are following their family Buddhist traditions as a source of strength and meaning making is important. The practitioner should also assess academic performance and peer relationships. Internal risk factors may be present if either Jenny or Gary express a loss of meaning and connection as they work to respect the cultural values of their family while simultaneously strive to be teenagers in a North American context. Given the current information, a psychoeducational intervention with Gary would be useful to help him cope with peer pressure as he makes important choices about sex.

Family

As noted in Chapter 5, the adolescent's family plays a role in both preventing problems and intervening when the teen enters rocky territory. Some families surround their teenager with solid protective factors such as positive discipline strategies, monitoring of behavior and activities, high expectations for achievement, racial pride, strong spiritual values, and extended family bonds (Jenson & Fraser, 2006). Other teens have families that are rife with risks such as family conflict and divorce, lack of parental involvement, inaccurate expectations for developmental capacities, cultural mismatch, and parental substance abuse. However, most adolescents' families offer a mix of protective and risk factors as the typical family responds to multiple contexts from which it draws both strength and hardship.

The Nguyen family is negotiating several tasks in the family life cycle, launching their eldest son into university studies, negotiating the ins and outs of balancing structure and freedom for their two teenagers at home, assisting their 9-year-old through the tasks of middle childhood, and caring for their aging parents/in-laws. The fact that Mr. Nguyen built a successful business from the ground up after arriving in the United States and that the family has launched one child to university studies demonstrate the protective factor of expectations for high achievement. Additional protective factors include the parental concern and involvement in the issue surrounding the condoms, their cultural link with other Vietnamese families, and their link to extended family through Mrs. Nguyen's parents. Family risk includes the cultural mismatch that results from parents who grew up in one culture raising their children who were born and growing up in a different culture. This is a common risk factor for all immigrant and refugee families that struggle to maintain their home culture and values within the context of a new country where their children are born and educated. In addition, there is the history of family loss from having to escape their war-torn home country, the deaths due to the war, and enduring separation from Mr. Nguyen's sister whom they believe is still in Vietnam.

The ecological theory encourages assessment of all the contexts in which the family lives. For example, the family's cultural and religious values represent the macro environment of Vietnam; however, the parents are working to transmit those in the macro environment of North American cultures. Within these two macro environments there are different expectations for the role of school in the lives of children, how children and parents ought to interact, and norms for sexuality. These differing macro contexts filter into the family relationships and interactions because of the dual cultures: the Vietnamese culture of their parents and grandparents and the U.S. culture of southern California. The practitioner who views the family from the contextual lens of the ecological theory can gain a deeper assessment of family resilience and can develop interventions that not only work to help family members negotiate among themselves, but also to negotiate within systems beyond the household door.

A family-level intervention would be useful for addressing Mr. and Mrs. Nguyen's fear that they have lost hold of their children and the presenting concern about the condoms. The form this intervention takes depends on the family's view of who will best be able to assist them. In other words, the parents may not think that North American remedies for family issues, such as family counseling, are useful or culturally relevant. However, the school principal may direct Mrs. Nguyen to the school social worker or counselor when she calls to complain about the condoms. Given this, it is incumbent upon the practitioner to talk with Mrs. Nguyen about how he or she can best serve the family. If the family believes they can benefit from family counseling, then the following intervention may be helpful.

Given the history of traumatic family loss, the genogram can serve as a foundation for a narrative intervention. The practitioner works with the family to create the genogram. During this activity, Mr. and Mrs. Nguyen and Mrs. Nguyen's parents can tell stories about the losses and the joys of their lives in Vietnam prior to the war. Then the family can create a new and different story about their current losses, for example, launching Jimmy to university and Mrs. Nguyen's father's dementia, so as not to have them serve as a reflection of the traumatic historical losses that are part of the family story prior to their lives in the United States.

School

Chapter 6 presented the school microsystem as a complex venue where youth spend at least 6 hours a day. Within this structure teens attempt to carve out a social life where they meet people of their own age and interests. School can be a place of great comfort for some teens and a place of great pain for other teens. In this context their peers admire, despise, emulate, or shun them. It is also the place where they may gain notoriety for their academic ability, their athletic or artistic prowess, their ability to make and keep friends, or for less positive behaviors that are just as noteworthy: their ability to be disruptive or angry, their ability to use drugs and alcohol, and their sexual escapades.

The teenage children in the Nguyen family exemplify the challenges of negotiating adolescence within the school setting. Many teens face difficulty as they learn to navigate high school where they attempt to express their independence from adults simultaneous to their continued dependence on them. Jenny and Gary Nguyen are trying to fit in with their peers at school as well as a school culture that is more permissive than that of the family. When the school hands out condoms, Gary takes them in order to be like the others, even though he is probably aware that his parents would not approve.

However, a full assessment from the M-E approach would allow the practitioner to make a clearer assessment of the family's concerns. Additionally, an assessment of the family risk and protective and risk factors will allow the practitioner to gain insights about their resilience. Depending on the result of these assessments, interventions for only one of the family members or for several or all family members may be developed. For example, the practitioner may want to engage Mr. and Mrs. Nguyen in a meeting with the teacher or the school social worker so they can share their concerns and learn more about the school culture. On the other hand, the practitioner may want to encourage the Nguyen's to talk together about the stresses of having their children educated with U.S. cultural norms that are different from those of the family. Additionally, the Nguyen's may have a spiritual leader who can be of assistance to the family.

Neighborhood

Chapter 7 addressed the impact of neighborhood context on adolescent development. The M-E approach impels us to assess for how neighborhoods influence the adolescents we serve. In fact, neighborhood opportunities that allow for mastery and control contribute to cognitive and social competence (David & Weinstein, 1987). Key concepts discussed in Chapter 7 are neighborhood social cohesion (social ties that promote trust and cooperation), neighborhood collective socialization (norms or expected behaviors found among residents and shaped by micro-, macro-, and exosystems), and neighborhood disorganization (positive or negative social and physical conditions in a neighborhood). When teen behaviors and complaints are not amenable to individual-, family-, peer-, or school-level interventions the practitioner needs to consider how the neighborhood context is affecting his or her client. However, practitioners who work from the M-E approach will not wait to assess neighborhood protective and risk factors.

Further assessment of the Nguyen family's neighborhood is appropriate because the practitioner knows only that the neighborhood is middle class and ethnically diverse. Exploring questions such as these might be helpful: Does Mrs. Nguyen have close ties with her neighbors who may be able to lend support as she cares for her aging parents? Does the ethnic diversity of the neighborhood include other Vietnamese families who can commiserate with Mr. and Mrs. Nguyen about raising teens in a North American context? Practitioners who practice from the M-E approach and who understand the importance of neighborhood social cohesion will be able to intervene with an adolescent client and his or her family to build social ties among neighbors who may assist in reducing loneliness that can lead to depressive symptoms.

Media

Chapter 8 discussed the media as an influence on the adolescent and its role in creating problems for teens and their families. Recent studies indicate that teenagers in the United States spend about 6 to 7 hours each day interacting with various media sources (Roberts et al., 2004, as cited in

L'Engle et al., 2006). The media represents a "significant other" (Cooley, 1902; G. Mead, 1934; M. Mead, 1965) in the teenager's world such that it can serve as a place for behavior rehearsal and social contacts beyond one's family, school, and neighborhood. New technologies have surpassed traditional media (television, radio, video games). More recent interactive Internet media such as text messaging, online gaming, Facebook, and MySpace add complexity to adolescent development. Traditional media represent macro- and exosystems because adolescents do not interact with them; however, the interactive nature of newer technologies bring media into the meso- and microsystems of young people. Stokols (1999) points out that these interactive media opportunities "blur" the "boundaries among one's micro-, meso-, and exosystems" (p. 343). Traditional media provide a place for a teen to witness how characters act and make choices and try those on in cognitive rehearsal. However, interactive social media present an immediacy of communication. Rehearsal of options for how to behave in real life disappears when communications are immediate and may result in mistakes or even tragedies. E-mails and blog postings are like the spoken word; they are not retractable.

Media-level risks can aggravate mental health issues, such as depression or eating disorders. Therefore, assessment of a teen's media diet should be a regular part of one's practice. Applying the M-E approach will keep the practitioner on target for assessment and interventions that incorporate all of the systems that play a role in clients' symptoms including the media.

The media can have positive influences on adolescents, and practitioners should view it not only as a source of problems but as a resource for intervention as well. For example, Loader (2007) discusses the positive ramifications of the Internet on political, civic, and community engagement of young people. Additionally, Thomas (2007), who interviewed teens about their cyber experiences, provides examples of how they build cyberspace communities and learn social-emotional skills as a result. For example, she describes how youth work out conflicts that develop as a result of online role playing. Thomas's interviews also demonstrate that teens are well aware of the fact they create online identities as one teen noted, "You *have* to change the way you are depending on which space you're in at any given moment. Although I am always 'me' underneath, I present my words and actions very differently depending what space or place or window or whatever you like to call it, that I am in" (p. 43). In this sense, teens use media in a positive way to regulate their presentation of self. This is similar to how they change the way they talk when they are with peers versus adults.

Further assessment of the Nguyen family's relationship to the media is important. Recall that Mr. Nguyen owns and runs a media store. Given this fact, he will be knowledgeable about the different kinds of media available and most likely have opinions about them, especially in reference to his children. The practitioner also knows that Gary has had his head buried in his computer and is texting his friends from his cell phone. This extends the face-to-face peer pressure. Given his father's knowledge and connection with varying types of media he will play an important role if an intervention into Gary's media use is necessary.

A Context-Dependent View of Adolescent Concerns

The application of resilience theory and ecological theory is integral to assessment and intervention of the concerns addressed in Chapters 10–14. For example, Chapter 14 presents the social ecology of protection from and risk for delinquent behaviors. We note that youth do not simply wake up one morning and look in the mirror and state, "I think I will be a juvenile delinquent." Instead, delinquency is the result of risks found at the individual level, as well as in the key contexts where adolescents spend much of their time including the family, peer group, school, media, and neighborhood (Fergusson & Horwood, 2003; Luster & Small, 1997; Ungar, 2004; Werner & Smith, 1998).

The M-E approach also helps us to understand that adolescents who engage in delinquent behavior or experience depression are a heterogeneous group and comprise teens that represent all genders, ethnicities, races, sexual orientations, religious affiliations, and social class statuses. Social structures that empower some social identity statuses over others effect the way society treats and labels these behaviors. For example, the justice system treats the suburban, upper-middle-class teenager who steals a neighbor's car while downing a six-pack of beer differently than the central city, working-class teenager acting the same way. Hence, the importance of assessing the macrosystem effects on adolescent outcomes and societal reactions to those outcomes. The M-E approach leads to these deeper assessments and interventions.

The Joys of Working with Adolescents

Practitioners' primary contact with adolescents involves those who have issues as troubling as, or even more troubling than, those presented by the teens discussed in this book. This can leave the practitioner weary and wondering about the "joys" of working with teenagers. However, teens *are* acting positively, even those whom adults view as troubled or troubling, as illustrated in the following example of a teen-leadership group in a public high school. The college students were teaching high school youth about community organizing. The youth in the group represented multiple cultures and felt ostracized from a school system that did not honor their home languages and cultures. Thus they

> had been withdrawing their consent to be part of the public school system for a long time, and by [the college student] making a point to help them discover the power to control their education, their views changed. Katie mentioned a game she wanted to play for a warm-up (and the next week we played it), and Maria, always the tangent-taker, somehow began a discussion about where everyone was from, and though it was not quite on topic, it was apparent to me that the girls had understood what I wanted to stress to them, so I let them run with the discussion and we began to get to know each other on a new level. . . . Eventually, not only would they talk about what I wanted and I would talk about what they wanted, but we also began to talk *together*. The girls had insightful comments and would prompt the other kids. They would ask the younger kids to stop goofing around and pay attention, a habit that only two months earlier they were being told to quit themselves. The process was like that of watching a flower bloom; one does not realize that small, individual changes are occurring, but one realizes the full beauty of the flower once it is fully open (Washburn, 2008, pp. 9–10).

Practitioners who apply the M-E approach may become overly aware of neighborhood deficits and their negative influences on clients. Therefore, we point out the positive actions adolescents take to build protective behavioral norms (collective socialization) and neighborhood social cohesion. The following example of youth neighborhood involvement conveys the strengths youth have to offer.

> Adult members of the housing association management attended the youth presentations. In their presentations, youth addressed the "bad words" graffitied on the slides in their playground and asked that places in the neighborhood be better for kids. As a result of the presentations, the maintenance supervisor, committed to having a daily graffiti cleanup crew, in fact returned to the neighborhood himself to remove graffiti that same day while the youth were working on their "good graffiti" project. For their project, the students painted the backs of benches with designs in bright colors with themes of "things that make us happy in the community . . . " and "peace is. . . . " The benches are part of a local urban garden. A neighborhood improvement council located in the neighborhood maintains the garden. The youth also worked on a bright yellow "Welcome to the Neighborhood" sign. The youth attached the benches to their bases in the garden and helped to put the Welcome to the Neighborhood sign in the ground. The youth also passed out door

hangers to tell people what to do if they see graffiti. The youth action not only created *good graffiti* where youth will be able to see themselves represented in the public art of the community, but also took action with the housing association management and community to insist that graffiti is an issue that needs to be addressed. (Nicotera & Matera, 2010, as compiled by Nola Miguel & Laurie Walker)

Practitioners who work with teens are at risk of forgetting about the joys and strengths they offer. Examples such as the ones presented here are a reminder that teens are in a discovery mode as they experiment with new power to influence adults and peers and the world.

Chapter Summary

This chapter reviewed the M-E approach to working with adolescents as they face the critical issues of their development. It also focused on the practitioner's attitude about the work and especially on the benefits of having a positive view about the potential of the adolescent client. An attitude of mutual respect can make a huge difference in the nature and outcome of the helping process.

Practitioners typically encounter adolescent clients with a variety of challenges from learning disabilities and acting out in school or the neighborhood, to experimenting with or abusing drugs, or coping with families in the midst of divorce or domestic violence. We expect that the knowledge and skills emphasized in this book will temper the challenges of assisting teens. We trust that practitioners will discover a deeper understanding of clients' concerns based on knowledge of protective and risk factors as well as about how contexts beyond peers and family influence behavior. Assessments and interventions based on the M-E approach must move beyond tradition to include the neighborhood, the media, and cultural or macro contexts that affect a clients' racial, gender, and sexual orientation identity statuses.

Our expectation is that this book has given you a clearer understanding of both the challenges of working with adolescent clients, and some helpful approaches for intervening. We anticipate that practitioners who have deeper understanding about the push–pull of adolescence will be able to apply theory, research, and practice strategies for successfully assisting their clients through the ups and downs of the adolescent years. Since the days when G. Stanley Hall (1904) coined adolescence as a period of "stress and storm," practitioners and parents alike have dreaded the teen years, perhaps even more than the "terrible two's" that depict the toddler years of the lifespan. There are parallels between these two phases of the lifespan because increased power for expression, choices, and movement at both stages creates bumps and bruises. It is the excitement of discovery that leads teens to meander the wrong way down "one-way streets" or to ignore signs such as "do not enter" and "dangerous curves ahead, slow down!" They rely on adults to express empathy and listen, to set limits, and to assist them as they develop their own inner controls for setting boundaries as they navigate the lives that lie ahead of them.

In conclusion, we have faith that practitioners will come to know and appreciate the amazing group of individuals who straddle the chasm between childhood and adulthood. We hope that practitioners will enjoy and sometimes laugh with their teenage clients. Most of all we hope that practitioners will provide both compassion and warmth to these individuals who are seeking to understand who they are and how they fit into the adult world. This worthy goal can bring immense satisfaction to the practitioner even as it fosters the growth of the next generation.

References

Abada, T., Hou, F., & Ram, B. (2007). Racially mixed neighborhoods, perceived neighborhood social cohesion, and adolescent health in Canada. *Social Science and Medicine, 65,* 2004–2017.

Aber, M., & Nieto, M. (2000). Suggestions for the investigation of psychological wellness in the neighborhood context: Toward a pluralistic neighborhood theory. In D. Cicchetti, J. Rappaport, I. Sardler, & R. Weissberg (Eds.), *The promotion of wellness in children and adolescents* (pp. 185–219). Washington, DC: CWLA Press.

Acoca, L. A., & Dedel, K. (1998). *No place to hide: Understanding and meeting the needs of girls in the California juvenile justice system.* Oakland, CA: National Council on Crime and Delinquency.

Adams, K., Sargent, R., Thompson, S., Richter, D., Corwin, S., & Rogan, T. (2000). A study of body weight concerns and weight control practices of 4th and 7th grade adolescents. *Ethnicity and Health, 5,* 79–94.

Agger, B. (2004). *The virtual self.* Malden, MA: Blackwell.

Allen, J. P. (2008). The attachment system in adolescence. In J. Cassidy & P. R. Shaver, *Handbook of attachment: Theory, research, and clinical applications* (2nd ed., pp. 698–717). New York: Guilford Press.

Allen, J. P., McElhaney, K. B., Kupermine, G. P., & Jodl, K. M. (2004). Stability and change in attachment security across adolescence. *Child Development, 75,* 1792–1805.

Allison, B. N., & Schultz, J. B. (2004). Parent–adolescent conflict in early adolescence. *Adolescence, 39,* 101–119.

American Academy of Child and Adolescent Psychiatry. (2004). *Facts for families: No. 33. Conduct disorder.* Washington, DC: Author.

American Association of Marriage and Family Therapy. (n.d.). *Board of director statement: The issue of reparative or conversion therapy and journal independence.* Retrieved March 21, 2009, from *www.aamft.org/about/boardletter.asp.*

American Psychiatric Association. (1998). *Psychiatric treatment and sexual orientation.* Retrieved March 21, 2009, from *www.psych.org/Departments/EDU/Library/APAOfficialDocumentsandRelated/PositionStatements/199820.aspx.*

American Psychiatric Association. (2000). *Diagnostic and statistical manual of mental disorders* (4th ed., text rev.). Washington, DC: Author.

American Psychological Association. (2004). *Guidelines for therapy with lesbian, gay, and bisexual clients.* Retrieved March 21, 2009, from *www.apa.org/pi/lgbc/guidelines.html.*

American School Counselors Association. (2004). *Ethical standards for school counselors.* Retrieved March 21, 2009, from *www.schoolcounselor.org/content.asp?contentid=173.*

American Social Health Association. (2005). *State of the nation: Challenges facing STD prevention in youth.* Triangle Park, NC: Author.

Anthony, E., & Nicotera, N. (2008). Youth perceptions of neighborhood hassles and resources: A mixed method analysis. *Children and Youth Services Review, 30*(11), 1246–1255.

Armey, M., & Crowther, J. (2008). A comparison of linear versus non-linear models of aversive self-awareness, dissociation, and non-suicidal self-injury among young adults. *Journal of Consulting and Clinical Psychology, 76*(1), 9–14.

Asher, S. R., & Coie, J. D. (1990). *Peer rejection in childhood.* New York: Cambridge University Press.

Ata, R., Ludden, A., & Lally, M. (2007). The effects of gender and family, friend, and media influences on eating behaviors and body image during adolescence. *Journal of Youth and Adolescence, 36*(8), 1024–1038.

Attar-Schwartz, S., Tan, J-P., Buchanan, A., Flouri, E., & Griggs, J. (2009). Grandparenting and adolescent adjustment in two-parent biological, lone-parent, and stepfamilies. *Journal of Family Psychology, 23,* 67–75.

Austin, E. (1993). Exploring the effects of active parental mediation of television content. *Journal of Broadcast Electronic Media, 37,* 147–158.

Aymer, S. (2005). *Exposure: An exploratory study of adolescent males' coping responses to domestic violence.* Unpublished doctoral dissertation, New York University.

Baer, J., & Maschi, T. (2003). Random acts of delinquency: Trauma and self-destructiveness in juvenile offenders. *Child and Adolescent Social Work Journal, 20* (2), 85–89.

Baird, A., & Grieve, F. (2006). Exposure to male models in advertisements leads to decrease in men's body dissatisfaction. *North American Journal of Psychology, 8,* 115–122.

Ballard, S., & Morris, M. (1998). Sources of sexuality information for university students. *Journal of Sex Education and Therapy, 23*(4), 278–287.

Bandura, A. (1964). The stormy decade: Fact or fiction? *Psychology in the Schools, 1,* 224–231.

Bandura, A. (1982). The psychology of chance encounters and life paths. *American Psychologist, 37*(7), 747–755.

Bandura, A. (1989). Human agency in social cognitive theory. *American Psychologist, 44*(9), 1175–1184.

Bandura, A. (1995). *Self-efficacy in changing societies.* New York: Cambridge University Press.

Bandura, A. (1997). *Self-efficacy: The exercise of control.* New York: Freeman.

Bandura, A., Ross, D., & Ross, S. (1963). Imitation of film-mediated aggressive models. *Journal of Abnormal and Social Psychology, 66,* 3–11.

Barkley, R. (1990). *Attention deficit/hyperactivity disorder: A handbook for diagnosis and treatment.* New York: Guilford Press.

Barkley, R. A., Edwards, G. H., & Robin, A. L. (1997). *Defiant teens: A clinician's manual for assessment and family intervention.* New York: Guilford Press.

Barnes, G. M., Hoffman, J. H., Welte, J. W., Farrell, M. P., & Dintcheff, B. A. (2007). Adolescents' time use: Effects on substance use, delinquency and sexual activity. *Journal of Youth Adolescence, 36,* 697–710.

Barratt, M., Roach, M., Morgan, K., & Colbert, K. (1996). Adjustment to motherhood by single adolescents. *Family Relations, 45*(2), 209–215.

Barrows, A. (1995). The ecopsychology of child development. In T. Roszak, M. Gomes, & A. Kanner (Eds.), *Ecopsychology* (pp. 101–110). San Francisco: Sierra Club Books.

Bates, L., Baird, D., Johnson, D. J., Lee, R. E., Luster, T., & Rehagen, C. (2005). Sudanese refugee youth in foster care: The Lost Boys in America. *Child Welfare, 84*(5), 631–648.

Baumrind, D. (1991). Effective parenting during the early adolescent transition. In. P. A. Cowan & E. M. Hetherington (Eds.), *Advances in family research* (Vol. 2, pp. 111–163). Hillsdale, NJ: Erlbaum.

Beck, A. (1995). *Cognitive therapy: Basics and beyond.* New York: Guilford Press.

Benson, P. L., Leffert, N., Scales, P. C., & Blyth, D. A. (1998). Beyond the "village" rhetoric: Creating healthy communities for children and adolescents. *Applied Developmental Science, 2*(3), 138–159.

Beveridge, R. M., & Berg, C. A. (2007). Parent–adolescent collaboration: An interpersonal model for understanding optimal interactions. *Clinical Child and Family Psychology Review, 10,* 25–52.

Blos, P. (1978). The concept of acting out in relation to the adolescent process. In E. Rexford (Ed.), *A developmental approach to the problem of acting out* (pp. 153–174). New York: International Universities Press.

Blos, P. (1979). *The adolescent passage.* New York: International Universities Press.

Blumer, H. (1969). *Symbolic interactionism: Perspective and method.* Englewood Cliffs, NJ: Prentice-Hall.

Bogenschneider, K. (1998). What youth need to succeed: The roots of resiliency. In K. Bogenschneider & J. Olson (Eds.), *Building resiliency and reducing risk: What youth need from families and communities to succeed* (Wisconsin Family Impacts Seminars Briefing Report). Madison: University of Wisconsin, Center for Excellence in Family Studies.

Bogle, K. (2008). *Hooking up: Sex, dating, and relationships on campus.* New York: New York University Press.

Boies, S. C., Knudson, G., & Young, J. (2004). The Internet, sex, and youth: Implications for sexual development. *Sexual Addiction and Compulsivity, 11,* 343–363.

Borg, M. (1998). The emotional reactions of school bullies and their victims. *Educational Psychology, 18*(4), 433–444.

Boss, P. (2006). *Loss, trauma, and resilience: Therapeutic work with ambiguous loss.* New York: Norton.

Botta, R. (2000). The mirror image of television: A comparison of black and white adolescents' body image. *Journal of Communication, 50,* 144–159.

Botvin, G., & Griffin, K. W. (2007). School-based programmes to prevent alcohol, tobacco and other drug use. *International Review of Psychiatry, 19*(6), 607–615.

Bouchard, T. J. (2004). Genetic influences on human psychological traits: A survey. *Current Directions in Psychological Science, 13*(4), 148–151.

Boutelle, K., Eisenberg, M. E., Gregory, M. L., & Neumark-Sztainer, D. (2009). The reciprocal relationship between parent–child connectedness and adolescent emotional functioning over 5 years. *Journal of Psychosomatic Research, 66,* 309–316.

Bowen, N., Bowen, G., & Ware, W. (2002). Neighborhood social disorganization, families, and the educational behavior of adolescents. *Journal of Adolescent Research, 17*(5), 468–490.

Bowlby, J. (1969). *Attachment and loss: Vol. 1. Attachment.* New York: Basic Books.

Bowlby, J. (1973). *Attachment and loss: Vol. 2. Separation.* New York: Basic Books.

Boxer, A., Cook, J., & Herdt, G. (1991). Double jeopardy: Identity transitions and parent–child relations among gay and lesbian youth. In K. Pillemer & K. McCartney (Eds.), *Parent–child relations throughout life* (pp. 59–92). Hillsdale, NJ: Erlbaum.

Boyer, D., & Fine, D. (1992). Sexual abuse as a factor in adolescent pregnancy and child maltreatment. *Family Planning Perspectives, 24*(1), 4–19.

Boylan, J. (2004). *She's not there: A life in two genders.* New York: Bantam Books.

Bradner, C., & Lindberg, L. (2000). Older, but not wiser: How men get information about AIDS and sexually transmitted diseases after high school. *Family Planning Perspectives, 32,* 33–38.

Brewster, K. L. (1994). Neighborhood context and the transition to sexual activity among young black women. *Demography, 31,* 603–614.

Brodsky, A. (1996). Resilient single mothers in risky neighborhoods: Negative psychological sense of community. *Journal of Community Psychology, 24*(4), 347–363.

Brody, L. R. (1996). Gender, emotional expression, and parent–child boundaries. In R. D. Kavanaugh, B. Zimmerberg, & S. Fein (Eds.), *Emotion: Interdisciplinary perspectives* (pp. 139–170). Hillsdale, NJ: Erlbaum.

Bronfenbrenner, U. (1979). *The ecology of human development.* Cambridge, MA: Harvard University Press.

Bronfenbrenner, U. (1986). Ecology of the family as a context for human development: Research perspectives. *Developmental Psychology, 22*(6), 723–742.

Bronfenbrenner, U. (1989). Ecological systems theory. *Annals of Child Development, 6,* 723–742.

Brooks-Gunn, J. (1988). Antecedents and consequences of variations in girl's maturational timing. *Journal of Adolescent Health Care, 9,* 365–373.

Brooks-Gunn, J., & Paikoff, J. (1997). Self, others and meaning: Sexual transitions in adolescence. In J. Schulenberg, J. Maggs, & K. Hurrelman (Eds.), *Health risks and developmental transitions during adolescence* (pp. 190–219). New York: Cambridge University Press.

Brosky, B., & Lally, S. (2004). Prevalence of trauma, PTSD, and dissociation in court-referred adolescents. *Journal of Interpersonal Violence, 19*(7), 801–814.

Brown, B., Clasen, D., & Eicher, S. (1986). Perceptions of peer pressure, peer conformity dispositions, and self-reported behavior among adolescents. *Developmental Psychology, 22,* 521–530.

Brown, B., Eicher, S., & Petrie, S. (1986). The importance of peer group affiliation in adolescence. *Journal of Adolescence, 9,* 73–96.

Brown, J., Halpern, C., & L'Engle, K. (2005). Mass media as a sexual super peer for early maturing girls. *Journal of Adolescent Health, 36,* 420–427.

Brown, J., & Keller, S. (2000). Can the mass media be healthy sex educators? *Family Planning Perspectives, 32*(5), 255–256.

Brown, J., L'Engle, K., Pardun, C., Guo, G., Kenneavy, K., & Jackson, C. (2006). Sexy media matter: Exposure to sexual content in music, movies, television, and magazines predicts black and white adolescents' sexual behavior. *Pediatrics, 117,* 1018–1027.

Browning, C. R., Leventhal, T., & Brooks-Gunn, J. (2005). Sexual initiation in early adolescence: The nexus of parental and community control. *American Sociological Review, 70,* 758–778.

Bubolz, M., & Sontag, S. (1993). Human ecology theory. In P. Boss, W. Doherty, R. LaRossa, W. Schumm, & S. Steinmetz (Eds.), *Sourcebook of family theories and methods: A contextual approach* (pp. 419–448). New York: Plenum Press.

Bunting, C. (1996). The middle school theme: What works, what needs reconsidering. *American Secondary Education, 24*(3), 23–26.

Burrow-Sanchez, J. J. (2006). Understanding adolescent substance abuse: Prevalence, risk factors, and clinical implications. *Journal of Counseling and Development, 84,* 283–290.

Burton, L., & Price-Spratlen, T. (1999). Through the eyes of children: An ethnographic perspective on neighborhoods and child development. In A. S. Hasten (Ed.), *Cultural processes in child development* (pp. 77–96). Mahwah, NJ: Erlbaum.

Bushman, B., & Anderson, C. (2001). Media violence and the American public: Scientific fact versus media misinformation. *American Psychologist, 56,* 477–489.

Butler, J., & Burton, L. (1990). Rethinking teenage childbearing: Is sexual abuse a missing link? *Family Relations, 39,* 73–80.

Butler, K. (1997). The anatomy of resilience. *Networker, 2,* 22–31.

Califano, J. (2003). The formative years: Pathways *to Substance Abuse among Girls and Young Women Ages 8–22* (National Center on Addiction and Substance Abuse [CASA]). New York: Columbia University.

Carrion, V., & Steiner, H. (2000). Trauma and dissociation in delinquent adults. *Journal of the American Academy of Child and Adolescent Psychiatry, 39*(3), 353–359.

Carver, J. M. (2009). *Attention-deficit hyperactivity disorder (ADHD).* Retrieved March 29, 2009, from *www.enotalone.com/article/4121.html.*

Caspi, A., McClay, J., Moffitt, T., Mill, J., Martin, J., Craig, I., et al. (2002). Role of genotype in the cycle of violence in maltreated children. *Science, 297*(2), 851–854.

Cass, V. (1979). Homosexual identity development: A theoretical model. *Journal of Homosexuality, 4*(3), 219–235.

Catalano, R. F., Kosterman, R., Hawkins, J. D., Newcomb, M. D., & Abbott, R. D.

(1996). Modeling the etiology of adolescent substance use: A test of the social development model. *Journal of Drug Issues, 26,* 429–455.

Celentano, D. D., Sifakis, F., Hylton, J., Torian, L. V., Guillin, V., & Koblin, B. A. (2005). Race/ethnic differences in HIV prevalence and risks among adolescent and young adult men who have sex with men. *Journal of Urban Health: Bulletin of the New York Academy of Medicine, 82*(4), 610–621.

Centers for Disease Control and Prevention. (2000). *Tracking the hidden epidemics: Trends in STDs in the United States.* Retrieved from *www.cdc.gov/std/Trends2000/.*

Centers for Disease Control and Prevention. (2005). Mental health in the United States: Prevalence of diagnosis and medication treatment for attention-deficit/hyperactivity disorder—United States, 2003. *MMWR Weekly, 54*(34), 842–849.

Centers for Disease Control and Prevention. (2007a). *Health risk behaviors by race/ethnicity, National Youth Risk Behavior Survey YRBS:2007.* Retrieved from *www.cdc.gov/HealthyYouth/yrbs/pdf/yrbs07_us_disparity_race.pdf.*

Centers for Disease Control and Prevention. (2007b). *Trends in reportable sexually transmitted diseases in the United States, 2007: National surveillance data for chlamydia, gonorrhea, and syphilis.* Retrieved from *www.cdc.gov/std/stats07/trends.htm.*

Centers for Disease Control and Prevention. (2008). *HIV/AIDS among youth.* Retrieved from *www.cdc.gov/hiv/resources/factsheets/youth.htm.*

Centers for Disease Control and Prevention. (2009). Adolescent reproductive health: About teen pregnancy. Retrieved from www.cdc.gov/eproductive-health/AdolescentReproHealth/AboutTP.htm.

Chadha, G. (2000). *What's cooking?* (DVD). UK: Lionsgate.

Chandra, A., Martino, S., Collins, R., Elliott, M., Berry, S., Kanouse, D., et al. (2008). Does watching sex on television predict teen pregnancy? Findings from a National Longitudinal Survey of Youth. *Pediatrics, 122,* 1047–1054.

Cherulnik, P., & Souders, S. (1984). The social contents of place schemata: People are judged by the places where they live and work. *Population and Environment, 7*(4), 211–233.

Chess, S., & Thomas, A. (1996). *Temperament: Theory and practice.* New York: Brunner/Mazel.

Child Trends. (2001). *Facts at a glance.* Retrieved from *www.childtrends.org.*

Child Trends. (2002). *Facts at a glance.* Retrieved from *www.childtrends.org.*

Cicchetti, D., Toth, S., & Rogosch, F. (2000). The development of psychological wellness in maltreated children. In D. Cicchetti et al. (Eds.), *The promotion of wellness in children and adolescents* (pp. 395–426). Washington, DC: Child Welfare League of America Press.

Ciro, D., Surko, M., Bhandarkar, K., Helfgott, N., Peake, K., & Epstein, I. (2005). Lesbian, gay, bisexual, sexual-orientation questioning adolescents seeking mental health services: Risk factors, worries, and desire to talk about them. *Social Work in Mental Health, 3*(3), 213–234.

Clark, D. B. (2004). The natural history of adolescent alcohol use disorders. *Addiction, 99,* 5–22.

Cleary, S. (2000). Adolescent victimization and associated suicidal and violent behaviors. *Adolescence, 35*(140), 671–682.

Cloninger, C. R., Christiansen, K., Reich, T., & Gottesman, I. (1978). Implications of sex differences in the prevalence of antisocial personality, alcoholism, and criminality for familial transmission. *Archives of General Psychiatry, 35*(8), 941–951.

Cohen, J., Mannarino, A., Zhitova, A., & Capone, M. (2003). Treating child abuse-related posttraumatic stress and comorbid substance abuse in adolescents. *Child Abuse and Neglect, 27*, 1345–1365.

Coleman, J., & Hagell, A. (2007). *Adolescence risk and resilience.* Chichester, UK: Wiley.

Coley, R. L., Morris, J. E., & Hernandez, D. (2004). Out-of-school care and problem behavior trajectories among low-income adolescents: Individual, family, and neighborhood characteristics as added risks. *Child Development, 75*, 948–965.

Collins, R., Elliott, M., Berry, S., Kanouse, D., Kunkel, D., Hunter, S., et al. (2004). Watching sex on television predicts adolescent initiation of sexual behavior. *Pediatrics, 114*, 280–289.

Collins, R. L., Elliott, M. N., Berry, S. H., Kanouse, D. E., & Hunter, S. B. (2003). Entertainment television as a healthy sex educator: The impact of condom-efficacy information in an episode of *Friends. Pediatrics,* 112, 1115–1121.

Collins, W. A. (1997). Relationships and development during adolescence: Interpersonal adaptation to individual change. *Personal Relationships, 4*, 1–14.

Collins, W. A., & Laursen, B. (2006). Parent–adolescent relationships. In P. Noller & J. A. Feeney (Eds.), *Close relationships* (pp. 112–125). New York: Psychology Press.

Collins, W. A., & Steinberg, L. (2006). Adolescent development in interpersonal context. In N. Eisenberg (Ed.), *Handbook of child psychology: Vol. 3. Social, emotional, and personality development* (6th ed., pp. 1003–1067). New York: Wiley.

Compas, B., Connor-Smith, J., & Jaser, S. (2004). Temperament, stress, reactivity, and coping: Implications for depression in childhood and adolescence. *Journal of Clinical Child and Adolescent Psychology, 33*, 21–31.

Cooley, C. (1902). *Human nature and the social order.* New York: Scribner.

Cooper, M., & Lesser, J. (2008). Clinical social work practice: An integrated approach. Boston: Allyn & Bacon.

Corcoran, J., & Walsh, J. (2006). *Clinical Assessment and Diagnosis in Social Work Practice.* New York: Oxford University Press.

Coulton, C. (1996). The effects of neighborhoods on families and children: Implications for services. In A. J. Kahn & S. B. Kamerman (Eds.), *Children and their families in big cities* (pp. 87–120). New York: Columbia University School of Social Work.

Coyle, K. K., Kirby, D. B., Robin, L. E., Benspach, S. W., Baumler, E., & Glassman, J. R. (2006). All4you! A randomized trial of an HIV, other STDs, and pregnancy prevention intervention for alternative school students. *AIDS Education and Prevention, 18*(3), 187–203.

Cross, W. (1991). *Shades of black: Diversity in African-American identity.* Philadelphia: Temple University Press.

Crowder, K., & South, S. (2003). Neighborhood distress and school dropout: The variable significance of community context. *Social Science Research, 32,* 659–698.

Currie, D. (1997). Decoding femininity: Advertisements and their teenage readers. *Gender and Society, 11*(4), 453–477.

D'Augelli, A., Hershberger, S., & Pilkington, N. (1998). Lesbian, gay, and bisexual youth and their families: Disclosure of sexual orientation and its consequences. *American Journal of Orthopsychiatry, 68*(3), 361–371.

David, C., Cappella, J., & Fishbein, M. (2006). The social diffusion of influence among adolescents: Group interaction in chat room environment about anti-drug advertisements. *Communication Theory, 16,* 118–140.

David, T., & Weinstein, C. (1987). The built environment and children's development. In C. Weinstein (Ed.), *Spaces for children: The built environment and child development* (pp. 3–20). New York: Plenum Press.

De Goede, I., Branje, S., & Meeus, W. (2009). Developmental changes in adolescents' perceptions of relationships with their parents. *Journal of Youth and Adolescence, 38,* 75–88.

Denizet-Lewis, B. (2004). Friends, friends with benefits and the benefits of the local mall. Retrieved from *www.nytimes.com/2004/05/30/magazine/30NONDATING. html?scp=1&sq=Friends,%20friends%20with%20benefits%20and%20the%20 benefits%20of%20the%20local%20mall&st=cse.*

Derib, A. (1998). *Group care and fostering of Sudanese children in Pignudo and Kakuma refugee camps: The experience of Save the Children Sweden from 1990 to 1997.* Stockholm: Save the Children Sweden.

Deslandes, R., Royer, E., & Turcotte, D. (1997/Fall). School achievement at the secondary level: Influence of parenting style and parent involvement in schooling. *McGill Journal of Education, 32,* 191–207.

Deutsch, N. (2008). *Pride in the projects: Teens building identities in urban contexts.* New York: New York University Press.

Diamond, G. M., Diamond, G. S., & Liddle, H. A. (2000). The therapist–parent alliance in family-based therapy for adolescents. *JCLP/In Session: Psychotherapy in Practice, 56,* 1037–1050.

Diamond, G. S. (2005). Attachment-based family therapy for depressed and anxious adolescents. In J. L. Lebow (Ed.), *Handbook of clinical family therapy* (pp. 17–41). New York: Wiley.

Dietz, T., & Dettlaff, A. (1997). The impact of membership in a support group for gay, lesbian, and bisexual students. *Journal of College Student Psychotherapy, 12,* 57–72.

Dishion, T. J., & Connell, A. (2006). Adolescents' resilience as a self-regulatory process: Promising themes for linking intervention with developmental science. In B. M. Lester, A. S. Masten, & B. S. McEwen (Eds.), *Resilience in children* (pp. 125–138). Boston: Annals of the New York Academy of Sciences, Volume 1094.

Dishion, T. J., & Loeber, R. (1985). Male adolescent marijuana and alcohol use: The role of parents and peers revisited. *American Journal of Drug and Alcohol Abuse, 11,* 11–25.

Dishion, T. J., McCord, J., & Poulin, F. (1999). When interventions harm: Peer groups and problem behavior. *American Psychologist, 54,* 755–764.

Dishion, T. J., & McMahon, R. J. (1998). Parental monitoring and the prevention of child and adolescent problem behavior: A conceptual and empirical formulation. *Clinical Child and Family Psychology Review, 1,* 61–75.

Dishion, T. J., & Owen, L. D. (2002). A longitudinal analysis of friendship and substance abuse: Bi-directional influence from adolescence to adulthood. *Developmental Psychology, 38,* 480–491.

Dobson, K. (2002). *Handbook of cognitive–behavioral therapies* (2nd ed.). New York: Guilford Press.

Dodge, K., Dishion, T., & Lansford, J. (2006). Deviant peer influences in intervention and public policy for youth. *Social Policy Report, SRCD, 20*(3), 3–19.

Dodge, K. A., & Pettit, G. S. (2003). A biopsychosocial model of the development of chronic conduct problems in adolescence. *Developmental Psychology, 39*(2), 349–371.

Donnerstein, E., & Smith, S. (1997). Impact of media violence on children, adolescents, and adults. In S. Kirschner & D. Kirschner (Eds.), *Perspectives on psychology and the media* (pp. 29–68). Washington, DC: American Psychological Press.

Drabman, R., & Thomas, M. (1975). The effects of television on children and adolescents: Does T.V. violence breed indifference? *Journal of Communication, 25*(4), 86–89.

Dryfoos, J. G., & Barkin, C. (2006). Adolescence: Growing up in America today. New York: Oxford University Press.

Du Bois, W. E. B. (1903, 1996). *The souls of black folks.* New York: Random House.

Duggal, S., Carlson, E., Sroufe L. A., & Egeland, B. (2001). Depressive symptomatology in childhood and adolescence. *Development and Psychopathology, 13*(1), 143–164.

Duncan, J. (2000, January). Overview and mental health findings for UAM and separated children. Interviews as part of the UNHCR best interest determinations, Kakuma Refugee Camp.

Duncan, J. (2001, May). Sudanese "Lost Boys" in the United States: Adjustment after six months. Paper presented at the United States Catholic Conference, Washington, DC.

Duncan, R. (1999). Maltreatment by parents and peers: The relationship between child abuse, bully victimization, and psychological distress. *Child Maltreatment, 4*(1), 45–55.

Dunn, J., & Plomin, R. (1990). *Separate lives: Why siblings are so different.* New York: Basic Books.

Dunphy, D. (1963). The social structure of urban adolescent peer groups. *Society, 26,* 230–246.

East, P., & Jacobson, L. (2001). The younger siblings of teenage mothers: A follow-up of their pregnancy risk. *Developmental Psychology, 37*(2), 254–264.

Eckenrode, J., Powers, J., & Garbarino, J. (1997). *Youth in trouble are youth who have been hurt.* San Francisco: Jossey-Bass.

Eisenberg, M. E., Sieving, R. E., Bearinger, L. H., Swain, C., & Resnick, M. D.

(2006). Parents' communication with adolescents about sexual behavior: A missed opportunity for prevention? *Journal of Youth Adolescence, 35*, 893–902.

Eisenberg, N. (2000). Emotion, regulation, and moral development. *Annual Review of Psychology, 51*, 665–697.

Elder, G. (1974). *Children of the great depression.* Chicago: University of Chicago Press.

Eliason, M. (1995). Accounts of sexual identity formation in heterosexual students. *Sex Roles, 32*(11/12), 821–834.

Elkind, D. (1984). *All grown up and no place to go.* Reading, MA: Addison-Wesley.

Elliott, D. S., Huizinga, D., & Ageton, S. S. (1985). *Explaining delinquency and drug use.* Beverly Hills, CA: Sage.

Ellis, A., & Wilde, J. (2001). *Case studies in rational emotive behavior therapy with children and adolescents.* Upper Saddle River, NJ: Merrill/Prentice-Hall.

Emery, R., & Forehand, R. (1996). Parental divorce and children's well-being: A focus on resilience. In R. Haggerty, L. Sherrod, N. Garmezy, & M. Rutter (Eds.), *Stress, risk, and resilience in children and adolescents* (pp. 64–99). Cambridge, UK: Cambridge University Press.

Emery, R., & Laumann-Billings, L. (1998). An overview of nature, causes and consequences of abusive family relationships. *American Psychologist, 53*(2), 121–135.

Epps, K. (1997). The use of secure accommodations for adolescent girls who engage in severe and repetitive self-injurious behavior. *Clinical Child Psychology and Psychiatry, 2*(4), 539–552.

Epstein, D., & White, D. (1990). *Narrative means to therapeutic ends.* New York: Norton.

Epstein, M., & Ward, M. (2008). "Always use protection": Communication boys receive about sex from parents, peers, and the media. *Journal of Youth and Adolescence, 37* (2), 113–126.

Erikson, E. (1959). *Identity and the life cycle.* New York: Norton.

Erikson, E. (1968). *Identity: Youth and crisis.* New York: Norton.

Evans, A. S., Spirito, A., Celio, M., Dyl, J., & Hunt, J. (2007). The relation of substance use to trauma and conduct disorder in an adolescent psychiatric population. *Journal of Child and Adolescent Substance Abuse, 17*(1), 29–49.

Fantuzzo, J., & Mohr, W. (1999). Prevalence and effects of child exposure to domestic violence. *The Future of Children, 9*(3), 21–32.

Farrington, D. (1995). The development of offending and antisocial behaviour from childhood: Key findings from the Cambridge Study in Delinquent Development. *Journal of Child Psychology and Psychiatry, 360*, 929–964.

Fassler, D., & Papolo, D. (2009). Could there be a problem? Retrieved *www.msnbc.com/id 4156151.*

Feeney, B. C., & Cassidy, J. (2003). Reconstructive memory related to adolescent–parent conflict interactions: Influence of attachment-related representations on immediate perceptions and changes in perception over time. *Journal of Personality and Social Psychology, 85*, 945–955.

Feldstein, S., & Miller, W. (2007). Does subtle screening for substance abuse work? A review of the Substance Abuse Subtle Screening Inventory (SASSI). *Addiction, 102*(1), 41–50.

Felix-Ortiz, M., Newcomb, M., & Myers, H. (1994). A multidimensional measure of cultural identity for Latino and Latina adolescents. *Hispanic Journal of Behavior Sciences, 16*, 99–115.

Fergusson, D., & Horwood, L. (2003). Resilience to childhood adversity: Results of a 21 year study. In S. Luthar (Ed.), *Resilience and vulnerability: Adaptation in the context of childhood adversities.* New York: Cambridge University Press.

Fergusson, D., Horwood, L., & Lynskey, M. (1994). The childhoods of multiple problem adolescents: A 15-year longitudinal study. *Journal of Child Psychology and Psychiatry, 35*, 1123–1140.

Field, A., Camargo, C., Taylor, C., Berkey, C., Roberts, S., & Colditz, G. (2001). Peer, parent and media influences on the development of weight concerns and frequent dieting among preadolescent and adolescent girls and boys. *Pediatrics, 107*, 54–60.

Field, T., Lang, C., & Yando, R. (1995). Adolescents' intimacy with parents and friends. *Adolescence, 30*, 133–140.

Finkelhor, D. (2008). *Child victimization: Violence, crime and abuse in the lives of young people.* New York: Oxford University Press.

Finkelhor, D., Turner, H., & Ormrod, R. (2007). Poly-victimization and trauma in a national longitudinal cohort. *Development and Psychopathology, 19*, 149–166.

Fish L., & Harvey R. (2005). *Nurturing queer youth: Family therapy transformed.* New York: Norton.

Foster, S. L., & Robin, A. L. (1989). Parent–adolescent conflict. In E. J. Mash & R. A. Barkley (Eds.), *Treatment of childhood disorders* (pp. 493–528). New York: Guilford Press.

Frankl, V. (1963). *Man's search for meaning.* New York: Pocket Books.

Frankl, V. (1969). *The will to meaning: Foundations and applications of logotherapy.* New York: New American Library.

Frankl, V. E. (1962). Man's search for meaning: An introduction to logotherapy. Boston: Beacon Press.

Franson, J. (2000). Prescription for bullying and bullies: An effective intervention strategy. *Schools in the Middle, 9*(8), 32–34.

Fraser, M. W. (2004). *Risk and resilience in childhood: An ecological perspective* (2nd ed.). Washington, DC: National Association of Social Workers Press.

Freeman, H., & Brown, B. B. (2001). Primary attachment to parents and peers during adolescence: Differences by attachment style. *Journal of Youth and Adolescence, 30*, 653–674.

Frick, P. (1998). *Conduct disorders and severe antisocial behavior.* New York: Plenum.

Friedrich, W., Jaworski, T., Huxsahl, J., & Bengston, B. (1997). Dissociative and sexual behaviors in children and adolescents with sexual abuse and psychiatric histories. *Journal of Interpersonal Violence, 12*(2), 155–171.

Fuller, M., & Olsen. G. (1998). *Home–school relations: Working successfully with parents and families.* Boston: Allyn & Bacon.

Funk, S. (1999). Risk assessment for juveniles on probation. *Criminal Justice and Behavior, 26*(1), 44–68.

Furstenberg, F. (1993). How families manage risk and opportunity in dangerous neighborhoods. In W. J. Wilson (Ed.), *Sociology and the public agenda* (pp. 231–258). Newbury Park, CA: Sage.

Galambos, N., Leadbeater, B., & Barker, E. (2004). Gender differences in and risk factors for depression in adolescence: A 4-year longitudinal study. *International Journal of Behavioral Development, 28*(1), 16–25.

Garbarino, J. (1995). *Raising children in a socially toxic environment.* New York: Wiley.

Garbarino, J. (1999). *Lost boys: Why our sons turn violent and how we can save them.* New York: Free Press.

Garbarino, J. (2001). *Parents under siege: Why you are the solution, not the problem, in your child's life.* New York: Free Press.

Garbarino, J., Dubrow, N., Kostelny, K., & Pardo, C. (1992). *Children in danger: Coping with the consequences of community violence.* San Francisco: Jossey-Bass.

Garber, J., & Little, S. (1999). Predictors of competence among offspring of depressed mothers. *Journal of Adolescent Research, 14*(1), 44–71.

Garcia-Coll, C., Lamberty, G., Jenkins, R., McAdoo, H., Crnic, K., Wasik, B., et al. (1996). An integrative model for the study of developmental competencies in minority children. *Child Development, 67,* 1891–1914.

Gardner, H. (1993). *Multiple intelligences: The theory in practice.* New York: Basic Books.

Garmezy, N. (1985). *Stress-resistant children: The search for protective factors.* Elmsford, NY: Pergamon Press.

Garmezy, N. (1993). Children in poverty: Resilience despite risk. *Psychiatry, 56,* 127–136.

Garmezy, N., Masten, A., & Tellegen A. (1984). The study of stress and competence in children: A building block for developmental psychopathology. *Child Development, 55*(1), 97–111.

Gay, Lesbian, Straight Educators Network (2009) Climate Survey, 2007. Retrieved October 7, 2009, from *www.glsen.org/cgi-bin/iowa/all/news/record/2340.html.*

Geltman, P. L., Grant-Knight, W., Mehta, S. D., Lloyd-Travaglini, C., Lustig, S., Landgraf, J. M., et al. (2005). The "Lost Boys" of Sudan: Functional and behavioral health of unaccompanied refugee minors resettled in the United States. *Archives of Pediatric and Adolescent Medicine, 159,* 585–591.

Gentles, K., & Harrison, K. (2006). Television and perceived peer expectations of body size among African American adolescent girls. *The Howard Journal of Communications, 17,* 39–55.

Giles, D. (2002). Parasocial interaction: A review of the literature and a model for future research. *Mediapsychology, 4,* 279–305.

Giles, D., & Maltby, J. (2004). The role of media figures in adolescent development: Relations between autonomy, attachment, and interest in celebrities. *Personality and Individual Differences, 36,* 813–822.

Gillham, J., & Reivich, K. (2004). Cultivating optimism in childhood and adolescence. *Annals of the American Academy of Political and Social Science, 591*(1), 146–163.

Gilligan, C., Lyons, N., & Hamer, T. (1990). *Making connections: The relational world of adolescent girls at Emma Willard School.* Cambridge, MA: Harvard University Press.

Goffman, E. (1959). *The presentation of self in everyday life.* Garden City, NY: Doubleday.

Goldstein, T., Collins, A., & Halder, M. (2007). Anti-homophobia education in public schooling: LA Canadian case study. *Journal of Gay and Lesbian Social Services: Issues in Practice, Policy, and Research, 19*(3/4), 47–65.

Goleman, D. (1995). *Emotional intelligence: Why it can matter more than IQ.* New York: Bantam Books.

Goleman, D. (1998). *Working with emotional intelligence.* New York: Bantam Books.

Goleman, D. (2001). *The emotionally intelligent workplace.* San Francisco: Jossey-Bass.

Golumb, M., Fava, M., Abraham, M. & Rosenbaum, J. (1995). Gender differences in personality disorders. *American Journal of Psychiatry, 152,* 579–582.

Gore, S., & Eckenrode, J. (1996). Context and process in research on risk and resilience. In R. Haggerty, L. Sherrod, N. Garmezy, & M. Rutter (Eds.), *Stress, risk, and resilience in children and adolescents* (pp. 19–63). Cambridge, UK: Cambridge University Press.

Gottlieb, H., & Sylvestre, S. (1994). Social support relationships between older adolescents and adults. In F. Nestmann & K. Hurrlemann (Eds.), *Social support networks and social support in childhood and adolescence* (pp. 53–73). New York: Walter de Gruyter.

Gottman, J. M., & Notarius, C. I. (2000). Decade review: Observing marital interaction. *Journal of Marriage and the Family, 62,* 927–947.

Gowen, L. K., Feldman, S., Diaz, R., & Yisrael, D. S. (2004). A comparison of the sexual behaviors and attitudes of adolescent girls with older vs. similar-aged boyfriends. *Journal of Youth and Adolescence, 33*(2), 167–175.

Green, J. (2004). *Becoming a visible man.* Norman, OK: Vanderbilt University Press.

Greenberg, M. T., Weissberg, R. P., O'Brien, M. U., Zins, J. E., Fredericks, L., Resnik, H., et al. (2003). Enhancing school-based prevention and youth development through coordinated social, emotional, and academic learning. *American Psychologist, 58,* 466–474.

Greenberger, E., Chen, C., Tally, S., & Dong, Q. (2000). Family, peer, and individual correlates of depressive symptomology among U.S. and Chinese adolescents. *Journal of Consulting and Clinical Psychology, 68*(2), 209–219.

Greenwald, R. (2002). *Trauma and juvenile delinquency: Theory, research, and interventions.* New York: Haworth.

Griffore, R., & Phenice, L. (2001). *The language of human ecology.* Dubuque, IA: Kendall/Hunt.

Grossman, A., & D'Augelli, A. (2006). Transgender youth: Invisible and vulnerable. *Journal of Homosexuality, 51*(1), 11–128.

Grossman, A., D'Augelli, A., Howell, T., & Hubbard, S. (2005) Parents' reactions to transgender youths' gender nonconforming expression and identity. *Journal of Gay and Lesbian Social Services, 18*(1), 3–16.

Gump, P. (1981). Big school, small school. In E. Hetherington & R. Parke (Eds.), *Contemporary readings in child psychology* (2nd ed., pp. 315–320). New York: McGraw-Hill.

Gurian, M. (2006). *Wonders of boys: What parents, mentors and educators can do to shape exceptional men.* New York: Tarcher/Penguin.

Hagan, J., & Foster, H. (2003). S/He's a rebel: Toward a sequential stress theory of delinquency and gendered pathways to disadvantage in emerging adulthood. *Social Forces, 82*(1), 53–86.

Hair, E. C., Moore, K. A., Garrett, S. B., Ling, T., & Cleveland, K. (2008). The continued importance of quality parent–adolescent relationships during late adolescence. *Journal of Research on Adolescence, 18*, 187–200.

Haley, J. (1976). *Problem solving therapy.* New York: Harper & Row.

Hall, G. S. (1904). *Adolescence: Its psychology, anthropology, sociology, sex, crime religion and education.* New York: Appleton.

Hall, J., Smith, D., Easton, S., Hyonggin A., Williams, J., Godley, S., et al. (2008). Substance abuse treatment with rural adolescents: Issues and outcomes. *Journal of Psychoactive Drugs. 40*(1), 109–120.

Halpern, C., Hallifors, D., Bauer, D., Iritini, B., Waller, M., & Cho, H. (2004). Implications for racial and gender differences in patterns of adolescent risk behavior for HIV and other sexually transmitted diseases. *Perspectives on Sexual and Reproductive Health, 36*, 239–247.

Hamilton, B. E., Martin, J. A., & Ventura, S. J. (2009). Births: Preliminary data for 2007. *National Vital Statistics Reports, 57*(12). Hyattsville, MD: National Center for Health Statistics.

Hanson, D. (2008). *The chemical carousel: What science tells us about beating addiction.* Booksurge.

Hardiman, R. (1994). White racial identity development in the United States. In E. P. Salett & D. R. Koslow (Eds.), *Race, ethnicity, and self: Identity in multicultural perspectives* (pp. 117–140). Washington, DC: National Multicultural Institute.

Hardy, S. A., & Raffaelli, M. (2003). Adolescent religiosity and sexuality: An investigation of reciprocal influences. *Journal of Adolescence, 26*, 731–739.

Harris, J. R. (1995). Where is the child's environment?: A group socialization theory. *Psychological Review, 102*, 458–489.

Harrison, K. (2000). The body electric: Thin ideal media and eating disorders in adolescents. *Journal of Communication, 50*, 119–143.

Harter, S. (1999). *The construction of self: A developmental perspective.* New York: Guilford Press.

Harter, S. (2004). *The cognitive and social construction of the developing self.* New York: Guilford Press.

Harvard Mental Health Letter. (2010, January). *Addiction in women.* Boston: Harvard Health Publications.

Harvard School of Public Health. (2003). Dating violence against adolescent girls linked with teen pregnancy, suicide attempts, and other health risk behaviors (Press Release). Retrieved September 29, 2009, from *www.hsph.harvard.edu/news/press-releases/archives/2001–releases/press07312001.html.*

Hatchett, S. J., & Jackson, J. S. (1999). African American extended *kin* systems: An empirical assessment in the National Survey of Black Americans. In H. P. McAdoo (Ed.), *Family ethnicity: Strength in diversity* (pp. 171–190). Thousand Oaks, CA: Sage.

Hawke, J., Hennen, J., & Gallione, P. (2005). Correlates of therapeutic involvement among adolescents in residential drug treatment. *American Journal of Drug and Alcohol Abuse, 31*(1), 163–177.

Hawkins, J., Catalano, R., & Miller, J. (1992). Risk and protective factors for alcohol and other drug problems in adolescence and early adulthood: Implications for substance abuse prevention. *Psychological Bulletin, 112*, 64–105.

Hayward, C., Killen, J., Wilson, D., Hammer, L., Litt, I., Kraemer, H., et al. (1997).

Psychiatric risk associated with early puberty in adolescent girls. *Journal of the American Academy of Child and Adolescent Psychiatry, 36,* 255–262.

Hayward, T. (1994). *Ecological thought.* Cambridge, UK: Polity Press.

Heatherington, L., & Lavner, J. (2008). Coming to terms with coming out: Review and recommendations for family systems-focused research. *Journal of Family Psychology, 22*(3), 329–343.

Heise, D., & Weir, B. (1999). A test of symbolic interactionist predictions about emotions in imagined situations. *Symbolic Interaction, 22,* 139–161.

Helms, J. (1990). *Black and white racial identity: Theory, research, and practice. Contributions in Afro-American and African studies, 129.* New York: Greenwood Press.

Helms, J. (1995). *Handbook of multicultural counseling.* New York: Sage.

Henderson, N., & Milstein, M. (1996). *Resiliency in schools: Making it happen for children and educators.* Thousand Oaks, CA: Sage.

Henggeler, S. (1999). Multisystemic therapy: An overview of clinical procedures, outcomes, and policy implications. *Child Psychology and Psychiatry Review, 4,* 2–10.

Henggeler, S. W., Clingempeel, W. G., Brondino, M. J., & Pickrel, S. G. (2002). Four-year follow up of multisystemic therapy with substance-abusing and substance dependent juvenile offenders. *Journal of the American Academy of Child and Adolescent Psychiatry, 41,* 868–874.

Henggeler, S. W., & Lee, T. (2003). Multisystemic treatment of serious clinical problems. In A. E. Kazdin & J. R. Weisz (Eds.), *Evidence-based psychotherapies for children and adolescents* (pp. 301–322). New York: Guilford Press.

Henry, B., Caspi, A., Moffitt, T., & Silva, P. (1996). Temperamental and familial predictors of violent and nonviolent convictions: Age 3 to 18. *Developmental Psychology, 32*(4), 614–623.

Hensel, J., & Anderson, J. (2006). *Comparing trends in sexual risk taking among rural and non-rural high school students: 1997–2003.* Paper presented at the annual meeting of the American Sociological Association, Montreal Convention Center, Montreal, Quebec, Canada.

Hernandez, A. (1999). *Peace on the streets: Breaking the cycle of gang violence.* Washington, DC: CWLA Press.

Higgins, G. (1994). *Resilient adults: Overcoming a cruel past.* San Francisco: Jossey-Bass.

Holloway, S., & Mulherin, S. (2004). The effect of adolescent neighborhood poverty on adult employment. *Journal of Urban Affairs, 26*(4), 427–454.

hooks, b. (1981). *Ain't I a woman: Black women and feminism.* Boston: South End Press.

Hogue, A., Dauber, S., Samuolis, J., & Liddle, H. A. (2006). Treatment techniques in multidimensional family therapy for adolescent behavior problems. *Journal of Family Psychology, 20,* 535–543.

Hogue, A., Dauber, S., Stambaugh, L. F., Cecero, J. J., & Liddle, H. A. (2006). Early therapeutic alliance and treatment outcome in individual and family therapy for adolescent behavior problems. *Journal of Consulting and Clinical Psychology, 74,* 121–129.

Hotz, V. J., McElroy, S. W., & Sanders, S. G. (1997). The impacts of teenage childbearing on the mothers and the consequences of those impacts for government. In R. A. Maynard (Ed.), *Kids having kids: Economic costs and social consequences of teen pregnancy* (pp. 55–94). Washington, DC: Urban Institute Press.

Howard, D. E., Wang, M. Q., & Yan, F. (2007). Prevalence and psychosocial correlates of forced sexual intercourse among U.S. high school adolescents. *Adolescence, 42*(168), 629–643.

Howard, M. O., & Jenson, J. M. (1999). Inhalant use among antisocial youth: Prevalence and correlates. *Addictive Behaviors, 24*, 59–74.

Howard, S., Dryden, J., & Johnson, B. (1999). Childhood resilience: Review and critique of literature. *Oxford Review of Education, 25*(3), 307–324.

Hung, N., & Rabin, L. (2009). Comprehending childhood bereavement by parental suicide: A critical review of research on outcomes, grief processes, and interventions. *Death Studies, 33*, 781–814.

Hussong, A. M., Curran, P. J., Moffitt, T. E., Caspi, A., & Carrig, M. M. (2004). Substance abuse hinders desistance in young adults' antisocial behavior. *Development and Psychopathology, 16*, 1029–1046.

Jaffee, S., Caspi, A., Moffitt, T. E., Belsky, J., & Silva, P. (2001). Why are children born to teen mothers at risk for adverse outcomes in young adulthood? Results from a 20-year longitudinal study. *Development and Psychopathology, 13*, 377–397.

James, A., Taylor, A., Winmill, L., & Alfoadari, K. (2007). A preliminary community study of dialectical behavior therapy (DBT) with adolescent females demonstrating persistent, deliberate self-harm. *Child and Adolescent Mental Health, 13*(3), 148–152.

Jaycox, L., Ebener, P., Damesek, L., & Becker, K. (2004). Trauma exposure and retention in adolescent substance abuse treatment. *Journal of Traumatic Stress, 17*(2), 113–121.

Jenson, J. (2004). Risk and protective factors for alcohol and other drug use in childhood and adolescence. In M. W. Fraser (Ed.), *Risk and resilience in childhood: An ecological perspective* (pp. 183–208). Washington, DC: NASW Press.

Jenson, J., & Fraser, M. (2006). *Social policy for children and families: A risk and resilience perspective.* Thousand Oaks, CA: Sage.

Jenson, J., & Howard, M. (1998). Correlates of gang involvement among juvenile probationers. *Journal of Gang Research, 5*, 7–15.

Jessor, R., Turbin, M., & Costa, F. (1998). Protective factors in adolescent health behavior. *Journal of Personality and Social Psychology, 75*, 788–800.

Jessor, R., Van Den Bos, J., Vanderryn, J., Costa, F., & Turbin, M. (1995). Protective factors in adolescent problem behavior: Moderator effects in developmental change. *Developmental Psychology, 31*(6), 923–933.

Johnston, L. D., O'Malley, P. M., Bachman, J. G., & Schulenberg, J. E. (2008). *Monitoring the future national results on adolescent drug use: Overview of key findings, 2007* (NIH Publication No. 08-6418). Bethesda, MD: National Institute on Drug Abuse.

Jones, R., Darroch, J., & Henshaw, S. (2002). Contraceptive use among U.S. women having abortions in 2000–2001. *Perspectives on Sexual and Reproductive Health, 34*, 294–303.

Kahn, J. R., & Anderson, K. E. (1992). Intergenerational patterns of teenage fertility. *Demography, 29*, 39–57.

Kaiser Family Foundation. (2005). *U.S. teen sexual activity*. Retrieved from *www.kff. org/womenshealth/3040.cfm*.

Kaiser Family Foundation. (2006). *Sexual health statistics for teenagers and young adults in the United States*. Retrieved from *www.kff.org/womenshealth/3040.cfm*.

Kaplowitz, P., Slora, E., Wasserman, R., Pedlow, S., & Herman-Giddens, M. E. (2001). Earlier onset of puberty in girls: Relation to increased body mass index and race. *Pediatrics, 108*, 347–353.

Katz, L., Cox, B., Gunasekara, S., & Miller, A. (2004). Feasibility of dialectical behavior therapy for suicidal adolescent inpatients. *Journal of the American Academy of Child and Adolescent Psychiatry, 43*(3), 276–282.

Kelley, P., Blankenburg, L., & McRoberts, J. (2002). Girls' fighting struggle: Restorying young lives. *Families in Society: The Journal of Contemporary Human Services, 83*(5/6), 530–561.

Kessler, R. C., Berglund, P. A., Foster, C. L., Saunders, W. B., Stang, P. E., & Walters, E. E. (1997). Social consequences of psychiatric disorders II: Teenage parenthood. *American Journal of Psychiatry, 154*, 1405–1411.

Kilpatrick, D., Acierno, R., Resnick, H., Saunders, B., & Best, C. (1997). A 2–year longitudinal analysis of the relationships between violent assault and substance use in women. *Journal of Consulting and Clinical Psychology, 65*(5), 834–847.

Kindlon, D. (2006). *Alpha girls: Understanding the new American girl and how she is changing the world*. New York: Rodale.

Kindlon, D., & Thompson, M. (1999). *Raising Cain: Protecting the emotional life of boys*. New York: Ballantine.

Kirby, D. (2007). *Emerging answers 2007: Research findings on programs to reduce teen pregnancy and sexually transmitted diseases*. Washington, DC: National Campaign to Prevent Teen and Unplanned Pregnancy. Retrieved from *www.thenationalcampaign.org/EA2007*.

Kisiel, C., & Lyons, J. (2001). Dissociation as a mediator of psychopathology among sexually abused children and adolescents. *American Journal of Psychiatry, 158*(7), 1034–1039.

Kistner, J., David, C., & White, B. (2003). Ethnic and sex differences in children's depressive symptoms: The mediating role of academic and social competence. *Journal of Clinical Child and Adolescent Psychology, 36*, 171–181.

Kohlberg, L. (1963). The development of children's orientation toward a moral order: I. Sequence in the development of moral thought. *Vita Humana, 6*, 13–35.

Kohler P. K., Manhart, L. E., & Lafferty, W. E. (2008). Abstinence-only and comprehensive sex education and the initiation of sexual activity and teen pregnancy. *Journal of Adolescent Health, 42*(4), 344–351.

Kotlowitz, A. (1991). *There are no children here: The story of two boys growing up in the other America*. New York: Anchor Books.

Kovacs, M., Krol, R. M., & Voti, L. (1994). Early onset psychopathology and the risk for teenage pregnancy among clinically referred girls. *Journal of the American Academy of Child and Adolescent Psychiatry, 33*, 106–113.

Kravitz, H., Cavanaugh, J., & Rigsbee, S. (2002). A cross-sectional study of psychosocial and criminal factors associated with arrest in mentally ill female detainees. *Journal of the American Academy of Psychiatry and the Law, 30*(3), 380–390.

Kumpfer, K. (1999). Factors and processes contributing to resilience: The resilience framework. In M. Glantz & J. Johnson (Eds.), *Resilience and development: Positive life adaptations* (pp. 179–224). New York: Kluwer.

Kuperman, S., Schlosser, S. S., Kramer, J. R., Bucholz, K., Hesselbrock, V., Reich, T., et al. (2001). Developmental sequence from disruptive behavior diagnosis to adolescent alcohol dependence.

La Greca, A. M., Prinstein, M. J., & Fetter, M. D. (2001). Adolescent peer crowd affiliation: Linkages with health-risk behaviors and close friendships. *Journal of Pediatric Psychology, 26*(3), 131–143.

Laird, R. D., Criss, M. M., Pettit, G. S., Dodge, K. A., & Bates, J. E. (2008). Parents' monitoring knowledge attenuates the link between antisocial friends and adolescent delinquent behavior. *Journal of Abnormal Child Psychology, 36,* 299–310.

Lam, T., Stewart, S., Leung, G., Lee, P., Wong, J., & Ho, L. (2004). Depressive symptoms among Hong Kong adolescents: Relation to atypical sexual feelings and behaviors, gender dissatisfaction, pubertal timing, and family peer relationships. *Archives of Sexual Behavior, 33*(5), 487–496.

Larson, R. (1995). Secrets in the bedroom: Adolescents' private use of media. *Journal of Youth and Adolescence, 24,* 535–550.

Larson, R. (2000). Toward a psychology of positive youth development. *American Psychologist, 55*(1), 170–183.

Larson, R. (2001). How US children and adolescents spend their time: What it does (and doesn't) tell us about their development. *Current Directions in Psychological Sciences, 10*(5), 160–164.

Laser, J. (2003). *Everyday resiliency in Japanese youth: Individual and ecological protective factors and risk factors.* Unpublished dissertation, Michigan State University.

Laser, J. (2006). Residual effects of repeated bully victimization before the age of 12 on adolescent functioning. *Journal of School Violence, 5*(2), 37–52.

Laser, J. (2008). Resilience in Japanese youth. In L. Leibenberg & M. Ungar (Eds.), *Resilience in action: Working with youth across cultures and contexts* (pp. 321–334). Toronto: University of Toronto Press.

Laser, J., Luster, T., & Oshio, T. (2007a). Promotive and risk factors related to deviant behavior in Japanese youth. *Criminal Justice and Behavior, 34*(11), 1463–1480.

Laser, J., Luster, T., & Oshio, T. (2007b). Risk and promotive factors related to depressive symptoms among Japanese youth. *American Journal of Ortho Psychiatry, 77*(4), 523–533.

Lau, R., Quadrel, M., & Hartman, K. (1990). Development and change of young adults' preventive health beliefs and behaviors: Influence from parents and peers. *Journal of Health and Social Behavior, 31,* 240–259.

Law, J., & Barber, B. (2006). Neighborhood conditions, parenting, and adolescent functioning. *Journal of Human Behavior in the Social Environment, 14*(4), 91–118.

Leibowitz, G., Laser, J., & Burton, D. (in press). Exploring the relationships between dissociation, victimization, and juvenile sexual offending. *Journal of Trauma and Dissociation.*

Leit, R., Gray, J., & Pope, H. (2002). The media's representation of the ideal male body: A cause for muscle dysmorphia? *International Journal of Eating Disorders, 31*, 334–338.

Lemoire, J., & Chen, C. (2005). Applying person-centered counseling to sexual minority adolescents. *Journal of Counseling and Development, 83*, 146–154.

L'Engle, K., Brown, J., & Kenneavy, K. (2006). The mass media are an important context for adolescents' sexual behavior. *Journal of Adolescent Health, 38*, 186–192.

Lerner, R., Brentano, C., Dowling, E., & Anderson, P. (2002). Positive youth development: Thriving as a basis of personhood and civic society. *New Directions for Youth Development, 95*, 11–33.

Lickona, T. (1991). *Educating for character: How our schools can teach respect and responsibility*. New York: Bantam Books.

Liddle, H. A., Rodriguez, R. A., Dakof, G. A., Kanzki, E., & Marvel, F. A. (2005). Multidimensional family therapy: A science-based treatment for adolescent drug use. In J. L. Lebow (Ed.), *Handbook of clinical family therapy* (pp. 128–163).

Liddle, H. A., & Schwartz, S. J. (2002). Attachment and family therapy: Clinical utility of adolescent–family attachment research. *Family Process, 41*, 455–476.

Lindberg, L., Jones, R., & Santelli, J. (2007). Non-coital sexual activities among adolescents. *Journal of Adolescent Health, 42*(2), 44–45.

Linehan, M. (1993). *Cognitive-behavioral treatment of borderline personality disorder*. New York: Guilford Press.

Lloyd, B. (2002). A conceptual framework for examining adolescent identity, media influence, and social development. *Review of General Psychology, 6*(1), 73–91.

Loader, B. (2007). *Young citizens in the digital age: Political engagement, young people, and the new media*. New York: Routledge, Taylor & Francis Group.

Loeber, R., & Dishion, T. (1983). Early predictors of male delinquency: A review. *Psychological Bulletin, 94*(1), 68–99.

Loeber, R., Farrington, D. P., Stouthamer-Loeber, M., & Van Kammen, W. B. (1998). Multiple risk factors for multiproblem boys: Co-occurrence of delinquency, substance use, attention deficit, conduct problems, physical aggression, covert behavior, depressed mood, and shy/withdrawn behavior. In R. Jessor (Ed.), *New perspectives on adolescent risk behavior* (pp. 90–149). New York: Cambridge University Press.

Loeber, R., & Hay, D. (1997). Key issues in the development of aggression and violence from childhood to early adulthood. *Annual Review of Psychology, 48*, 371–410.

Long, P. W. (2008). Internet mental health: Alcohol dependence. Retrieved August 25, 2008, from *www.mentalhealth.com/dis/p20–sb01.html*.

Luker, K. (1991, Spring). Dubious conceptions: The controversy over teen pregnancy. *The American Prospect*, 73–83.

Luster, T. (1998). Individual differences in the care giving behavior of teenage mothers: An ecological perspective. *Clinical Child Psychology and Psychiatry, 3*, 341–360.

Luster, T., Bates, L., & Johnson, D. (2004). The lost boys of Sudan: A study of resilience and adaptation. *NCFR Family Focus, 24*, 10–11.

Luster, T., & Small, S. (1997). Sexual abuse history and number of sex partners among female adolescents. *Family Planning Perspectives, 29*(5), 204–211.

Luthar, S., Cicchetti, D., & Becker, B. (2000). The construct of resilience: A critical evaluation and guideline for future work. *Child Development, 71*, 543–562.

Luthar, S., Cushing, G., Merikangas, K., & Rounsaville, B. (1998). Multiple jeopardy: Risk and protective factors among addicted mothers' offspring. *Development and Psychopathology, 10*, 117–136.

Maag, C. (2007, December 16). When bullies turned faceless. *New York Times.*

Mackey, S. K. (2003). Adolescence and attachment: From theory to treatment implications. In P. Erdman & T. Caffery (Eds.), *Attachment and family systems: Conceptual, empirical, and therapeutic relatedness* (pp. 79–113). New York: Brunner-Routledge.

Madsen, W. C. (2009). Collaborative helping: A practice framework for family-centered services. *Family Process, 48*, 103–116.

Mahler, M. S., Pine, F., & Bergman (1975). *The psychological birth of the human infant.* New York: Basic Books.

Main, M., Kaplan, N., & Cassidy, J. (1985). Security in infancy, childhood and adulthood: A move to the level of representation. In I. Bretherton & E. Waters (Eds.), *Growing points of attachment theory and research. Monographs of the Society for Research in Child Development, 50*(1–2, Serial No. 209), 66–106.

Mallon, J. (1999). *Social services with transgendered youth.* Binghamton, NY: Haworth Press.

Marcia, J. (1966). Development and validation of ego identity status. *Journal of Personality and Social Psychology, 3*, 551–558.

Marcia, J. (1987). Identity in adolescence. In J. Adelson (Ed.), *Handbook of adolescent psychology.* New York: Wiley.

Marcia, J. (1991). Identity and self-development. In R. Lerner, A. C. Petersen, & J. Brooks-Gunn (Eds.), *Encyclopedia of adolescence*(Vol. 1, pp. 529–533). New York: Garland.

Marcia, J. (1993). *Ego identity: A handbook for psychosocial research.* New York: Springer Verlag.

Martin, C. S., & Winters, K. C. (1999). Diagnosis and assessment of alcohol use disorders among adolescents. *Alcohol Health and Research World, 22*, 95–105.

Maschi, T. (2006). Unraveling the link between trauma and male delinquency: The cumulative versus differential risk perspective. *Social Work, 51*(1), 59–70.

Masten, A., & Coatsworth, J. (1998). The development of competence in favorable and unfavorable environments: Lessons from research on successful children. *American Psychologist, 53*(5), 205–220.

Masten, A. A., & Powell, J. L. (2003). A resilience framework for research, policy, and practice. In S. S. Luthar (Ed.), *Resilience and vulnerabilities: Adaptation in the context of childhood adversities* (pp. 1–25). New York: Cambridge University Press.

Masters, J., & Burish, T. (1987). *Behavior therapy: Techniques and empirical findings* (3rd ed.). San Diego, CA: Harcourt Brace Jovanovich.

Matthews, R., Matthews, J., & Speltz, K. (1989). *Female sexual offenders: An exploratory study.* Orwell, VT: Safer Society Press.

Maughan, B. (1992). School experiences as risk/protective factors. In B. Tizard &

V. Varma (Eds.), *Vulnerability and resilience in human development: Festschrift for Ann and Alan Clarke* (pp. 201–220). London: Jessica Kingsley.

Mayeux, L., Sandstrom, M., & Cillessen, A. (2008). Is being popular a risky proposition? *Journal of Research on Adolescence, 18*, 49–74.

Maylon, A. (1982). Biphasic aspects of homosexual identity formation. *Psychotherapy: Theory, Research, and Practice, 19*, 335–340.

Mayseless, O., & Scharf, M. (2009). Too close for comfort: Inadequate boundaries with parents and individuation in late adolescent girls. *American Journal of Orthopsychiatry, 79*, 191–202.

McAdoo, H. P. (2001). Parent and child relationships in African American families. In N. B. Webb (Ed.), *Culturally diverse parent-child and family relationships* (pp. 89–105). New York: Columbia University Press.

McCabe, M., & Ricciardelli, L. (2005). A prospective study of pressure from parents, peers, and the media on extreme weight change behaviors among adolescent boys and girls. *Behavior Research and Therapy, 43*, 653–668.

McCaskell, T., & Russell, V. (2000). Anti-homophobia initiatives at the former Toronto Board of Education. In T. Goldstein & D. Selby (Eds.), *Weaving connections: Educating for peace, social, and environmental justice* (pp. 27–56). Toronto, Canada: Sumach.

McCave, E. L. (2007). Comprehensive sexuality education vs. abstinence-only sexuality education: The need for evidence-based research and practice. *School Social Work Journal, 32*(1), 14–28.

McGee, R.,Wolfe, D.,& Wilson, S. (1997). Multiple maltreatment experiences and adolescent behavior problems: Adolescent perspectives. *Development and Psychopathology, 9*, 131–149.

McGue, M., & Bouchard, T. J. (1998). Genetic and environmental influences on human behavioral differences. *Annual Review of Neuroscience, 21*, 1–24.

McGue, M., Elkins, I., Walden, B., & Iacono, W. G. (2005). Perceptions of the parent–adolescent relationship: A longitudinal investigation. *Developmental Psychology, 41*, 971–984.

McIntyre, T., & Von Ornsteiner, J. (2001). What do we do about Alberto? Providing a safe haven for youngsters with gender identity disorder. *Reclaiming Children and Youth, 9*(4), 219–223.

McLoyd, V. (1998). Socioeconomic disadvantage and child development. *American Psychologist, 53*(2), 185–204.

McMillan, J., & Reed, D. (1994). At-risk students and resiliency: Factors contributing to academic success. *Clearing House, 67*(3), 137–140.

McNally, R. (2003). Progress and controversy in the study of posttraumatic stress disorder. *Annual Review of Psychology, 54*, 229–252.

Mead, G. (1934). *Mind, self, and society: From the standpoint of a social behaviorist.* Chicago: University of Chicago Press.

Mead, M. (1965). *And keep your powder dry: An anthropologist looks at America.* New York: Morrow.

Mednick, S. A., Gabrielli, W. F., & Hutchings, B. (1984). Genetic influence in criminal convictions: Evidence from an adoption cohort. *Science, 224*, 891–894.

Merrell, K. (2003). *Behavioral and social emotional assessments of children and adoelscents.* Mahwah, NJ: Earlbaum.

Meschke, L., & Silbereisen, R. (1997). The influence of puberty, family processes, and leisure activities on the timing of first sexual experience. *Journal of Adolescence, 20*, 403–418.

Meschke, L. L., Bartholomae, S., & Zentall, S. R. (2000). Adolescent sexuality and parent–adolescent process: Promoting healthy teen choices. *Family Relations, 49*(2), 143–154.

Mihlalic, S., Fagan, A., Irwin, K., Ballard, D., & Elliot, D. (2002). *Blueprints for violence prevention replications: Factors for implementation success.* Boulder: University of Colorado, Center for the Study and Prevention of Violence.

Miller, K. E., Farrell, M. P., Barnes, G. M., Melnick, M. J., & Sabo, D. (2005). Gender/racial difference in jock identity, dating, and adolescent sexual risk. *Journal of Youth and Adolescence, 34*(2), 123–136.

Miller, W. (1995). *Motivational enhancement therapy with drug users.* Albuquerque: University of New Mexico, Department of Psychology and Center on Alcoholism, Substance Abuse, and Addictions (CASAA).

Miller, W., & Rollnick, S. (1991). *Motivational interviewing: Preparing people to change addictive behavior.* New York: Guilford Press.

Miller-Johnson, S., Winn, D. M., Coie, J., Maumary-Gremaud, A., Hyman, C., Terry, C., et al. (1999). Motherhood during the teen years: A developmental perspective on risk factors for childbearing. *Development and Psychopathology, 11*, 85–100.

Minuchin, S. (1974). *Families and family therapy.* Cambridge, MA: Harvard University Press.

Moffitt, T. (1993). Adolescence-limited and life course-persistent antisocial behavior: A developmental taxonomy. *Psychological Review, 100*, 674–701.

Moffitt, T., Caspi, A., Rutter, M., & Silva, P. (2001). *Sex differences in anti-social behavior: Conduct disorder, delinquency, and violence in the Dunedin Longitudinal Study.* New York: Cambridge University Press.

Mohr, J. (2002). Heterosexual identity and the heterosexual therapist. *Counseling Psychologist, 30*, 532–566.

Molidor, C., Nissen, L., & Watkins, T. (2002). The development of theory and treatment with substance abusing female juvenile offenders. *Child and Adolescent Social Work Journal, 19*(3), 209–225.

Moore, K., & Lippman, L. H. (2005). *What do children need to flourish?: Conceptualizing and measuring indicators of positive development.* New York: Springer.

Moore, K. A., Miller, B. C., Glei, D., & Morrison, D. R. (1995). *Adolescent sex, contraception, and childbearing: A review of recent research.* Washington, DC: Child Trends.

Moore, R. (1986). *Children's domain: Play and place in child development.* London: Croom Helm.

Moran, G., Diamond, G. M., & Diamond, G. S. (2005). The relational reframe and parents' problem constructions in attachment-based family therapy. *Psychotherapy Research, 15*, 226–235.

Moreno, A., & Thelen, M. (1995). Eating behavior in junior high females. *Adolescence, 30*(117), 171–174.

Morita, Y., Soeda, H., Soeda, K., & Taki, M. (1998). Japan. In P. K. Smith, Y. Morita,

J. Junger-Tas, D. Olweus, R. Catalano, & P. Slee (Eds.), *The nature of school bullying: A cross national perspective* (pp. 309–323). London: Routledge.

Morrison, D. M., Casey, E. A., Beadnell, B. A., Hoppe, M. J., Gillmore, M. R., Wilsdon, A., et al. (2007). Effects of friendship closeness in an adolescent group HIV prevention intervention. *Prevention Science, 8*(4), 274–284.

Morrow, D. (2006). Gay, lesbian, bisexual, and transgender adolescents. In D.Morrow & L. Messinger (Eds.), *Sexual orientation and gender expression in social work practice: Working with gay, lesbian, bisexual, and transgender people* (pp. 177–195). New York: Columbia University Press.

Mota, J., Almeida, M., Santos, P., & Ribeiro, J. (2005). Perceived neighborhood environments and physical activity in adolescents. *Preventative Medicine, 41,* 834–836.

MSNBC. (2005). *Tackling the topic of teen sex.* Retrieved from *www.msnbc.msn.com/id/5344844.*

Murray, B. (1998). Does "emotional intelligence" matter in the workplace? *APA Monitor, 29*(7), 5–15.

Musick, J. S. (1993). *Young, poor, and pregnant: The psychology of teenage motherhood.* New Haven, CT: Yale University Press.

Nansel, T., Overpeck, M., Pilla, R., Ruan, W., Simons-Morton, B., & Scheidt, P. (2001). Bullying behaviors among US youth: Prevalence and association with psychological adjustment. *Journal of the American Medical Association, 285*(16), 2094–2100.

Nappi, C. M., McBride, C. K., & Donenberg, G. R. (2007). HIV/AIDS communication among adolescents in psychiatric care and their parents. *Journal of Family Psychology, 21*(4), 637–644.

National Association of Social Workers. (2000). *"Reparative" and "conversion" therapies for lesbians and gay men.* Retrieved March 21, 2009, from *www.socialworkers.org/diversity/lgb/reparative.asp.*

National Campaign to Prevent Teen and Unplanned Pregnancy. (2008). *Sex and tech: What is really going on?* Retrieved September 25, 2009, from *www.thenationalcampaign.org/sextech.*

Nebbitt, V., & Lombe, M. (2007). Environmental correlates of depressive symptoms among African American adolescents living in public housing. *Journal of Human Behavior in the Social Environment, 15*(2/3), 435–454.

Nettles, S., & Pleck, J. (1996). Risk, resilience, and development: The multiple ecologies of black adolescents in the United States. In R. Haggerty, L. Sherrod, N. Garmezy, & M. Rutter (Eds.), *Stress, risk, and resilience in children and adolescents* (pp. 147–181). Cambridge, UK: Cambridge University Press.

Newcomb, M. D., & Bentler, P. M. (1989). Substance use and abuse among children and teenagers. *American Psychologist, 22,* 242–248.

Nickerson, A. B., & Nagle, R. J. (2005). Parent and peer attachment in late childhood and early adolescence. *Journal of Early Adolescence, 25,* 223–249.

Nicotera, N. (2003). *Children and their neighborhoods: A mixed methods approach to understanding the construct neighborhood.* Unpublished dissertation, University of Washington, Seattle.

Nicotera, N. (2005). The neighborhood as resource for family health social work practice. In F. K. Yuen (Ed.), *Family health social work practice with children and families* (pp. 219–251). New York: Haworth Press.

Nicotera, N. (2008). Children speak about neighborhoods: Using mixed methods to measure the construct neighborhood. *Journal of Community Psychology, 36*(3), 333–351.

Nicotera, N., & Matera, D. (2010, January). *Building civic leadership through neighborhood-based afterschool programming*. Paper presented at the Society for Social Work and Research Conference, San Francisco, CA.

Nock, M., & Mendes, W. (2008). Physiological arousal, distress tolerance, and social problem-solving deficits among adolescent self-injurers. *Journal of Consulting and Clinical Psychology, 76*, 28–38.

Nolin, M. J., Davies, E., & Chandler, K. (1996). Student victimization at school. *Journal of School Health, 66*, 216–221.

Novak, S., Reardon, S., & Buka, S. (2002). How beliefs about substance use differ by socio-demographic characteristics, individual experiences, and neighborhood environments among urban adolescents. *Journal of Drug Education, 32*(4), 319–342.

Novick, R. (1998). The comfort corner: Fostering resiliency and emotional intelligence. *Childhood Education, 74*(4), 200–204.

O'Donnell, J., Hawkins, J., Catalano, R., Abbott, R., & Day, L. (1995). Preventing school failure, drug use, and delinquency among low-income children: Long-term intervention in elementary schools. *American Journal of Orthopsychiatry, 65*, 87–100.

O'Koon, J. (1997). Attachment to parents and peers in late adolescence and their relationship with self-image. *Adolescence, 32*, 471–482.

Oliver, R., Hoover, J., & Hazler, R. (1994). The perceived roles of bullying in small town midwestern schools. *Journal of Counseling and Development, 72*(4), 416–421.

Olson, D. H. (1996). Clinical assessment and treatment interventions using the family circumplex model. In F. W. Kaslow, *Handbook of relational diagnosis and dysfunctional family patterns* (pp. 59–80). Hoboken, NJ: Wiley.

Olweus, D. (1993). *Bullying at school*. Oxford, UK: Blackwell.

Olweus, D. (2001a). Health consequences of bullying and its prevention in schools. In J. Juvonen & S. Graham (Eds.), *Peer harassment in school: The plight of the vulnerable and victimized* (pp. 3–12). New York: Guilford Press.

Olweus, D. (2001b). Peer harassment: A critical analysis and some important issues. In J. Juvonen & S. Graham (Eds.), *Peer harassment in school: The plight of the vulnerable and victimized* (pp. 310–331). New York: Guilford Press.

Paley, B., Conger, R. D., & Harold, G. T. (2000). Parents' affect, adolescent cognitive representations, and adolescent social development. *Journal of Marriage and the Family, 62*, 761–776.

Parham, T. (1989). Cycles of psychological nigrescence. *Counseling Psychologist, 17*(2), 187–226.

Parker, H. (1992). *The ADHD hyperactivity handbook for schools*. Plantation, FL: Impact.

Parker, J., & Herrera, C. (1996). Interpersonal processes in friendships: A comparison of maltreated and non-maltreated children's experiences. *Developmental Psychology, 32,* 1025–1038.

Patterson, G. (1995). Coercion—A basis for early age of onset for arrest. In J. McCord (Ed.), *Coercion and punishment in long term perspective* (pp. 81–105). New York: Cambridge University Press.

Patterson, G., DeBaryshe, B., & Ramsey, E. (1989). A developmental perspective on antisocial behavior. *American Psychologist, 44*(2), 329–335.

Paul, P. (2003, September 1). We're just friends. Really! *Time.* Retrieved September 25, 2009, from *www.time.com/time/magazine/articles/0,9171,1005599,00.html.*

Perkins, D., Meeks, J., & Taylor, R. (1992). The physical environment of street blocks and residential perceptions of crime and disorder: Implications for theory and measurement. *Journal of Environmental Psychology, 12,* 21–34.

Perrin, E. C., and the Committee on Psychosocial Aspects of Child and Family Health. (2002). Technical report: Coparent or second-parent adoption by same-sex parents. *Pediatrics, 109,* 341–344.

Perry, B. (2001a). *The cost of maltreatment: Who pays? We all do* (K. Franey, R. Geffner, & R. Falconer (Eds.). San Diego, CA: Family Violence and Sexual Assault Institute.

Perry, B. (2001b). The neuroarcheology of childhood maltreatment: The neurode-velopmental costs of adverse childhood events. In K. Franey, R. Geffner, & R. Falconer (Eds.), *The cost of maltreatment: Who pays? We all do* (pp. 15–37). San Diego, CA: Family Violence and Sexual Assault Institute.

Perry, B. (2008). Child maltreatment: A neurodevelopmental perspective on the role of trauma and neglect in psychopathology. In T. Beauchaine & S. Hinshaw (Eds.), *Child and adolescent psychopathology* (pp. 93–129). Hoboken, NJ: Wiley.

Perry, B. D. (1997). Incubated in terror: Neurodevelopmental factors in the "cycle of violence." In J. Osofky (Ed.), Children, youth, and voilence: Searching for solutions (pp. 124–148). New York: Guilford Press.

Peterson, K., Paulson, S., & Williams, K. (2007). Relations of eating disorder symptomology with perceptions of pressures from mother, peers, and media in adolescent girls and boys. *Sex Roles, 57*(9/10), 629–640.

Petraitis, J., Flay, B. R., & Miller, T. Q. (1995). Reviewing theories of adolescent substance use: Organizing pieces in the puzzle. *Psychological Bulletin, 117*(1), 67–86.

Phenice, L., & Griffore, R. (2000). Social identity of ethnic minority families: An ecological approach for the new millennium. *Michigan Family Review, 5,* 29–39.

Piaget, J. (1952). *The origins of intelligence in children.* New York: International Universities Press.

Piaget, J. (1970, May). Conversations. *Psychology Today, 3,* 25–32.

Pilkington, N. W., & D'Augelli, A. R. (1995). Victimization of lesbian, gay, and bisexual youth in community settings. *Journal of Community Psychology, 23,* 34–56.

Pipher, M. (1994). *Reviving Ophelia.* New York: Random House.

Plybon, L., Edwards, L., Butler, D., Belgrave, F., & Allison, K. (2003). Examining the link between neighborhood cohesion and school outcomes: The role of support coping among African American adolescent girls. *Journal of Black Psychology, 29*(4), 393–407.

Pollack, W. (1999). *Real boys.* New York: Henry Holt.

Pope, H., Philips, K., & Olivardia, R. (2000). *The Adonis complex: How to identify, treat and prevent body obsession in men and boys.* New York: Touchstone.

Popkin, B., & Urdery, R. (1998, April). Adolescent obesity increases significantly in second and third generation U.S. immigrants. *Journal of Nutrition, 128,* 701–706.

Prochaska, J., Norcross, J., & DiClemente, C. (1994). *Changing for good.* New York: Morrow.

Quinton, D., Rutter, M., & Liddle, C. (1984). Institutional rearing, parenting difficulties, and marital support. *Psychological Medicine, 14,* 107–124.

Randall, J., & Henggeler, S. (1999). Multisystemic therapy: Changing the social ecologies of youths presenting serious clinical problems and their families. In S. Russ & T. Ollendick (Eds.), *Handbook of psychotherapies with children and families* (pp. 405–418). New York: Plenum Press.

Raneri, L. G., & Wiemann, C. M. (2007). Social ecological predictors of repeat adolescent pregnancy. *Perspective on Sexual and Reproductive Health, 39*(1), 39–47.

Rathus, S. A., Nevid, J. S., & Fichner-Rathus, L. (2000). *Human sexuality in a world of diversity* (4th ed.). Needham Heights, MA: Allyn & Bacon.

Rauch-Elnekave, H. (1994). Teenage motherhood: Its relationship to undetected learning problems. *Adolescence, 29,* 91–103.

Remafedi, G., Farrow, J., & Deischer, R. (1991). Risk factors for attempted suicide in gay and bisexual youth. *Pediatrics, 87,* 869–895.

Repetti, R., Taylor, S., & Seeman, T. (2002). Risky families: Family social environments and the mental and physical health of the offspring. *Psychological Bulletin, 128*(2), 330–366.

Ricciardelli, L., & McCabe, M. (2003). Sociocultural and individual influences on muscle gain and weight loss strategies among adolescent boys and girls. *Psychology in Schools, 40*(2), 209–224.

Ricciardelli, L., McCabe, M., & Banfield, S. (2000). Body image and body change methods in adolescent boys: Role of parents, friends, and the media. *Journal of Psychosomatic Research, 49*(3), 189–197.

Richardson, G. Neiger, B. Jensen, S., & Kumpfer, K. (1990). The resiliency model. *Health Education, 21*(6), 33–39.

Rigby, K., Cox, I., & Black, G. (1997). Cooperativeness and bully/victim problems among Australian schoolchildren. *Journal of Social Psychology, 137*(3), 357–368.

Riggs, P. D. (2003). Treating adolescents for substance abuse and comorbid psychiatric disorders. *Science and Practice Perspectives, 2*(1), 18–29.

Robins, L., & McEvoy, L. (1990). Conduct problems as predictors of substance abuse. In L. Robbins & M. Rutter (Eds.), *Straight and devious pathways from childhood to adulthood* (pp. 182–204). New York: Cambridge University Press.

Robinson, S. (2009). The core assessment of young females who sexually abuse. In M. C. Calder (Ed.), *Sexual abuse assessments: Using and developing frameworks for practice* (pp. 146–177). Dorset, UK: Russell House.

Roehlkepartain, E. C., Benson, P. L., & Sesma, A. Jr. (2003). *Signs of progress in putting children first: Developmental assets among youth in St. Louis Park, 1997–2001.* Minneapolis: Search Institute.

Rohde, P., Lewinson, P., Kahler, C., Seeley, J., & Brown, R. (2001). Natural course of alcohol use disorders from adolescence to young adulthood. *Journal of the American Academy of Child and Adolescent Psychiatry, 40,* 83–90.

Rolande, D., Royer, E., & Turcotte, D. (1997, Fall). School achievement at the secondary level: Influence of parenting style and parent involvement in schooling. *McGill Journal of Education, 32*(3), 191–207.

Rose, E., DiClemente, R. J., Wingood, G. M., Sales, J. M., Latham, T. P., Crosby R. A., et al. (2009). The validity of teens' and young adults' self-reported condom use. *Archives of Pediatric and Adolescent Medicine, 163*(1), 61–64.

Rose, H., Boyce Rodgers, K., & Small, S. (2006). Sexual identity confusion and problem behaviors in adolescents: A risk and resilience approach. *Marriage and Family Review, 40*(2/3), 131–150.

Roth, J., & Brooks-Gunn, J. (2000). What do adolescents need for healthy development?: Implications for youth policy. *Society for Research in Child Development Policy Report, 14*(1), 1–19.

Rotheram-Borus, M., Rosario, M., Van Rossem, R., Reid, H., & Gillis, R. (1995). Prevalence, course, and predictors of multiple problem behaviors among gay and bisexual male adolescents. *Developmental Psychology, 31,* 75–85.

Rotter, J. B. (1966). Generalized expectancies for internal versus external control of reinforcement. *Psychological Monographs, 80*(1), 1–28.

Rubin, L. (1996). *The transcendent child: Tales of triumph over the past.* New York: Harper.

Ruiz, S. A., & Silverstein, M. (2007). Relationships with grandparents and the emotional well-being of late adolescent and young adult grandchildren. *Journal of Social Issues, 63,* 793–808.

Rutter, M. (1981). The city and the child. *American Journal of Orthopsychiatry, 51*(4), 610–625.

Rutter, M. (1987). Psychosocial resilience and protective mechanisms. *American Journal of Orthopsychiatry, 57,* 316–331.

Rutter, M. (1989). Pathways from childhood to adult life. *Journal of Child Psychology and Psychiatry, 30*(1), 23–51.

Rutter, M. (1999). Resilience concepts and findings: Implications for family therapy. *Journal of Family Therapy, 21*(2), 119–144.

Rutter, M. (2001). Psychosocial adversity: Risk, resilience and recovery. In M. W. Fraser, & J. M. Richman (Eds.), *The context of youth violence: Resilience, risk and protection* (pp. 13–41). Wesport, CT: Praeger.

Rutter, M. (2006a). *Genes and behavior: Nature-nurture interplay explained.* London: Blackwell.

Rutter, M. (2006b). Implications of resilience concepts for scientific understanding. In B. M. Lester, A. S. Masten, & B. S. McEwen (Eds.), *Resilience in children* (pp. 1–12). Boston: Annals of the New York Academy of Sciences.

Rutter, M., Giller, H., & Hagell, A. (1998). *Antisocial behavior by young people.* Cambridge, UK: Cambridge University Press.

Rutter, M., & Sroufe, L. (2000). Developmental psychopathology: Concepts and challenges. *Development and Psychopathology, 12*, 265–296.

Ryan, S., Franzetta, K., Manlove, J., & Holcombe, E. (2007). Adolescents' discussion about contraception or STDs with partners before first sex. *Perspectives on Sexual and Reproductive Health, 39*(3), 149–157.

Saldana, L., Swenson, C., & Letourneau, E. (2006). Multisystemic therapy with juvenile sexual offenders. In R. Longo & D. Prescott (Eds.), *Current perspectives: Working with sexually aggressive youth and youth with sexual behavior problems* (pp. 563–579). Holyoke, MA: NEARI Press.

Saltzburg, S. (2004). Learning that an adolescent child is gay or lesbian: The parent experience. *Social Work, 49*(1), 109–118.

Sameroff, A. (2000). Ecological perspectives on developmental risk. In J. Osofsky & H. Fitgerald (Eds.), *WAIMH handbook of infant mental health* (Vol. 4, pp. 1–33). New York: Wiley.

SAMHSA. (2008). National survey on drug use and health report. Retrieved September 26, 2009, from *www.oas.samhsa.gov/2k8/stimulants/depression.pdf*.

Sampson, R., Raudenbush, S., & Earls, F. (1997). Neighborhoods and violent crime: A multilevel study of collective efficacy. *Science, 277*, 918–924.

Sandefur, G. (1998). Race, ethnicity, families and education. In H. McCubbin, E. Thompson, A. Thompson, & J. Fromer (Eds.), *Resiliency in Native American and immigrant families* (pp. 49–70). Thousand Oaks, CA: Sage.

Sanson, A., Hemphill, S. A., & Smart, D. (2004). Connections between temperament and social development: A review. *Social Development, 13*(1), 142–170.

Santelli, J. S., Lowry, R., Brener, N. D., & Robin, L. (2000). The association of sexual behaviors with socioeconomic status, family structure, and race/ethnicity among US adolescents. *American Journal of Public Health, 90*(10), 1582–1588.

Santrock, J. (1998). *Adolescence.* New York: McGraw-Hill.

Santrock, J. W. (2005). *Adolescence* (10th ed.). New York: McGraw-Hill.

Savin-Williams, R. (1994). Verbal and physical abuse as stressors in the lives of sexual minority youth: Association with school problems, running away, substance abuse, prostitution, and suicide. *Journal of Counseling and Clinical Psychology, 62*, 261–269.

Savin-Williams, R., & Diamond, L. (1999). Sexual orientation. In W. K. Silverman & T. H. Ollendick (Eds.), *Developmental issues in the clinical treatment of children* (pp. 241–258). Needham Heights, MA: Allyn & Bacon.

Scales, P. C., & Leffert, N. (1999). *Developmental assets: A synthesis of the scientific research on adolescent development.* Minneapolis, MN: Search Institute.

Scarr, S., & McCartney, K. (1983). How people make their own environments: A theory of genotype environment effects. *Child Development, 54*, 424–435.

Scharrer, E., & Leone, R. (2006). I know you are but what am I? Young people's perceptions about video game influence. *Mass Communication and Society, 9*(3), 215–238.

Schradley, P., Turner, R., & Gotlib, I. (2002). Stability of retrospective reports in depression: Traumatic events, past depressive episodes, and parental psychopathology. *Journal of Health and Social Behavior, 43*, 307–316.

Schulenberg, J., Maggs, J., Steinman, K., & Zucker, R. (2001). Developmental matters: Taking the long view on substance abuse etiology and intervention during adolescence. In P. Monti, S. Colby, & T. O'Leary (Eds.), *Adolescents, alcohol, and substance abuse: Reaching teens through brief interventions* (pp. 19–57). New York: Guilford Press.

Seilhamer, R., & Jacob, T. (1990). Family factors and adjustment of children of alcoholics. In M. Windle & J. Searles (Eds.), *Children of alcoholics: Critical perspectives* (pp. 168–186). New York: Guilford Press.

Seligman, M. (1995). *The optimistic child.* New York: Houghton Mifflin.

Sheafor, B., & Horejsi, C. (2003). *Techniques and guidelines for social work practice.* Boston: Allyn & Bacon.

Shedler, J., & Block, J. (1990). Adolescent drug use and psychological health: A longitudinal inquiry. *American Psychologist, 45*(5), 612–630.

Sieverding, J., Boyer, C. B., Siller, J., Gallaread, A., Krone, M., & Chang, Y. J. (2005). Youth united through health education: Building capacity through a community collaborative intervention to prevent HIV/STD in adolescents residing in a high STD prevalent neighborhood. *Aids Education and Prevention, 17*(4), 375–385.

Simmons-Morton, B., & Haynie, D. (2008). *Preventing problem behavior among middle school students.* National Institute of Child Health and Human Development. Retrieved Septemember 29, 2009, from *nichd.nig.gov/about/org/despr/studies/behavior/goplaces.cfm.*

Sinkkonen, J., Anttila, R., & Siimes, M. (1998). Pubertal maturation and changes in self-image in early adolescent Finnish boys. *Journal of Youth and Adolescence, 27,* 209–218.

Small, S., & Covalt, B. (2006). Adolescence and the family: Myths and realities. In F. Villarruel & T. Luster (Eds.), *The crisis in mental health: Critical issues and effective programs: Vol. 2. Issues in adolescence* (pp. 1–25). Westport, CT: Greenwood Press.

Smetana, J. G. (1989). Adolescents' and parents' reasoning about actual family conflict. *Child Development, 60,* 1052–1067.

Smith, C., Lizotte, A., Thornberry, T., & Krohn, M. (1995). Resilient youth: Identifying factors that prevent high-risk youth from engaging in delinquency and drug use. In J. Hagan (Ed.), *Delinquency and disrepute in the life course* (pp. 217–247). Greenwich, CT: JAI Press

Smith, P. (1997). Bullying in life-span perspective: What can studies of school bullying and workplace bullying learn from each other? *Journal of Community and Applied Social Psychology, 7,* 249–255.

Snyder, H., & Sickmund, M. (2006). *Juvenile offenders and victims: 2006 National Report.* Washington, DC: Office of Juvenile Justice and Delinquency Prevention, U.S. Department of Justice.

Spencer, M. (1999). Social and cultural influences on school adjustment: The application of identity-focused cultural ecological perspective. *Educational Psychologist, 34,* 43–57.

Spoth, R., Redmond, C., Shin, C., Greenberg, M., Clair, S., & Feinberg, M. (2007). Substance-use outcomes at 18 months past baseline: The PROSPER community-university partnership trial. *American Journal of Preventive Medicine, 32*(5), 395–402.

Sroufe, L. A., Egeland, B., Carlson, E. A., & Collins, W. A. (2005). *The development of the person: The Minnesota study of risk and adaptation from birth to adulthood.* New York: Guilford Press.

St. John, W. (2007, January 21). The fugees: Adjusting to America: Outcasts united. *New York Times.*

Steinberg, L. (1990). Autonomy, conflict, and harmony in the family relationship. In S. S. Feldman & G. R. Elliot (Eds.), *At the threshold: The developing adolescent* (pp. 255–276). Cambridge, MA: Harvard University Press.

Steinberg, L. (2009, April). A social neuroscience perspective on adolescent risk-taking. Paper presented as part of a symposium entitled "Current Theories of Adolescent Risk Taking" at the biennial meeting of the Society for Research in Child Development, Denver, CO.

Steinberg, L., & Silk, J. S. (2002). Parenting adolescents. In M. H. Bornstein (Ed.), *Handbook of parenting* (pp. 103–133). Mahwah, NJ: Erlbaum.

Steinberg, L., & Steinberg, W. (1994). *Crossing paths: How your child's adolescence triggers your own crisis.* New York: Simon & Schuster.

Stepp, L. S., & Shaver, K. (2008). *STD data comes as no surprise, area teenagers say.* Retrieved February 9, 2009, from *www.washingtonpost.com/wp-dyn/content/article/2008/03/11/AR2008031101342_pf.html.*

Stocker, C. M., Richmond, M. K., Rhoades, G. K., & Kiang, L. (2007). Family emotional processes and adolescents' adjustment. *Social Development, 16,* 310–325.

Stodghill, R. (1998). Where'd you learn that? *Time,* June 15, 52–59.

Stokols, D. (1999). Human development in the age of the Internet: Conceptual and methodological horizons. In S. Friedman & T. Wachs (Eds.), *Measuring environment across the lifespan* (pp. 327–356). Washington, DC: American Psychological Association.

Surko, M., Ciro, D., Blackwood, C., Nembhard, M., & Peake, K. (2005). Experience of racism as a correlate of developmental health outcomes among urban adolescent mental health clients. *Social Work in Mental Health, 3*(3), 235–260.

Sweet, M., & DesRoches, S. (2007). Citizenship for somer: Heteronormativity as cloaked bullying. *Journal of Gay and Lesbian Social Services, 19*(3/4), 173–187.

Swenson, C., Henggler, S., Taylor, I., & Addison, O. (2005). *Multisystemic therapy and neighborhood partnerships: Reducing adolescent violence and substance abuse.* New York: Guilford Press.

Taffel, R. (2005). *Breaking through to teens: A new psychotherapy for the new adolescence.* New York: Guilford Press.

Tarter, R. E. (2002). Etiology of adolescent substance abuse: A developmental perspective. *American Journal on Addictions, 11*(3), 171–191.

Tatum, B. (2003). *"Why are all the black kids sitting together in the cafeteria?": And other conversations about race.* New York: Basic Books.

Taylor, C. (2007). A human rights approach to stopping homophobic bullying in schools. *Journal of Gay and Lesbian Social Services: Issues in Practice, Policy, and Research, 19*(3/4), 157–172.

Taylor, C., Lerner, R., & von Eye, A. (2001). *Developmental assets and positive youth development: 2001 annual report for phase II of the "Overcoming the Odds" project: Understanding successful development among African American and Latino male adolescents.* Hoboken, NJ: William T. Grant Foundation.

Thomas, A. (2007). *Youth online: Identity in the digital age.* New York: Peter Wang.

Tietjen, A. (1989). The ecology of children's social support networks. In D. Belle (Ed.), *Children's social networks and social supports* (pp. 37–69). New York: Wiley & Sons.

Timmons-Michell, J., Brown, C., Shultz, S., Webster, S., Underwood, L., & Semple, W. (1997). *Final report: Results of a three year collaborative effort to assess the mental health needs of youth in the juvenile justice system in Ohio.* Columbus, OH: Ohio Department of Youth Services.

Tubman, J. G., Gil, A. G., & Wagner, E. F. (2004). Co-occurring substance use and delinquent behavior during early adolescence: Emerging relations and intervention strategies. *Criminal Justice and Behavior, 31*(4), 463–488.

Ungar, M. (2004). The importance of parents and other caregivers to resilience of high-risk adolescents. *Family Process, 43*, 23–41.

Urschel, H. (2009). *Healing the addicted brain.* Naperville, IL: Sourcebooks.

Valente, T., & Pumpuang, P. (2007). Identifying opinion leaders to promote behavior change. *Health Education and Behavior, 34*(6), 881–896.

Vitaro, F., Brendgen, M., & Tremblay, R. E. (2000). Influence of deviant friends on delinquency: Searching for moderator variables. *Journal of Abnormal Child Psychology, 28*, 313–325.

Vowell, P. (2007). A partial test of an integrative control model: Neighborhood context, social control, self-control, and youth violent behavior. *Western Criminology Review, 8*(2), 1–15.

Wachs, T. D. (2006). Contributions of temperament to buffering and sensitization processes in children's development. In B. M. Lester, A. S. Masten, & B. S. McEwen (Eds.), *Resilience in children* (pp. 28–39). Boston: Annals of the New York Academy of Sciences.

Waldner-Haugrud, L., & Magruder, B. (1996). Homosexual identity expression among lesbian and gay adolescents: An analysis of perceived structural associations. *Youth & Society, 27*, 313–333.

Wall, A. E., & Kohl, P. L. (2007). Substance use in maltreated youth: Findings from the National Survey of Child and Adolescent Well-Being. *Child Maltreatment, 12*(1), 20–30.

Walsh, J., & Lantz, J. (2007). *Short-term existential intervention in clinical practice.* Chicago: Lyceum Books.

Wang, M., Haertel, G., & Walberg, H. (1994). Educational resilience in inner cities. In M. Wang & E. Gordon (Eds.), *Educational resilience in inner-city America: Challenges and prospects* (pp. 45–72). Hillsdale, NJ: Erlbaum.

Ward, L. (2003). Understanding the role of entertainment media in the sexual socialization of American youth: A review of empirical research. *Development Review, 23*, 347–388.

Ward, L., & Friedman, K. (2006). Using TV as a guide: Associations between television viewing and adolescents' sexual attitudes and behavior. *Journal of Research on Adolescence, 16*, 133–156.

Washburn, E. (2008). *Building a relationship, creating empowerment.* Public Achievement Coaches Handbook, University of Denver, Center for Community Engagement and Service Learning. Retrieved February 19, 2009, from *www.du.edu/ccesl/docs/Students/PA_Coach_Reflections.pdf.*

Weierich, M. R., & Nock, M. K. (2008). Posttraumatic stress symptoms mediate the relation between childhood sexual abuse and nonsuicidal self-injury. *Journal of Consulting and Clinical Psychology, 76*, 39–44.

Weiner, M., Pentz, M., Skara, S., Li, C., Chou, C., & Dwyer, J. (2004). Relationships of substance use and associated predictors of violence in early, middle and late adolescence. *Journal of Child and Adolescent Substance Abuse, 13*(4), 97–117.

Werner, E. (1985). Stress and protective factors in children's lives. In A. R. Nicol (Ed.), *Longitudinal studies in child psychology and psychiatry* (pp. 335–355). New York: Wiley.

Werner, E. (1986). Resilient offspring of alcoholics: A longitudinal study from birth to age 18. *Journal of Studies on Alcohol, 47*, 34–40.

Werner, E. (1989a). Children of the garden island. *Scientific American, 4*, 106–111.

Werner, E. (1989b). High risk children in young adulthood: A longitudinal study from birth to 32 years. *American Orthopsychiatric Association, 59*(1), 372–381.

Werner, E. (1994). Overcoming the odds. *Journal of Developmental and Behavioral Pediatrics, 15*(2), 131–136.

Werner, E. E., & Smith, R. S. (1982). *Vulnerable but invincible: A study of resilient children.* New York: McGraw-Hill.

Werner, E., & Smith, R. (1992). *Overcoming the odds: High risk children from birth to adulthood.* Ithaca, NY: Cornell University Press.

Werner, E., & Smith, R. (1998). *Vulnerable but invincible.* New York: Adams, Bannister and Cox.

Werner, E., & Smith, R. (2001). *Journeys from childhood to midlife.* Ithaca, NY: Cornell University Press.

Wessells, M., & Strang, A. (2006). Religion as resource and risk. In N. Boothby, A. Strang, & M. Wessells (Eds.), *A world turned upside down: Social ecological approaches to children in war zones* (pp. 199–222). Bloomfield, CT: Kumarian Press.

White, M., & Epston, D. (1990). *Narrative means to therapeutic ends.* New York: Norton.

Whitmore, E., Mikulich, S., Thompson, L., Riggs, P., Aarons, G., & Crowley, T. (1997). Influences on adolescent substance dependence: Conduct disorder, depression, attention deficit hyperactivity disorder, and gender. *Drug and Alcohol Dependence, 47*(2), 87–97.

Wight, R., Sepúlveda, J., & Aneshensel, C. (2004). Depressive symptoms: How do adolescents compare with adults? *Journal of Adolescent Health, 34*, 314–323.

Wilens, T., Biederman, J., Millstein, R., Wozniak, J., Hahesy, A., & Spencer, T. (1999). Risk for substance use disorders in youth with child and adolescent onset bipolar disorder. *Journal of the American Academy of Child and Adolescent Psychiatry, 38*(6), 680–685.

Williams, T., Connolly, J., Pepler, D., & Craig, W. (2005). Peer victimization, social support, and psychosocial adjustment of sexual minority adolescents. *Journal of Youth and Adolescence, 34*(5), 471–482.

Wilson, W. J. (1987). *The truly disadvantaged.* Chicago: University of Chicago Press.

Wilson, W. J. (1996). *When work disappears: The world of the new urban poor.* New York: Vantage Books.

Windle, R., & Windle, M. (1997). An investigation of adolescents' substance abuse behaviors, depressed affect, and suicidal behavior. *Journal of Child Psychology and Psychiatry, 38*(8), 921–929.

Winters, K. (2001). Assessing adolescent substance use problems and other areas of functioning. In P. M. Monti, S. M. Colby, & T. A. O'Leary (Eds.), *Adolescents, alcohol, and substance abuse: Reaching teens through brief interventions* (pp. 80–108). New York: Guilford Press.

Wiseman, R. (2003). *Queen bees and wannabes: Helping your daughter survive cliques, gossip, boyfriends, and other realities of adolescence.* New York: Three Rivers Press.

Woodberry, K., & Poepenoe, E. (2008). Implementing dialectical behavior therapy with adolescents and their families in a community outpatient clinic. *Cognitive and Behavioral Practice, 15*(3), 277–286.

Worthington, R., Savoy, H., Dillon, F., & Vernaglia, E. (2002). Heterosexual identity development: A multidimensional model of individual and society identity. *Counseling Psychologist, 30,* 496–531.

Yampolskaya, S., Brown, E. C., & Vargo, A. C. (2004). Assessment of teen pregnancy prevention interventions among middle school youth. *Child and Adolescent Social Work Journal, 21*(1), 69–83.

Yarhouse, M., & Tan, E. (2005). Addressing religious conflicts in adolescents who experience sexual identity confusion. *Professional Psychology: Research and Practice, 36*(5), 530–536.

Yates, T. M., Tracy, A. J., & Luthar, S. S. (2008). Nonsuicidal self-injury among "privileged" youths: Longitudinal and cross-sectional approaches to the developmental process. *Journal of Consulting and Clinical Psychology, 76,* 52–62.

Young, S. (1995). Sexual identity: The Cass model. Retrieved March 16, 2009, from *www.ecu.edu.au/equ/resources/docs/sexuality_cass_model.pdf.*

Yule, W. (1992). Resilience and vulnerability in child survivors of disasters. In B. Tizard & V. Varma (Eds.), *Vulnerability and resilience in human development* (pp. 182–197). London: Kingsley.

Zaff, J., & Hair, E. (2003). Positive development of the self: Self-concept, self-esteem, and identity. In M. Bornstein, L. Davidson, C. Keyes, & K. Moore (Eds.), *Well-being: Positive development across the life course* (pp. 235–251). Mahwah, NJ: Erlbaum.

Zimmerman, J., & Dickerson, V. (1996). *If problems talked: Narrative therapy in action.* New York: Guilford Press.

Zoccolillo, M., Meyers, J., & Assiter, S. (1997). Conduct disorder, substance dependence, and adolescent motherhood. *American Journal of Orthopsychiatry, 67,* 152–157.

Zoccolillo, M., & Rogers, K. (1991). Characteristics and outcomes of hospitalized adolescent girls with conduct disorders. *Journal of the American Academy of Child and Adolescent Psychiatry, 30,* 973–981.

Zurbriggen, E., & Morgan, E. (2006). Who wants to marry a millionaire? Reality dating television programs, attitudes toward sex, and sexual behaviors. *Sex Roles, 54,* 1–17.

Index